Selling Sexual Knowledge

Bringing together perspectives from the histories of medicine, sexuality, and the book, Sarah Bull presents the first study of how medical publications on sexual matters were made, promoted, and sold in Victorian Britain. Drawing on pamphlets, manuals, textbooks, periodicals, and more, this innovative book illustrates the free and unruly circulation of sexual information through a rapidly expanding publishing industry. Bull demonstrates how the ease with which print could be copied and claimed, recast and repurposed presented persistent challenges to those seeking to position themselves as authorities over sexual knowledge at this pivotal moment. Medical publishers, practitioners, and activists embraced allegations of obscenity and censorship to promote ideas, contest authority, and consolidate emergent collective identities. Layer by layer, their actions helped create and sustain one of the most potent myths ever made about the Victorians: their sexual ignorance. This title is also available as open access on Cambridge Core.

SARAH BULL is an Associate Professor in the Department of English at Toronto Metropolitan University.

Selling Sexual Knowledge

Medical Publishing and Obscenity in Victorian Britain

Sarah Bull

Toronto Metropolitan University

CAMBRIDGE
UNIVERSITY PRESS

CAMBRIDGE
UNIVERSITY PRESS

Shaftesbury Road, Cambridge CB2 8EA, United Kingdom

One Liberty Plaza, 20th Floor, New York, NY 10006, USA

477 Williamstown Road, Port Melbourne, VIC 3207, Australia

314–321, 3rd Floor, Plot 3, Splendor Forum, Jasola District Centre, New Delhi – 110025, India

103 Penang Road, #05–06/07, Visioncrest Commercial, Singapore 238467

Cambridge University Press is part of Cambridge University Press & Assessment, a department of the University of Cambridge.

We share the University's mission to contribute to society through the pursuit of education, learning and research at the highest international levels of excellence.

www.cambridge.org
Information on this title: www.cambridge.org/9781009578073

DOI: 10.1017/9781009578103

When citing this work, please include a reference to the DOI 10.1017/9781009578103

First published 2025

A catalogue record for this publication is available from the British Library

Library of Congress Cataloging-in-Publication Data
Names: Bull, Sarah, author.
Title: Selling sexual knowledge : medical publishing and obscenity in Victorian Britain / Sarah Bull.
Description: [New York] : Cambridge University Press, [2025] | Includes bibliographical references and index.
Identifiers: LCCN 2024050812 | ISBN 9781009578073 (hardback) | ISBN 9781009578080 (paperback) | ISBN 9781009578103 (ebook)
Subjects: LCSH: Sex – Great Britain – Public opinion – History – 19th century. | Sex – Information resources – Great Britain – History – 19th century. | Medical publishing – Great Britain – History – 19th century. | Great Britain – History – Victoria, 1837–1901.
Classification: LCC HQ18.G7 B85 2025 | DDC 306.770941/09034–dc23/eng/20250306
LC record available at https://lccn.loc.gov/2024050812

ISBN 978-1-009-57807-3 Hardback
ISBN 978-1-009-57808-0 Paperback

For Riley and Ralph

Contents

Figures

Acknowledgements

It took me a long time to write this book. Now that I'm wrapping it up, I feel lost for words to express my gratitude to those who made it possible. I'm especially grateful to two people without whom it definitely would not exist: Colette Colligan and Jim Secord. Both are kind and patient teachers. Colette took me on as a PhD student, introduced me to the study of print culture, and taught me the joys (and frustrations) of bibliographic detective work. Jim sponsored my postdoctoral fellowship, introduced me to the history of science, and helped me figure out how to shape my findings into a narrative. I couldn't have asked for better mentors.

Several organizations supported my work. A Joseph Armand Bombardier Canada Graduate Scholarship and a Michael Smith Foreign Study Supplement from the Social Sciences and Humanities Research Council of Canada [grant numbers 65151 and 78730] funded the early stages of my research, enabling me to spend an academic year in London and devote myself fully to my doctoral dissertation. A Research Fellowship in Medical Humanities from the Wellcome Trust [grant number 106548/Z/14/Z] enabled me to expand my research well beyond what I was able to accomplish during my doctoral work and write a first draft of the book. A start-up grant from Toronto Metropolitan University provided funding for the images, and supplemental funding from the Wellcome Trust enabled me to publish an open-access electronic version.

My research would not have been possible without staff at many libraries and archives who enabled me to locate, examine, and, in some cases, reproduce portions of the primary material discussed in the book, and access secondary sources. Special thanks to staff at the Archive of British Printing and Publishing (University of Reading), the British Library, Cambridge University Library, the London Metropolitan Archives, the National Archives, the Archives of the Royal College of Surgeons of England, Simon Fraser University Library, Toronto Metropolitan University Library, and the Wellcome Library, where I did most of my research. A special word of thanks also goes to Ann Hale, who visited the British Library on my behalf after I moved to Toronto and photographed several obscure items that I belatedly realized I needed to read.

Many colleagues read chapter drafts, discussed different aspects of the book with me, and cheered me on. Thanks especially to Maria Damkjær, who read and commented on an entire draft of the manuscript, and to Rich McKay, Jesse Olszynko-Gryn, and Charissa Varma for having lengthy discussions about the book with me at a crucial stage. More broadly, I'm grateful to the communities that sustained me across three institutions and two continents. In Vancouver and the surrounding area, Marc Acherman, Livia Chan, Sarah Creel, Amy De'Ath, Peter Dickinson, Kim O'Donnell, Michael Everton, Carole Gerson, Riley Kearns, Erin Keating, Mary Elizabeth Leighton, Carolyn Lesjak, Jennifer Anne Scott, Lisa Surridge, and Lise Jaillant all supported the work that informs this book in different ways. Along with Charissa, Jesse, and Rich, so, too, did Elizabeth Smith, Salim Al-Gailani, Leah Astbury, Jenny Bangham, Victoria Bartels, Mary Brazelton, Jack Dixon, Mike Drymoussis, Jo Edge, Meira Gold, Nick Hopwood, Tamara Hug, Boris Jardine, Josh Kaggie, Lauren Kassell, Josh Nall, Thea and Jon Reimer, Edwin Rose, Louisa Russell, Verity Smith, François Sherwood, Lesley Steinitz, James Poskett, and Michelle Wallis in Cambridge. These folks are great company and, just as importantly, helped me forget about the book from time to time and enjoy life off the page.

I'm thankful to have been able to attend the Media History Seminar at the University of London's Institute for Advanced Study while I was in the UK. Along with the invited speakers, seminar regulars, including Ann, Laurel Brake, Helena Goodwyn, Andrew King, Matthew Rubery, Mark Turner, and Liwen Zhang, helped me think about print culture in new and productive ways. I'm grateful, too, to Kate Fisher and Jana Funke for inviting me to events connected with their Rethinking Sexology project at the University of Exeter; to the scholars I met through those and other events connected with work in the histories of medicine and sexuality, including Jen Grove, Kate Davison, Agata Ignaciuk, Sarah Jones, Ina Linge-Granger, Claire Jones, Lesley Hall, Sally Shuttleworth, Jon Topham, Alison Moulds, and Sally Frampton; to Lisa Z. Sigel and Kathleen Lubey for their expert feedback on my work on the pornography trade; and to the community of academics on Twitter and, later, Bluesky, who I enjoyed chatting with about the highs and lows of research. When I moved to Toronto, I was welcomed by another delightful community. Thanks especially to Jason Boyd, Tina Young Choi, Joaney Cole-Abdul, Colleen Derkatch, Laura Fisher, Wendy Francis, Naomi Hamer, Afrina Hashem, Leslie Howsam, Lorraine Janzen-Kooistra, Craig Jennex, Lauren Kirshner, Melanie Knight, Anne-Marie Lee-Loy, Andrew O'Malley, Amy Peng, Simon Stern, Pamela Sugiman, Monique Tschofen, Justin Vanlieshout, and Olivia Wong for their support as I finished the book.

I was lucky to have great editorial support as I prepared to publish it, too. Many thanks to Lucy Rhymer, my editor at Cambridge University Press, for believing in the book and shepherding it into print with such grace and efficiency, and to editorial assistant Rosa Martin, who patiently answered a steady stream of queries. I'm also grateful to the anonymous readers for their engagement with the manuscript. Their suggestions made *Selling Sexual Knowledge* a better book. Jeremy Andriano, who worked as my research assistant in 2023–4, also left his mark: thanks to Jeremy for correcting some truly laughable typos, tracking down last-minute references, and noting places where clarification would be useful.

My family members must now know more than they ever cared to about nineteenth-century publishing or sexual culture. It's a testament to their love for me that I need to qualify that sentence: my parents, Mike and Anne Bull; my siblings, Martha, Jonathan, and Eve; my grandparents, Beverly and Arthur Bull; and my in-laws, Richard Ball and Mickey Guy, Seb and Erica Ball, and Mike Ball, never complained. Lastly, and above all, I'm grateful for the support of my funny, kind, and extraordinarily patient husband, Ralph Ball, and my son, Riley, who has never known a time when I was not working on this book. This book is dedicated to them.

Abbreviations

ABPP	Archive of British Printing and Publishing
RCS	Archives of the Royal College of Surgeons of England
BNF	Bibliothèque Nationale de France
BL	British Library
BMJ	*British Medical Journal*
UL	Cambridge University Library
HRC	Harry Ransom Center
HBM	Hoare's Bank Museum
KIL	Kinsey Institute Library and Special Collections
LMA	London Metropolitan Archives
LSE	London School of Economics
MSCE	Michael Sadleir Collection of Ephemera
ML	Morris Library
TNA	National Archives, UK
NLM	National Library of Medicine, USA
WL	Wellcome Library

Introduction

"Your last book goes off famously, Doctor . . . Nothing like a highly-seasoned work to sell," Mr. Quarto crows. Clerks are milling about behind him, carrying stacks of books to and fro. A customer samples the wares. Mr. Quarto and the Doctor are sitting at a table towards the back of the bookshop. Books and papers lie scattered carelessly at their feet. One is emblazoned with the words *Mysteries of Matrimony*. Another, *Manly Vigour*. "We can push the thing," Mr. Quarto continues, "because it is written by an M.D; the police authorities can't touch us, we are *beyond* all *law*; because we are privileged by the *law* to write obscene books, and call it *science*." "Capital, by Jove," the Doctor exclaims. He leans forward and smiles, satisfied with himself. "It's a jolly lark, though; isn't it? Licensed to write, publish, and sell, [*sic*] all the obscenities we can collect . . . The only thing which can knock up our trade is, Mr. Morison's system, by which *everyone becomes his own physician*."

This scene is staged in an 1852 advertisement for Hygeism, a holistic system of medicine invented by the Scottish pill-maker James Morison (Figure 0.1). Morison theorized that all diseases resulted from impurities in the blood and claimed that the sick could cure themselves of every malady by taking his purgative Hygeian Vegetable Universal Medicine. Consumed in the recommended quantities, the medicine was a powerful laxative: it caused diarrhoea, dehydration, and, in a few tragic cases, death. Sales went briskly anyway, thanks to the endless stream of propaganda that Morison's institution, an outfit called the British College of Health, issued against its competition. Through public lectures, illustration series, books, and, from 1842, a journal called the *Hygeist*, the College set Morison's theories against what it called the "Organic or Doctors' System," which it framed as hopelessly corrupted by its practitioners' self-interest. It accused M.D.s of experimenting on, poisoning, and molesting patients' bodies in many of these publications, and, in "The Obscene M.D.," of poisoning their minds.[1]

[1] For a more detailed account of Morison and the British College of Health, see Michael Brown, "Medicine, Quackery, and the Free Market: The 'War' against Morison's Pills and the Construction of the Medical Profession, c. 1830–c. 1850," in *Medicine and the Market in*

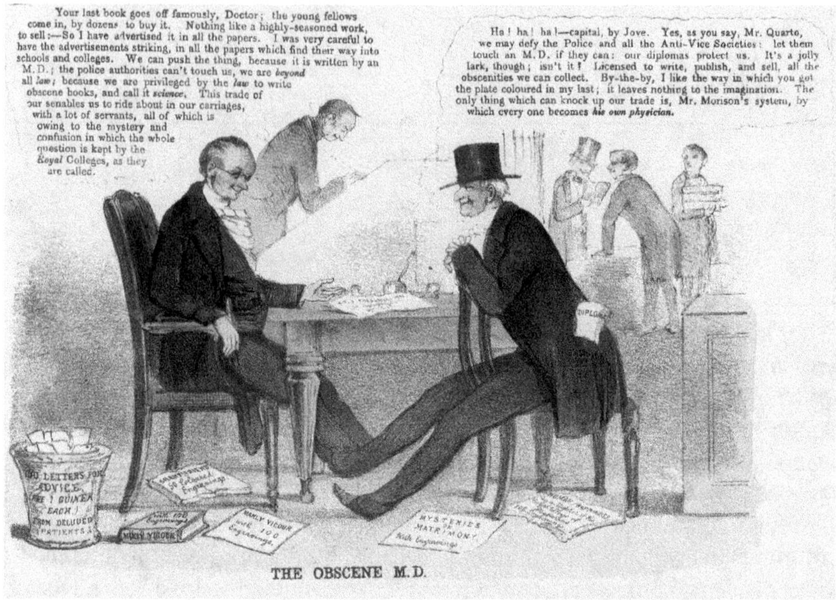

Figure 0.1 "The Obscene M.D." Coloured Lithograph. *Morality of Modern Medicine Mongers* (London: British College of Health, 1852). 563105i, Iconographic Collection, WL. Wellcome Collection, CC BY-NC 4.0.

"The Obscene M.D." exploits two familiar features of Victorian culture. One is the proliferation of medical works that described, analyzed, and theorized sex and reproduction. Premodern conceptions of sexual knowledge as pluralistic and experiential had begun to narrow in the previous century, giving way to a model that established sex centrally as a domain of medical expertise.[2] Sexual knowledge was increasingly regarded as a set of biological facts that could be discovered, ordered, and applied to managing bodies and populations. Many of these facts were contested. So were exactly how they should be used and who could speak of them with authority. But the idea that science had a singular power to make the most intimate workings of the body legible and tractable was

England and Its Colonies, c. 1450–c. 1850, ed. Mark S. R. Jenner and Patrick Wallis (Basingstoke: Palgrave Macmillan, 2007), 238–261.

2 Kate Fisher, "Modern Ignorance," in *Reproduction: Antiquity to the Present*, ed. Nick Hopwood, Rebecca Fleming, and Lauren Kassell (Cambridge: Cambridge University Press, 2018), 471–472. See also Mary Fissell and Roger Cooter, "Exploring Natural Knowledge: Science and the Popular," in *The Cambridge History of Science*, vol. 4, *Eighteenth-Century Science*, ed. Roy Porter (Cambridge: Cambridge University Press, 2003), 129–158; Ralph O'Connor, "Reflections on Popular Science in Britain: Genres, Categories, and Historians," *Isis* 100, no. 2 (2009): 333–345.

becoming more and more fixed. The bibliographic legacy of this paradigm's rise weighs down the shelves of academic libraries today and is rapidly filling digital space.

At the same time, the lithograph capitalizes on the politicization of access to sexual representations. The meanings and effects of all kinds of depictions of sex came under scrutiny during this period, including medical ones. Legal experts agreed that words and pictures that would render a novel or a newspaper indecent were necessities of medical communication. Authors of works on anatomy or obstetrics could not avoid discussions of sexual matters, nor, in most cases, could they bury the details in euphemism. Resorting to these common strategies of self-censorship risked misinterpretation, if not the destruction of a medical work's utility altogether. Yet, necessity did not ameliorate such works' potential to arouse dangerous thoughts and unseemly feelings. During a period that witnessed the passage of a raft of laws against the display and distribution of obscene material, medical works thus occupied a strange cultural position, traversing the categories of the scientific and the indecent, the licit and the illicit.

The proliferation of medical works about sex and reproduction and the debates about social effects of sexual representation that marked the Victorian period are now considered elements of the same transformation: an "explosion of discourse" that put sex – and its management – at the centre of modern life.[3] Each has been studied extensively within this framework. Less well-understood are the practical implications of their coexistence for the circulation of sexual knowledge and for those who sought to establish themselves as authorities over it. As "The Obscene M.D.'s" setting in a bookshop reminds us, medical books and pamphlets are not just discourse, or even just texts. They are also commercial objects, which had to be made, promoted, and moved into readers' hands. And as they moved through the marketplace, these objects did more than communicate medical information. They also acted as representatives of their makers, and of businesses, professions, and movements with which they were associated.

In a context in which M.D.s could be accused of being quasi-pornographers, and laws against the display and distribution of obscene material could, in fact, accommodate the arrest of figures like the fictive Mr. Quarto, what did trade in medical works on sexual matters really look like? And how did those most invested in medical publishing, practice, and knowledge sell themselves as trustworthy authorities? As the lithograph also suggests, the mobility of print

[3] This framework is elaborated from Michel Foucault's influential theories in *The History of Sexuality, Volume 1: The Will to Knowledge*, trans. Robert Hurley (1978; repr., New York: Vintage, 1990). For an overview of the historiography I refer to, see the introduction to Jeffrey Weeks, *Sex, Politics and Society: The Regulation of Sexuality since 1800*, 4th ed. (London: Routledge, 2017).

and the vagaries of interpretation could make communicating the right things to the right people hard to do. Medical works could fall into the wrong hands, and they could be used in the wrong ways. Readers could employ them as a kind of pornography, or as instruction manuals in how to have immoral sex. Disreputable entrepreneurs could capitalize on these uses of medical literature. The motivations of those who made and sold these works could also be misinterpreted, or deliberately misrepresented by hostile agents. How these possibilities were negotiated is the subject of this book.

Selling Sexual Knowledge examines the practices and politics of trade in medical works about sex and reproduction in Victorian Britain. Bringing perspectives from the history of the book together with conversations in the histories of medicine and sexuality, much of it explores how different sourcing strategies, publishing arrangements, marketing techniques, and distribution networks shaped how medical information about sexual matters reached the kinds of readers typically invoked in Victorian debates about obscenity: people who were not medical experts or other professionals who could claim to need such knowledge to do their jobs. Many scholars are used to thinking of a book's text and images as the main event, and of the details of its commercial history as background information. For a period in which print comprised an increasingly important way of sourcing knowledge, however, these kinds of details are vital to establishing how people acquired information that would have influenced their understandings of their own bodies and experiences. More broadly, I argue, paying attention to these details is essential to understanding the consolidation of movements, institutions, and narratives that have come to define how we think about the modern history of sexuality.

When I began the research for this book, I assumed that the biggest problem that sellers of sexual knowledge faced was opposition from people who sought to protect readers from moral corruption. Eventually, I had to concede that such opposition was more limited and, when it appeared, more ambivalent than I had anticipated. Legal experts debated medical works' obscene potential less out of concern for readers' morals than because they worried that vague obscenity laws endangered legitimate sexual discussion. State authorities and anti-vice crusaders were never invested in trying to suppress trade in even the cheapest, most lurid, or most radical medical works. Nor was there any sustained public opposition. Newspapers sometimes railed against trade in cheap manuals on venereal disease, but they advertised the same works that they complained about; and although parents hid midwifery manuals from their children, they owned them and wanted to read them. In fact, the most vocal and most consistent advocates of the idea that medical works could be obscene were medical publishers, practitioners, and activists themselves. With minor changes, "The Obscene M.D.'s" depiction of shady medical bookselling could have been ripped from the pages of the *Lancet*.

Charges of obscenity can have different aims, meanings, and effects. Victorian allegations of medical obscenity were often tactical and became imbricated in what sociologists of science call "boundary work": projects through which various groups sought to establish moral and epistemic authority at a time when the boundaries of legitimate medical knowledge and practice were ambiguous and contested.[4] In railing against M.D.s for writing obscene books and calling them science in an effort to establish Hygeism as a superior medical system, the British College of Health's "Obscene M.D." offers a helpfully transparent illustration of what this could look like. But allegations of obscenity, and later of censorship on the grounds of obscenity, also functioned as a means through which groups that considered themselves far more respectable promoted books and causes, contested authority, and consolidated emergent collective identities. Over time, relatively crude strategies to promote publications and attack rivals in the marketplace gave way to more subtle rhetorics that helped produce one of the most potent myths ever made about the Victorians: that of their sexual ignorance.

By tracing the evolution of these strategies in tandem with the changing infrastructures of medical publishing and bookselling, *Selling Sexual Knowledge* demonstrates how arguments about obscenity were deployed in contests for authority whose outcomes had far-reaching implications: the consolidation of medicine as a modern scientific profession and the positioning of sexual-scientific knowledge as a means of personal and societal liberation. At the same time, it exposes conditions of communication that made contesting authority in these ways feel necessary in the first place. The technology of print was essential to establishing sex as a field of medical expertise. However, the ease with which print could be copied and claimed, recast and repurposed presented persistent challenges for those who sought to position themselves as authorities over medical knowledge and direct its applications. Alongside the slippery meanings of medical representations themselves, their promiscuous movements through the marketplace constantly threatened to undo careful self-positioning. At its core, this book is about that potential for failure, the consequent struggle to manage interpretation, and its legacies.

Medical Publishing in the Age of Mass Print

A series of developments established the nineteenth century as a pivotal turning point in the histories of medicine, sexuality, and print. Initially a divided body ostensibly run by the Royal College of Physicians, the Royal College of Surgeons, and the Society of Apothecaries in London, medicine ended the

[4] Thomas F. Gieryn, *Cultural Boundaries of Science: Credibility on the Line* (Chicago: University of Chicago Press, 1999).

century as a legally regulated profession and a far more coherent social and scientific authority. Support for marriage reform, contraception, and same-sex relationships expanded and became more visible, and sexual science began to emerge as a field in its own right. Publishing and advertising transformed with these changes. Literacy rose rapidly from the 1830s, creating new audiences hungry for print. New printing and paper-making technologies made it faster and cheaper to publish. The expansion of the postal service, the introduction of the railway, and the extension of transnational transport networks made it easier to distribute books and pamphlets. The abolition of taxes on the press facilitated their promotion, and the emergence of advertising as a dedicated industry.

These transformations are staged in the history that *Selling Sexual Knowledge* traces. Trade in medical works was populated by a changing but always rather motley crew of players. Working out of tiny printshops and dockside warehouses, country houses and city offices, they harnessed the expanding infrastructures of the press and the post to sell works on subjects as diverse as anatomy, midwifery, venereal disease, "foreign" sexual practices, same-sex desire, and contraceptive techniques across the country and around the world. Many of these agents believed that the works they sold could decrease mortality and improve public health, heal communities scarred by poverty and shame, or bring about much-needed changes to law and public policy. But commerce in sexual knowledge was also an economic enterprise and a means of professional advancement. Trade in medical works facilitated the sale of contraceptives, patent medicines, and a crystallizing media form that was eventually dubbed pornography. It encouraged visits to museums, brothels, and doctors' consulting rooms. It made careers, and it made money on its own.

Reconstructing these activities can be challenging. The business records of many important players in the trade have not survived, nor have many of the cheapest medical works. For different reasons, some agents concealed their identities by publishing anonymously or under pseudonyms, and sometimes affixed false imprints, dates, and places of publication to their books and pamphlets. To address these issues and set the work of publishing and bookselling into its wider contexts, I have drawn on a diverse range of sources, including publishers' archives, newspapers and periodicals, advertisements, court, government, and bank records, private correspondence, and books and pamphlets themselves, which can reveal a great deal about their origins when subjected to different kinds of bibliographical analysis. Throughout the book, I have included notes on the methods as well as the sources that I used to track various elements of the trade in sexual knowledge and highlight aspects of activities under discussion that remain mysterious.

Given the diversity of the trade and the fragmentary state of the historical record, it is perhaps not surprising that previous work on this topic has been quite targeted. Historians have produced sprawling surveys of medical works on sexual matters, to which this book is indebted.[5] However, detailed accounts of their creation, publication, advertisement, and distribution during the Victorian period have mainly focused on single publications, such as Havelock Ellis and John Addington Symonds's landmark *Sexual Inversion* (1897), and occasionally kinds of publications, such as the contraception manual.[6] Disciplinary trends also shape historiography. Literary and scientific publishing have been the focus of serious scholarship for decades, and there now is a great deal of work on early modern medical print culture. Book-historical approaches to modern medical print culture have been slower to catch on. There is a growing body of scholarship on medical periodicals, and new research on medical publishing and bookselling after 1800 is emerging. Phoebe Gill's recent doctoral work on sexual advice literature, for instance, illuminates how aspects of the trade examined here developed over the twentieth century.[7] However, broad accounts of modern medical publishing are presently few and far between.[8]

While this book aims to cast a wider net than previous studies, it is not by any means a comprehensive survey. As will become clear, medical publishing and bookselling were global enterprises, integrated into the wider web of colonial and transnational traffic in goods, services, and information. Given my interest in the role that the law played in this history, a narrower geographic focus

[5] For instance, see Roy Porter and Lesley Hall, *The Facts of Life: The Creation of Sexual Knowledge in Britain, 1650–1950* (New Haven, CT: Yale University Press, 1995).

[6] Ivan Crozier, "Introduction: Havelock Ellis, John Addington Symonds and the Construction of Sexual Inversion," in *Sexual Inversion: A Critical Edition*, ed. Ivan Crozier (Basingstoke: Palgrave Macmillan, 2008), 1–95 and Ruth Richardson, *The Making of Mr. Gray's Anatomy: Bodies, Books, Fortune, Fame* (Oxford: Oxford University Press, 2009) offer rare accounts of the publishing histories of single medical books. Claire L. Jones, *The Business of Birth Control: Contraception and Commerce in Britain before the Sexual Revolution* (Manchester: Manchester University Press, 2020) offers a detailed account of the trade in contraception pamphlets, manuals, and catalogues after 1877. I gratefully cite such studies throughout the book.

[7] Phoebe Letitia Gill, "The Production, Circulation, and Reception of Sexual Knowledges in Published Advice Literature in Britain and Ireland, 1918–1987" (PhD thesis, University of Birmingham, 2023).

[8] Nancy Tomes discusses this divide in "'Not Just for Doctors Anymore': How the *Merck Manual* Became a Consumer Health 'Bible'," *Bulletin of the History of Medicine* 95, no. 1 (2021), 2–3. For broad accounts of medical periodicals, see W. F. Bynum, Stephen Lock, and Roy Porter, eds., *Medical Journals and Medical Knowledge: Historical Essays* (1992; repr., London: Routledge, 2019); Sally Frampton and Jennifer Wallis, eds., *Reading the Nineteenth-Century Medical Journal* (London: Routledge, 2020); Sally Frampton, "The Medical Press and Its Public," in *The Edinburgh History of the British and Irish Press*, vol. 2, ed. David Finkelstein (Edinburgh: Edinburgh University Press, 2022), 438–456. For broad overviews of medical publishing, see David McKitterick, "Publishing for the Trades and Professions," in *The Cambridge History of the Book in Britain*, vol. 6, ed. David McKitterick (Cambridge: Cambridge University Press, 2010), 500–530; Elizabeth Lake, "Medicine," in *The Oxford History of the Irish Book*, vol. IV, ed. James H. Murphy (Oxford: Oxford University Press, 2011), 576–584. There is some work that broadly addresses other medical genres, such as Claire L. Jones, *The Medical Trade Catalogue in Britain, 1870–1914* (London: Routledge, 2016).

seemed best. My strategy has been to focus on the intersecting activities of four loosely defined groups of players, mostly working in London, who brought medical works about sex and reproduction into non-expert readers' hands and, in different ways, became embroiled in debates about medical obscenity. These groups are *radicals*, or reformers and revolutionaries who sought to galvanize social change; *pornographers*, or entrepreneurs who specialized in making and selling sexual material; *regular practitioners*, or medical practitioners who were generally accepted by members of established medical institutions like the Royal Colleges, and the specialist publishers with whom they collaborated; and *irregular practitioners*, who published and practised medisine outside these institutions, or were expelled from them.

These kinds of figures have rarely marched through the pages of the same book. Their styles and aims diverged in important ways, and while outsiders often found it difficult or pointless to distinguish one from another, making their differences known was very important to members of some of these groups. This was especially true of regular practitioners, who were deeply preoccupied with establishing the boundaries of orthodox medical practice.[9] Troubled by dysfunctional hierarchies of governance, vast differences in training, and shaky public trust in medical expertise, successive waves of reformers sought to hammer medicine into a coherent "scientific" profession that could win the kind of social status and public regard afforded to the clergy and the legal profession. Establishing legislation to regulate medical practice was a major focus of this work. Distancing the profession from lower-status trades and rooting out "quackery," a term used for "a mode of conduct . . . that represented a loss of scientific restraint under the pressures of the capitalist profit motive," was another.[10] The practices of the irregular practitioners examined here embodied this loss of restraint, which medical reformers worried could infect the whole profession and undermine what credibility it enjoyed.

The development of what has retrospectively been called sex radicalism was similar in some important respects.[11] Over the course of the nineteenth century,

[9] Peter J. Bowler and Iwan Rhys Morus, *Making Modern Science: A Historical Survey* (Chicago: University of Chicago Press, 2005); Michael Brown, *Performing Medicine: Medical Culture and Identity in Provincial England, c. 1760–1850* (Manchester: Manchester University Press, 2011); W. F. Bynum, *Science and the Practice of Medicine in the Nineteenth Century* (Cambridge: Cambridge University Press, 1994); Anne Digby, *Making a Medical Living: Doctors and Patients in the English Market for Medicine, 1720–1911* (Cambridge: Cambridge University Press, 1994).

[10] Anat Rosenberg, *The Rise of Mass Advertising: Law, Enchantment, and the Cultural Boundaries of British Modernity* (Oxford: Oxford University Press, 2022), 197.

[11] I take this term from Elizabeth Carolyn Miller, *Slow Print: Literary Radicalism and Late Victorian Print Culture* (Stanford, CA: Stanford University Press, 2013). For explorations of different aspects of sex radicalism, see Jones, *Business*; Lesley A. Hall, *Sex, Gender and Social Change in Britain since 1880*, 2nd ed. (London: Bloomsbury, 2017); Laura Schwatz, *Secularism, Religion, and Women's Emancipation, England 1830–1914* (Manchester:

Britain witnessed the rise of a loose, diverse movement for sexual reform that was united only by its adherents' desire for change: it encompassed advocates of family planning, legal equality for illegitimate children, "free unions" outside marriage, more sympathetic treatments of same-sex relationships, and more. The movement's diversity presented considerable problems for it. Many sex radicals were affiliated with secularist, feminist, and socialist groups wary of engaging with causes associated with sex and reproduction, partly for fear of associating their views with sexual immorality. Seeking to reconcile these differences and fashion more coherent collective identities that could gain mainstream support, they worked to distance sexual causes that they believed in from promiscuity and vice. Pornographers, who shared the movement's origins in early nineteenth-century radical circles and intermittently claimed affiliation with social protest, brought these elements together.

It is a testament to the success of the efforts I have described that it does not necessarily feel intuitive to set an account of the activities of the pornographers who set up shop in London's Holywell Street alongside an account of the work of earnest social protestors like Annie Besant, or to study the practices of eminent medical publishers like John Churchill alongside the self-publishing activities of practitioners best known for hawking dubious patent medicines. Yet, this is precisely what is required if we want to understand the practices and politics of selling sexual knowledge during the nineteenth century. Scholars have remarked on how diverse trade in advice about sex and reproduction was, comprising a "polyphony" or "cacophony" of players clamouring for attention.[12] Studying how these groups operated in concert helps identify important elements of this history, such as the pornography trade's traffic in radical contraception pamphlets, that would benefit from closer attention. It also draws attention to serious challenges inherent in establishing coherent collective identities in a context in which print was a major vehicle through which all of these groups engaged the public.

Making Authority in a Convoluted Marketplace

To understand the fraught politics of selling sexual knowledge during this period, we need to move beyond thinking about the nature of the subject matter alone and consider what the messy conditions I have begun to sketch meant for making authority. For many of the agents examined in this book, the act of

Manchester University Press, 2015); Edward Royle, *Radicals, Secularists, and Republicans: Popular Freethought in Britain, 1866–1915* (Manchester: Manchester University Press, 1980); Sarah L. Jones, "'As though Miles of Ocean did not Separate us': Print and the Construction of a Transatlantic Free Love Community at the Fin de Siècle," *Journal of Victorian Culture* 25, no. 1 (2020): 95–109.

12 Porter and Hall, *Facts of Life*, 132; Fisher, "Modern Ignorance," 478.

publishing meant more than putting information into circulation or creating a product to sell. It was also a way of defining fields of expertise and of asserting some form of authority over them. In studying the relationship between print and authority, scholars have identified the mechanism of *association* as crucial to this process.[13] Classically, printed knowledge derives its authority from its association with authors or institutions. A publication's identification with their expertise guarantees the knowledge it contains. At the same time, authors and institutions establish authority by publishing. In offering knowledge to the public, they display their expertise. In an ideal situation, this associational loop is clear of obstacles. There is a single, legible group identified with a particular body of knowledge, and the act of putting it into circulation can only be interpreted in one way. The situation that concerns this book was far from ideal on either of these fronts.

Those who sought to position themselves as authorities in sexual matters had to negotiate three overlapping issues that they often worried would undermine their efforts. One issue – the one that has dominated previous accounts of the politics of presenting sexual information to the public – was the slippery meanings and multiple uses of sexual representations.[14] Some agents examined in this book drew attention to medical eroticism and openly encouraged medical works' supposedly immoral applications. However, many worried that their motives for publishing on sexual matters would be misunderstood, and their reputations compromised. Another persistent issue was the slippery meanings and multiple uses of publishing. The difference between publishing for the public benefit and publishing to generate publicity could be ambiguous. Many sellers of sexual knowledge cheerfully exploited this ambiguity. For regular practitioners, however, who were working within a profession obsessed with distancing itself from the market, the idea that their books could be interpreted as advertisements was often alarming.

The third issue was the convoluted physical and textual geography of the print marketplace itself. Especially during the first decades of the

13 Adrian Johns, *The Nature of the Book: Print and Knowledge in the Making* (Chicago: University of Chicago Press, 1998) examines the relationship between print's authority and its association with authors; Alex Csiszar, *The Scientific Journal: Authorship and the Politics of Knowledge in the Nineteenth Century* (Chicago: University of Chicago Press, 2018) examines the relationship between author's authority and publishing.

14 For instance, see Harry Newman, "'[P]rophane fidlers': Medical Paratexts and Indecent Readers in Early Modern England," in *Medical Paratexts from Medieval to Modern: Dissecting the Page*, ed. Hannah C. Tweed and Diane G. Scott (Cham: Palgrave Macmillan, 2018), 15–42; Sarah Toulalan, "Pornography, Procreation and Pleasure in Early Modern England," in *The Cambridge Companion to Erotic Literature*, ed. Bradford K. Mudge (Cambridge: Cambridge University Press, 2017), 105–122; Ludmilla J. Jordanova, *Sexual Visions: Images of Gender in Science and Medicine between the Eighteenth and Twentieth Centuries* (Madison, WI: University of Wisconsin Press, 1993); Gowan Dawson, *Darwin, Literature, and Victorian Respectability* (Cambridge: Cambridge University Press, 2007).

Victorian period, radicals, pornographers, and regular and irregular practitioners could look awfully similar in print. They advertised their publications in many of the same venues, and those publications were often sold in the same places. They routinely addressed the same subject matter, in similar language, and often shared pages of verbatim text. Sometimes, there were few, or no, discernible differences between publications that these groups offered. They were copies of the same works. Some of these overlaps were deliberate. Others were just a result of the way the book trade worked. The Victorian publishing industry relied heavily on economies of reproduction. Most the works that were published, sold, and read during this period were old works, not newly written ones.[15] This was especially true of manuals and pamphlets at the cheaper end of the market for medical literature. New and third-hand editions of *Aristotle's Masterpiece* (1684), a wildly popular midwifery manual, and *Onania: or, The Heinous Sin of Self-Pollution* (c. 1712), a screed against masturbation, mixed and mingled with Georgian and Victorian productions in bookshops and mail-order catalogues. Many publications migrated from producer to producer, and some became staple products of very differently identified players.

The same texts also revolved around and around the marketplace in parts. Compilation is a traditional way of organizing and synthesizing knowledge, and has a long history in medicine.[16] Although it is typically associated with older textual cultures, it remained a common method of making books throughout the nineteenth century.[17] Many of the agents examined in this book habitually disassembled writing intended for one audience, edited it, and combined it with material from other sources to make a book for a different audience, often without any kind of attribution. Others borrowed from their compilations, and others borrowed from them. As a result, medical text weaved in and out of contexts that we now associate with the categories of the popular and the professional, the orthodox and the fringe, the respectable and the unrespectable. The corollary of this is that medical text had no fixed identity of its own. Rarely did any aspect of the text itself reliably distinguish an

[15] Leah Price, *How to Do Things with Books in Victorian Britain* (Princeton, NJ: Princeton University Press, 2012), 219–257. Although it focuses on the American context, Meredith McGill, *American Literature and the Culture of Reprinting, 1834–1853* (Philadelphia: University of Pennsylvania Press, 2013) is helpful for understanding the culture of reprinting during this period.

[16] Angela N. H. Creager, Mathias Grote, and Elaine Leong, "Learning by the Book: Manuals and Handbooks in the History of Science," *BJHS Themes* 5 (2020): 1–13.

[17] See Sarah Bull, "Content Generation in the Age of Mechanical Reproduction," *Book History* 26, no. 2 (2023): 324–361 for an overview of recent scholarship on compilation in the nineteenth-century context.

"original" medical work issued by one of the groups examined in this book from a work issued by another.

These features of the Victorian print marketplace had some important implications for readers, which I primarily explore in the first chapters of the book. They also have wider implications for the history of knowledge that may interest my own audience. Historians of science have long maintained that knowledge does not simply trickle down from experts to lay readers but circulates in all kinds of directions.[18] Patterns of text reuse examined in *Selling Sexual Knowledge* suggest that this was true at the textual level for much of the nineteenth century. The fact that the agents I examine rarely discussed the legal implications of these practices also affirms a growing understanding among historians that the unsettled nature of copyright laws and ideas about what constituted intellectual property supported the continuation of some cultures of text reuse typically associated with the early modern period well past 1800 and facilitated the development of new ones. Acts of copying considered immoral or illegal today were widely practised and often not considered remarkable.[19]

Where these features gain their significance for the politics of selling sexual knowledge is that they magnified problems that regular practitioners and sex radicals faced as they sought to establish themselves as recognized and trusted authorities. How could any group establish a coherent collective identity through print when others sold the same knowledge it claimed, in the same words, down the street? How could any group claim to be trustworthy and respectable, or that the knowledge it claimed was beneficial to the public, when others used it in advertorials for dubious nostrums or sold it alongside pornographic photographs? These issues were an object of particularly deep anxiety for regular practitioners, and their rivals were more than happy to take advantage of the fact. It is no coincidence that "The Obscene M.D.," which attacks members of the Royal Colleges, attributes *Manly Vigour* to them. *Manly*

18 For an overview of these arguments, see Johan Östling, David Larsson Heidenblad, Erling Sandmo, Anna Nilsson Hammar, and Kari Nordberg, "The History of Knowledge and the Circulation of Knowledge," in *Circulation of Knowledge: Explorations in the History of Knowledge*, ed. Johan Östling, David Larsson Heidenblad, Erling Sandmo, Anna Nilsson Hammar, and Kari Nordberg (Lund: Nordic Academic Press, 2018), 9–33, especially 21–22.

19 For instance, see McGill, *American Literature*; Catherine Seville, *Literary Copyright Reform in Early Victorian England: The Framing of the 1842 Copyright Act* (Cambridge: Cambridge University Press, 1999); Will Slauter, *Who Owns the News? A History of Copyright* (Stanford, CA: Stanford University Press, 2020); Ryan Cordell and Avery Blankenship, "Reprinting Wright," prepublication release from *Going the Rounds: Virality in Nineteenth-Century Newspapers* (Minneapolis: University of Minnesota Press, forthcoming), https://manifold.umn.edu/projects/going-the-rounds; Petra S. McGillen, *The Fontane Workshop: Manufacturing Realism in the Industrial Age of Print* (London: Bloomsbury, 2019).

Vigour was a real title issued by an irregular firm whose practices members of these colleges felt deeply undermined medicine's credibility.[20]

There was no easy means of addressing these problems, least of all through print. Scholars of early modern Europe have shown how medical authors dealt with a context in which distinctions between medical and erotic writing could be even more ambiguous than they were in the nineteenth century by employing various devices to steer readers' interpretations in what they considered the "right" directions.[21] These devices frequently took the form of paratext, a term used in literary scholarship to refer to any material separate from, yet clearly associated with, the main text of a book, from titles, prefaces, epigraphs, and prefatory defences called *apologia*s to bindings and advertisements.[22] Literary scholars have shown that paratexts can act as powerful interpretive mechanisms, influencing readers' understanding of a work by providing them with a framework for comprehending it. A snippet from the surgeon William Burke's *apologia* for describing the generative organs in his *Popular Compendium of Anatomy* (1804) offers an early nineteenth-century example in action:

> While, however, the compiler of the present publication declaims with energy all idea of wishing to gratify the prurient curiosity of a polluted imagination, and is firmly persuaded that nothing will be found in it that will be in the least offensive to the delicacy of a chastened and correct mind, he is desirous of giving such a view of his subject as will best inform the reader, and illustrate the beautiful mechanism of the human frame.[23]

Here, Burke anticipates objections to his work's sexual content by defending its utility, and turns them back on the reader, suggesting that only hopeless leches (certainly not the reader!) will find it anything but enlightening.

[20] C. J. Lucas and Co., *Manly Vigour: A Popular Inquiry into the Concealed Causes of Its Premature Decline with Instructions for Its Complete Restoration* [. . .]. (London: Published by the Authors, 1841).

[21] Sarah Toulalan, *Imagining Sex: Pornography and Bodies in Seventeenth-Century England.* (Oxford: Oxford University Press, 2007) offers an extended analysis of these categories and their confusion in the seventeenth century. For work on how medical authors employed paratexts to negotiate this issue, see Harry Newman, "'[P]rophane fidlers'."; Toulalan, "Pornography, Procreation." Monica H. Green traces the emergence of some of these techniques to the late medieval period in "'Diseases of Women' to 'Secrets of Women': The Transformation of Gynecological Literature in the Later Middle Ages." *The Journal of Medieval and Renaissance Studies* 30, no. 1 (2000): 5–40.

[22] Gerard Genette, *Paratexts: Thresholds of Interpretation*, trans. Jane Lewin (Cambridge: Cambridge University Press, 1997). For insights into how paratexts are used in book marketing, I have found Clare Squires, *Marketing Literature: The Making of Contemporary Writing in Britain* (Basingstoke: Palgrave Macmillan, 2007) helpful.

[23] William Burke, *The Popular Compendium of Anatomy: or, A Concise and Clear Description of the Human Body* [. . .]. (London: S. Highley, 1804), 242.

Literary scholars emphasize that paratexts do not have to be as explicit as Burke's *apologia*, which bludgeons readers with his preferred interpretation of the sexual details in his book and his motives for including them, to be effective. Even the quality of a book's binding can speak volumes in a culture in which certain material features of a publication are thought to signify respectability. However, as episodes in this book illustrate, paratexts could not be counted on to function as desired – and this was doubly true in a marketplace teeming with competing players. Like the texts they framed, paratexts could be ignored or misinterpreted. They could be misrepresented, or contaminated by agents who co-opted them for their own purposes. And their powers could be overwhelmed: irregulars traded so much in information about venereal disease from the eighteenth century, for instance, that the topic became closely associated with commercialism and showmanship, while pornographers' regular traffic in contraception manuals from the 1830s intensified their identification with licentiousness.

Over time, regular practitioners addressed some of these issues by developing stricter, more distinctive conventions for writing, publishing, and advertising. Extrapolating from Alex Csiszar's study of the scientific journal, which explores how specialized publishing formats function as frameworks for legitimating knowledge and consolidating public trust in expertise, I argue that a variety of conventions came to operate in concert as a more robust framework than single paratexts for legitimating medical books and their producers.[24] Just as a physician's qualifications, social networks, dress, comportment, and sex traditionally combined to endorse him as a credible medical practitioner,[25] certain styles of writing, publishers' imprints, advertising methods, and distribution networks increasingly came together to mark a book out as a credible medical intervention – and relatively minor deviations from this set of conventions increasingly marked one out as dubious. These conventions included significant constraints on medical book advertising, one of several developments in medical publishing that I argue had important implications for public access to information on sexual matters and, initially, for emerging cross-disciplinary fields like sexology. They also coalesced so slowly and gained such uneven recognition with the public that they did not begin to present a meaningful resolution to the problems I have described until the end of the nineteenth century.

24 Csiszar, *The Scientific Journal*.

25 See Hannah Barker, "Medical Advertising and Trust in Late Georgian England," *Urban History* 36, no. 3 (2009): 379–398.

The Frame of Obscenity

The potentially obscene status of medical works on sexual matters offered alternative possibilities for contesting authority and consolidating collective identities, and much of the book focuses on how regular practitioners and sex radicals deployed them. When the British College of Health accused M.D.s of writing obscene books and calling them science, it referred to a legal as well as a moral offence. Initially derived from common laws against libel during England's Restoration, laws against the publication, display, and distribution of obscene material multiplied during the nineteenth century, largely as a result of lobbying from the Society for the Suppression of Vice, Britain's longest-running anti-vice society. The passage of the most famous of these laws, the 1857 Obscene Publications Act, was plagued by legislators' reservations about the ambiguous legal meaning of the term "obscene." Unlike "blasphemy" or "sedition," the term was not attached to any specific language, subject matter, media form, genre, style, or range of imagery. Even the first legal definition in Britain, formulated in 1868 by the Lord Chief Justice Alexander Cockburn, defined obscene material only by its effects (to "deprave and corrupt") on its likely audience ("those into whose hands it may fall").[26]

Obscenity was thus more of an argument about a work's social effects than a thing in its own right.[27] And it proved to be a highly portable argument that has been put to work for a wide variety of purposes: as a spectacular means of performing and justifying state power; as an "entrepreneurial gimmick" used to sell books, films, and lifestyles; as an aesthetic device in avant-garde literature; and more.[28] These diverse uses of the idea of obscenity are often implicitly characterized as post-Victorian innovations, with modernist sophistication replacing corseted prudery. However, a closer look at the Victorian context repudiates this view. Arguments and laws addressing obscene material were routinely used to advance goals that extended beyond, and sometimes had little to do with, concern about the specific works at issue.

26 Regina v. Hicklin, *Law Reports 3: Queen's Bench Division* (1868), 371. These developments are examined in detail in Chapter 4.

27 I am adapting an argument about the term "pornography" from Walter M. Kendrick, *The Secret Museum: Pornography in Modern Culture* (1987; repr., Berkeley: University of California Press, 1996), xiii.

28 Jordan S. Carroll, *Reading the Obscene: Transgressive Editors and the Class Politics of US Literature* (Stanford: Stanford University Press, 2021), 6. See also Adam Parkes, *Modernism and the Theater of Censorship* (Oxford: Oxford University Press, 1996); Leon Janssens, "Erotische censuur: De seksuele revolutie in gecensureerde pornografische filmposters in België (1971–1980)," *Tijdschrift voor Geschiedenis* 133, no. 2 (2020): 347–366; Loren Glass, *Counterculture Colophon: Grove Press, the Evergreen Review, and the Incorporation of the Avant-Garde* (Stanford: Stanford University Press, 2013); Allison Pease, *Modernism, Mass Culture, and the Aesthetics of Obscenity* (Cambridge: Cambridge University Press, 2000); Rachel Potter, *Obscene Modernism: Literary Censorship and Experiment, 1900–1940* (Oxford: Oxford University Press, 2013).

Claims about obscenity were commonly used as a marketing strategy. As we will see throughout this book, claims that a work had been suppressed, or was liable to be suppressed, reliably spurred sales. But different agents also made more sophisticated use of the argument to advance other interests. The state and anti-vice societies periodically exploited the ambiguous meaning of the term "obscene" to crack down on fraud, political organizing, and the sale of graphically explicit novels, prints, and photographs: items whose primary aim was considered sexual arousal, whose rapid refinement by a new body of specialized producers and increasing visibility in public spaces did attract consistent opposition. From the mid-1880s, this material would collectively be labelled "pornography." (I use the term for the entire period in this book because there was no stable term for this material before the 1880s.)[29] Finding pornography to seize could be difficult because sellers learned to conceal it. Fraudulent acts were hard to prove in court. Intervening in radical politics was a minefield. In some cases, authorities seized medical works from individuals involved in these activities even as they allowed the same works to circulate openly – and often on a much larger scale – in other hands.

In arguing that medical works could be obscene, state authorities and anti-vice crusaders relied on a contextual model of obscenity that Cockburn formalized in the 1868 case *R.* v. *Hicklin*. What made a work dangerous to the public was not the intent with which it had been written, they argued. The issue lay with the mode of its sale, which could expose vulnerable readers to dangerous material. Scholars have shown that these arguments relied on paternalistic models of reading that cast young men, women, children, and, in some contexts, racialized groups as especially vulnerable to the influences of print. However, their significance for this book lies largely in their insistence that a work's commercial context determined its legitimacy, to the point that the same work might be legitimate when sold in one context, and illegitimate when sold in another. Grounded in the idea that commercial context influences who engages with a text, and how, these arguments speak to Victorians' sophisticated understandings of interpretation, and reflected real cultural concerns about the social effects of an expanding media world. However, they also served transient interests of state authorities and anti-vice crusaders, and the longer-term interests of regular practitioners, who used language and laws against obscenity to attack rivals in the marketplace, distance medicine from "trade," and define its field of authority.

My interest in this history was initially aroused by the work of Alan Bates, who has argued that during the mid-nineteenth century medics opposed public

[29] My reasons for this choice of terminology are practical and generally align with Lisa Z. Sigel's in *Governing Pleasures: Pornography and Social Change in England, 1815–1914* (Rutgers, NJ: Rutgers University Press, 2001).

anatomical museums on the grounds that they were obscene because they threatened medicine's authority over anatomical knowledge.[30] This book shows that campaigns against so-called obscene quackery spanned a much longer period and often focused on publications, moving from relatively crude campaigns aimed at convincing newspaper editors to stop publishing advertisements for irregular health manuals to organized efforts to use obscenity laws to distance medicine from overtly commercial styles of practice and situate them as illegitimate. Like many of the publications examined in this book, these tactics were not very original. Medical practitioners had contested authority through allegations of various transgressions involving the misappropriation or misrepresentation of knowledge, including piracy, fraud, quackery, and indecency, for centuries.[31] I argue that an array of developments simply made allegations of obscenity look like an especially promising means of contesting authority in some contexts.

Sex radicals' uses of the idea of obscenity were also adaptations of earlier strategies, this time from radical politics. Many sex radicals were affiliated with political groups that had a long history of protesting restrictions on the freedom of the press and recognized that decrying restrictions on the circulation of knowledge could galvanize support for controversial causes and help consolidate collectives around them. In a context in which authorities seized progressive works on sexual matters in the interest of fighting the pornography trade, and, in one case, anarchist organizing, sex radicals made claims about their medical publications' vulnerability to destruction under obscenity laws to distance causes that they believed in from immorality and galvanize support from other activists, scientists, and members of the public. Under the evolving narratives that they constructed, sexual causes became free speech issues, sex reformers and sexual scientists became seekers of truths that could liberate society from sexual ignorance, and pornographers became exploiters of that ignorance.

This is not to say that no Victorian really thought that medical works on sexual matters endangered morality, nor that some sellers of these works did not genuinely worry about arrest. Although Victorians often resisted the idea that medical works could, or should, be criminally obscene, they accepted that people could misuse them, just as people had in earlier periods.[32] Tactical

[30] A. W. Bates, "Dr. Kahn's Museum: Obscene Anatomy in Victorian London," *Journal of the Royal Society of Medicine* 99 (2006): 618–624.

[31] Adrian Johns, *Piracy: The Intellectual Property Wars from Gutenberg to Gates* (Chicago: University of Chicago Press, 2009), 83–108, especially 98; Roy Porter, *Health for Sale: Quackery in England, 1660–1850* (Manchester: Manchester University Press, 1989). On the twentieth-century context, see Colleen Derkatch, *Bounding Biomedicine: Evidence and Rhetoric in the New Science of Alternative Medicine* (Chicago: University of Chicago Press, 2016).

[32] See Toulalan, "Pornography, Procreation," 107–109 for details about early modern perspectives.

actions, trade routes, and marketing techniques examined here repeatedly associated certain works with indecency, too. These actions influenced public perception, and in some cases increased the risks of prosecution for selling them. Overall, though, *Selling Sexual Knowledge* argues that language and laws about obscenity should be seen less as impediments to the work of selling sexual knowledge in either sense of the term than as means through which sexual knowledge was defined and promoted as a specialized field of expertise.[33] Allegations of obscenity were used by those most invested in medical publishing, practice, and knowledge to market medical books and pamphlets, define what constituted sexual knowledge, and promote its production and distribution as projects of vital importance. At the same time, such allegations were deployed to position certain kinds of figures as legitimate authorities over this knowledge, and others as mere exploiters of it.

Plan of the Book

Because collective identities are so important to this history, most of the chapters in this book focus on the activities of particular groups of players, though their stories become increasingly intermingled over the course of the narrative. The chapters proceed chronologically, but only roughly. The first three chapters examine the activities of three different groups in parallel, covering the first half of the Victorian period, from the mid-1830s to the early 1860s. The middle chapter examines important legal developments in the 1850s and 1860s, and their relation to conditions explored in the previous chapters. The last three chapters examine the activities of three different groups of players, again roughly in parallel, from the 1870s to the early 1900s.

The book begins with a chapter on the pornography trade. In "Holywell Street Medicine," I trace the trade's birth out of the collapse of revolutionary politics in the 1820s, and show how its reliance on scavenging for content fostered a vibrant mid-century traffic in cheap reprints and reworkings of works on contraception, venereal disease, procreation, and midwifery. While showing how pornographers harnessed the expanding infrastructures of the press and the post to sell these works across the nation, I demonstrate how they framed them through two different lenses. Pornographers followed a long line of disreputable booksellers in framing some medical works on sexual matters as voyeuristic *entrées* to "secret" knowledge that people could read for pleasure. However, they also adapted radical arguments for sex education, reproductive autonomy, and female pleasure to position medical knowledge as practical

[33] For an overview of recent work on the history of "sexual expertise," which influences the perspective I outline here, see Hannah Charnock, Sarah L. Jones, and Ben Mechen, "Sexpertise: Sexual Knowledge and the Public in the Nineteenth and Twentieth Centuries," *Social History of Medicine* 36, no. 4 (2024): 585–591.

information that readers could apply to support safe, pleasurable sex lives of their own.

Chapter 2, "Stereotyped Knowledge," examines another major route through which readers encountered sexual information: irregular practitioners' global trade in cheap manuals on venereal disease, sexual debility, and fertility problems. While historians have often focused on these manuals' lurid depictions of weakened male bodies, this chapter emphasizes their origins in respected publications: irregular practitioners combined verbatim sections from textbooks and treatises aimed at practising medics with snippets from works in other genres to construct their own "popular treatises." These productions offered readers an affordable means of acquiring up-to-date information about sexual health, and their authors a means of cultivating trust in their expertise and advertising more expensive products and services. By examining other practitioners' responses to these figures' publishing and advertising activities alongside the activities themselves, this chapter begins to demonstrate why these figures attracted virulent opposition in regular medical circles: the way they used print to commodify medical expertise was seen as both an economic and an existential threat to regular medicine.

Regular practitioners portrayed pornographers' and irregulars' uses of sexual knowledge as misuses. While exploring how specialist medical publishers and regular practitioners worked together to publish and advertise their own works, however, Chapter 3, "Publishing for Professional Advantage," shows that the boundaries between communicating knowledge, promoting expertise, and trading on medical eroticism were also blurry in regular medicine. Works issued by medical publishers were often textually similar to those issued by pornographers and irregulars; worked up using similar techniques; and advertised and distributed in similar ways, in the same venues. Building on Chapter 2, this chapter examines how and why overlaps between regular and irregular medical publishing aroused especially acute concern among medical reformers. Instead of concentrating on disciplining regular medical publishing, however, many reformers initially sought to remedy this situation by launching campaigns aimed at stamping out irregular practitioners' trade in sexual health manuals.

Chapter 4, "Obscene . . . in a Certain Sense," shows how charges of obscenity were used against pornographers and irregulars during the 1850s and 1860s, amid landmark changes to obscenity law. In doing so, it introduces one of the book's major arguments: that allegations of medical obscenity were usually tactical, and became increasingly imbricated in projects aimed at contesting moral and epistemic authority in a marketplace that invited troubling confusions of identity. Many Victorians did not believe that obscenity laws applied to medical works. However, anti-vice crusaders recognized that legal arguments could be made that they did, and capitalized on it as they attempted to destroy the pornography trade. I parallel these tactics with tactics in the medical press. With mixed success, anti-quackery campaigners sought to discredit irregulars and even bring about their prosecution by arguing that their sexual health manuals' low prices and wide circulation made them a threat to public morals. The chapter ends with the 1868 *Hicklin* judgement, which affirmed such arguments could justify charges for distributing obscene material.

Chapter 5, "Dull Instead of Light," examines increasing efforts to disambiguate "medicine" and "quackery" in *Hicklin*'s wake. The first section explores how regular practitioners experimented with using obscenity laws as alternatives to the Medical Act (1858) to regulate medical practice. These experiments foundered after a few years, but in some respects the work they did to collapse quackery and obscenity paid off: authorities now accepted that irregular trade in sexual health advice was illegitimate and introduced legislation to limit advertising for it. The rest of the chapter examines efforts to professionalize regular medical publishing. In advocating limitations on book advertising, the use of dry, technical language in professional writing, and other changes to medical print culture, regular practitioners again worked to disambiguate "medicine" from "quackery." The lines between popular and professional medical works had previously been blurry. The changes examined in this chapter helped cleave a growing chasm between the kinds of sexual knowledge accessible to medical and non-medical audiences.

Chapter 6, "Branding Birth Control," examines how sex radicals made claims about medical works' vulnerability to destruction to distance contraception from sex itself, frame its advocacy as a free speech issue, and generate publicity for the cause. Both social reformers and pornographers had long sold contraception pamphlets first published by radical agitators in the 1820s and 1830s. In 1876, a figure with feet in both worlds was arrested for selling one of them, Charles Knowlton's *Fruits of Philosophy* (1832). The following year, the Secularists Annie Besant and Charles Bradlaugh engineered their own trial for selling Knowlton's pamphlet. The chapter examines the selective publication history that Bradlaugh and Besant constructed to divorce *Fruits* from the pornography trade and promote contraception as both a respectable and a radical cause. It also examines their trial's afterlife. The trial attracted enormous publicity, and practical works on contraceptive techniques sold in huge volumes in the 1880s and 1890s. Although they encountered relatively little legal opposition during this period, birth controllers claimed that selling such works was incredibly risky. I argue that these claims operated as a way of generating further publicity for the cause and branding it as brave, modern, and progressive.

The book ends with a chapter on sexology. In "Be Careful about the Publisher," I examine how the diverse sources, distribution networks, and audiences associated with sexology undermined Havelock Ellis's attempts to frame *Sexual Inversion* as a serious medical work and led to its appearance in the obscenity trial *R. v. Bedborough* (1898). Authorities were aiming to break up a radical group when they charged George Bedborough for selling *Sexual Inversion*, but sexologists and their allies framed his arrest and trial as an ignorant attack on scientific progress. Elaborating on strategies pioneered by birth controllers, they argued that the censorship of "naturalistic" sexual expression had mired society in sexual ignorance, fostering "abnormal" sexual behaviour and appetite for pornography, the rightful target of obscenity laws. In doing so, they obfuscated sexology's debts to the pornography trade, which increasingly disseminated sexual-scientific publications and supplied material used in sex research. By examining sexologists' attempts to navigate these issues, the chapter further demonstrates how arguments about obscenity and censorship were used to sanitize sexual knowledge and promote a particular group's authority over it.

The conclusion, "Victorian Ignorance," places this history into conversation with the emergence of a new history of sexual knowledge at the turn of the twentieth century. Drawing on the work of Kate Fisher, it begins by considering how well publishing activities explored in the book served Victorian readers. The ways Victorians discussed their own reading experiences evince what Fisher calls an "epistemology of sexual ignorance," in which sexual knowledge is thought of as a set of facts that must be learned through interaction with an expert.[34] The conclusion reflects on how commercial practices and rhetorical strategies that the book examines not only encouraged this way of conceptualizing sexual knowledge but also helped foster the emergence of historical narrative about Victorian censorship that would serve as a powerful justification for sexual-scientific research and sex reform movements in the twentieth century. It would also obfuscate the extent to which Victorians enjoyed access to sexual information in the new age of mass print.

[34] Fisher, "Modern Ignorance," 484.

1 Holywell Street Medicine

The Secrets of Nature Revealed opens with an image of a nude woman. Lurid red drapes frame her body, lit by a candelabra suspended over her head. She is clutching a bedsheet, as if it has just slipped. A book – this book? – lies open on the table beside her. Mirroring her exposed body, its naked pages promise to give secrets away, to unveil, as the subtitle on the facing page suggests, "mysteries of human procreation and copulation." If you were to turn *Secrets of Nature* over and look at the back of its cheap paper cover, you would see a list of novels and illustration series that sound at least as racy as this image. *Woman of Pleasure. Voluptuarian Cabinet. Wanton Widow. Secrets of Nature*, however, is not that kind of fiction. It's a compilation of chapters from two old manuals on procreation, the anonymous *Aristotle's Masterpiece* (1684) and an English translation of the French physician Nicholas Venette's *La génération de l'homme, ou tableau de l'amour conjugal* (1675), which the publisher is passing off as a translation of the alchemist Michael Scot's (1175–c. 1232) much older treatise, *De physiognomia et de hominis procreatione* (Figure 1.1). Together, these remnants from early modern print culture form a manual that describes the structure of the reproductive organs and outlines the ebbs and flows of female desire, offers advice about how to conceive strong children, and suggests remedies for impotence and infertility. Only the frontispiece is original to the nineteenth century.[1]

The Secrets of Nature Revealed was first published in the 1830s by the printer, publisher, and bookseller William Dugdale (1800–68).[2] The deist

[1] To identify copied text in *Secrets of Nature* and all other publications discussed in this book, I made manual comparisons and used the computer-assisted method described in Sarah Bull, "Content Generation in the Age of Mechanical Reproduction," *Book History* 26, no. 2 (2023): 339. Although Scot's work did influence many early modern publications, including *Aristotle's Masterpiece*, *Secrets of Nature* was clearly created by compiling verbatim chapters from the later works. Compare the introduction to chapter VII of *Secrets of Nature* with chapters IV and VI–VIII of Nicolas Venette, *Conjugal Love; or, The Pleasures of the Marriage Bed Considered* [. . .]. (London: Printed for the Booksellers, c. 1750), 1174.a.32, BL and chapters VII–XV of *Secrets of Nature* with chapters II and IV–VI of Aristotle [pseud.], *The Works of Aristotle: In Four Parts* [. . .]. (London: Published for the Booksellers, 1790), RB.23.a.28545, BL.

[2] Holywell Street publishers routinely published anonymously or under pseudonyms, and often affixed their books with false imprints and dates of publication. My practice is to name the most

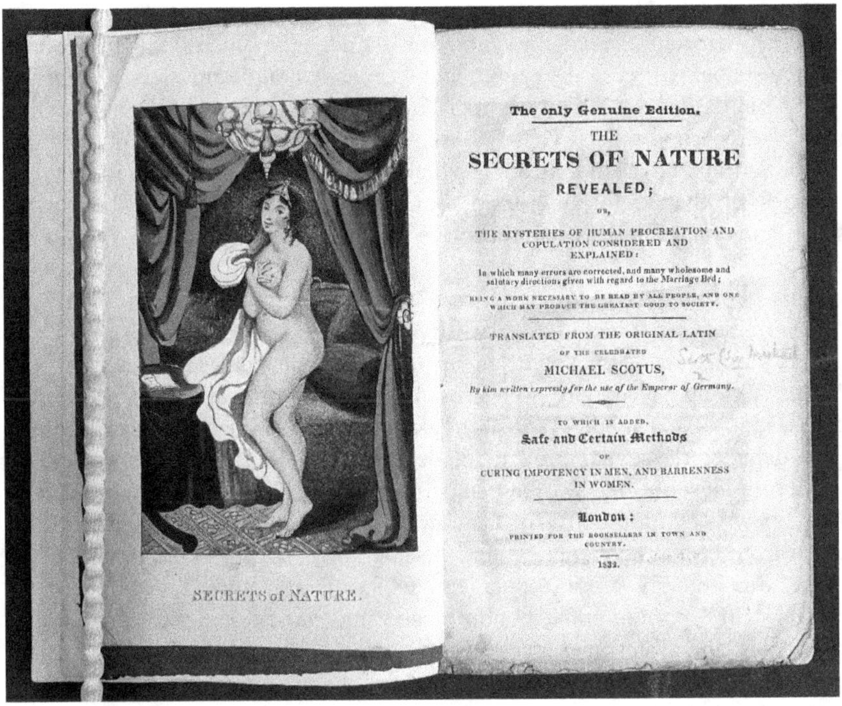

Figure 1.1 Frontispiece and title page, *The Secrets of Nature Revealed; or, The Mysteries of Human Procreation and Copulation Considered and Explained* (London: Printed for the Booksellers in Town and Country, 1832), Cup.365.a.36, BL. By courtesy of The British Library.

son of a Stockport Quaker, Dugdale moved to London in 1818 to agitate for revolution, where he became known, appropriately enough, as the Radical Quaker. By the time *Secrets of Nature* was published, he was well on his way to transforming himself into the Ogre of Holywell Street: the most notorious and successful of a number of publishers of sexual material who kept bookshops in Holywell Street and other thoroughfares near London's Strand. Publishers like Dugdale are best known for their trade in graphically explicit fiction and images, and widely considered Britain's first career

likely publisher, date, and place of publication given all available bibliographical and historical information. My research has benefitted from carefully documented lists of aliases and addresses in Peter Mendes, *Clandestine Erotic Fiction in English 1800–1930: A Bibliographical Study* (1993; repr., London: Routledge, 2016) and Sheryl Straight, *The Erotica Bibliophile*, accessed February 19, 2024, eroticabibliophile.com.

pornographers.[3] Yet, just as Holywell Street was a more diverse space than its Victorian usage as a synonym for indecency would suggest, home to newspaper offices and pubs, butcher shops and clothiers, Holywell Street publishers sold many works that do not fit neatly into most definitions of pornography. These works include books and pamphlets on reproduction and sexual health, which they hawked throughout the first decades of the Victorian period alongside salacious periodicals, bawdy song and joke books, contraceptive devices, and guides to London's nightlife.

This book begins at these shops where *Secrets of Nature* and *Woman of Pleasure* met. What look like very different modes of sexual representation to us today were less distinct at the dawn of the Victorian period. Just as *Secrets of Nature*'s frontispiece bore some resemblance to illustrations in Dugdale's clandestine novels, medical and pornographic literature shared a set of features. Both depicted the sexual body in detailed and sometimes lyrical ways. *Secrets of Nature*'s descriptions of "that rising hill which is called the Mount of Venus," the "sinewy and hard body" of the clitoris, the red flesh of the labia could be taken from early nineteenth-century pornography.[4] At the same time, neither genre was reliably erotic. Emergent, experimental, and "temperamentally inconsistent," pornographic fiction lapsed into narrative digressions, comic spectacles, and grotesque scenes.[5] Just as medical texts put the body's failures on display, pornography's heroes endured the ravages of venereal disease, were embarrassed by impotence, and suffered from incontinence.

Disreputable booksellers had a long tradition of drawing attention to medical eroticism, and Holywell Street publishers followed in that tradition. However, like most Victorians, they did not think of medical and pornographic works as identical. Publishers like Dugdale were actively working to refine pornography into a more distinctive, more potent media form, one more concentrated on sexual fantasy.[6] In this context, they recognized and capitalized on the fact that medical works offered something valuable that was harder to come by in fantasy narratives: practical information about the

[3] Colette Colligan, *The Traffic in Obscenity from Byron to Beardsley: Sexuality and Exoticism in Nineteenth-Century Print Culture* (Basingstoke: Palgrave Macmillan, 2006); Iain McCalman, *Radical Underworld: Prophets, Revolutionaries, and Pornographers in London, 1795–1840* (Cambridge: Cambridge University Press, 1988); Kathleen Lubey, *What Pornography Knows: Sex and Social Protest since the Eighteenth Century* (Stanford, CA: Stanford University Press, 2022); Lisa Z. Sigel, *Governing Pleasures: Pornography and Social Change in England, 1815–1914* (Rutgers, NJ: Rutgers University Press, 2001).

[4] *Secrets of Nature*, 19.

[5] Kathleen Lubey, "Making Pornography, 1749–1968: The History of *The History of the Human Heart*," *ELH* 82, no. 3 (2015): 900. See also Thomas J. Joudrey, "Penetrating Boundaries: An Ethics of Anti-perfectionism in Victorian Pornography," *Victorian Studies* 57, no. 3 (2015): 423–432.

[6] Lubey, *What Pornography Knows*.

body and its operations that could be readily applied to support active, satisfying sex lives. While tracing how Holywell Street publishers built a nationwide trade in sexual material, this chapter shows how they brought the medical and the erotic into conversation in new ways inspired by their roots in radical politics. By employing strategic editorial techniques and suggestive advertising, Holywell Street publishers encouraged Victorian readers to use even the most dated and most moralizing medical works according to a vision for modern life adapted from the libertine fictions of revolutionary France: one in which men and women educated themselves about the body and its failures, and used their knowledge to embrace the pleasures of the flesh.

The Holywell Street trade emerged in a changing print world, one in which new printing and paper-making technologies, falling taxes on advertising, and expanding press and postal infrastructures fostered the rapid growth of trade in cheap medical works. Publishers like Dugdale were fixtures in this trade through the mid-nineteenth century, and probably the most significant source of practical works on contraceptive techniques. Yet, their traffic in medical works has scarcely attracted scholarly notice. I begin with an account of their work partly to draw attention to a kind of business that uniquely interpolated Victorian readers of works on sexual matters as savvy, street-smart agents: interested in sexual pleasure, justifiably eager to take control of their reproductive lives, and, like Holywell Street publishers themselves, perfectly equipped to take what was useful from a rag-bag of printed knowledge and leave what was not behind.

Beginning with the Holywell Street trade also helps introduce historical developments and perspectives that are crucial to understanding the larger story that this book has to tell. By tracing the trade's development, we can witness the rapid expansion of a brash traffic in sexual material that brought the medical and the erotic into conversation on an unprecedented commercial scale. The eclectic catalogues that Holywell Street publishers developed and the applications of medical material that they drew attention to would galvanize debate about the boundaries of obscenity, and set in motion many events examined in this book. The history of the Holywell Street trade also offers a particularly concrete illustration of the Victorian publishing industry's reliance on old content, and the extent to which authors and publishers relied on context to steer interpretation in the directions they wanted. Although they were sometimes marketed as such, the medical works that Holywell Street publishers sold were not usually rare or novel works. Many could be found in bookshops and bookstalls all over the country. What made Holywell Street publishers' trade in medical material distinctive was how they framed it.

Medical Eroticism at the Birth of the Pornography Trade

Pornography's emergence as a distinct genre and the development of an industry focused on its distribution were intertwined processes. From the early modern period, a dispersed traffic in a variety of genres that depicted sex with varying degrees of explicitness gradually crystallized into a more concentrated trade in a more discrete range of material increasingly oriented around graphic depictions of sexual acts.[7] Radical politics and libertine philosophy played crucial roles in this history. The revolutionary foment of eighteenth-century France, in which *philosophes* used sexual allegation to undermine the monarchy and the Church, gave birth to works now considered landmarks in the genre's development – most famously, the writings of the Marquis de Sade. In Britain, early nineteenth-century radical print culture laid the groundwork for the Holywell Street trade, a key precursor to the modern pornography industry.

English Republican agitators famously used the humour and shock-value of smut to expose the hypocrisies of the clergy and aristocracy, press for their abolishment, and push for the expansion of the franchise.[8] For some of these agitators, though, obscene expression was more than just an arresting tool for critique: it was a revolt against blinkered sexual ideologies in its own right. Influenced by the Enlightenment ideals of revolutionary France, radical pressmen like Dugdale, William Benbow, and George Cannon advocated a class-conscious brand of libertinism that collapsed political, intellectual, and sexual freedom. Sexual desire, they maintained, was a "secret spring" implanted in man by Nature. By "yielding to the dictates of love, and in performing its joyous rites," they rejected the strictures of Christian morality in favour of a "religion of NATURE" that enabled piety without hypocrisy, "real instead of pretended inspiration," harmony instead of "wars, and jars, and brawls, and strife."[9] Publications from French and older English libertine traditions flowed from their presses alongside more straightforwardly revolutionary works.[10]

[7] See Lynn Hunt, *The Invention of Pornography: Obscenity and the Origins of Modernity, 1500–1800* (New York: Zone Books, 1993); James Grantham Turner, *Schooling Sex: Libertine Literature and Erotic Education in Italy, France and England, 1534–1685* (Oxford: Oxford University Press, 2003); Robert Darnton, *The Literary Underground of the Old Regime* (Cambridge, MA: Harvard University Press, 1982); Karen Harvey, *Reading Sex in the Eighteenth Century: Bodies and Gender in English Erotic Culture* (Cambridge: Cambridge University Press, 2004); Julie Peakman, *Mighty Lewd Books: The Development of Pornography in Eighteenth-Century England* (Basingstoke: Palgrave Macmillan, 2003); Lubey, *What Pornography Knows*; McCalman, *Radical Underworld*; Sigel, *Governing Pleasures*; Jamie Stoops, *The Thorny Path: Pornography in Early Twentieth Century Britain* (Montreal: McGill-Queens University Press, 2018).

[8] McCalman, *Radical Underworld*, 162–177.

[9] "On Love," *Rambler's Magazine*, January 1, 1822, 2.

[10] See Sigel, *Governing Pleasures*, 18; McCalman, *Radical Underworld*, 207–212; Colligan, *Traffic*, 23–35.

Other agitators rejected revolutionary libertinism but agreed that political change and sexual freedom went hand in hand. Inspired by the economic arguments of Thomas Robert Malthus, whose *Essay on the Principle of Population* (1798) predicted cataclysmic population growth, the social reformer Francis Place embraced contraception as the answer to some of Britain's most pressing political problems.[11] Place considered Malthus's solution to overpopulation – sexual abstinence – unrealistic, but he thought that in working-class hands, contraception could be transformative. As well as alleviating the economic pressures of population growth, knowledge of the practice could enable working people to force wage rises and end child labour. By 1823, Place was distributing pamphlets on contraceptive techniques in London's East End, which were quickly reprinted in radical periodicals.[12] In 1825, the printer and publisher Richard Carlile issued essays of his own in his radical periodical the *Republican*, which wove practical instruction on contraceptive techniques together with an argument for a sexually egalitarian society in which sex education was taken seriously, premarital sex was not looked down on, and women's pleasure was valued as much as men's. A stand-alone pamphlet, *Every Woman's Book*; *or, What is Love?*, followed in 1826.[13]

By the time Carlile published *Every Woman's Book*, radicalism was in crisis. The passage of the Six Acts in 1819 and the election of a suppressive Tory government the following year had made political publishing and demonstrating dangerous. Public appetite for revolution was also on the decline. Radical pressmen were struggling to sell their stock, and the circles that Carlile and Place ran in were shifting their focus away from confrontational politics in favour of a reformist approach focused on working-class education. This turn to compromise spurred efforts to distance the movement from immorality, and dealt a huge blow to Carlile's vision for sexual life. His pamphlet, and later two American pamphlets inspired by it – the social reformer Robert Dale Owen's *Moral Physiology* (1830) and the physician Charles Knowlton's *Fruits of Philosophy* (1832) – were charged with promoting promiscuity, blasphemy,

11 Norman F. Himes, *Medical History of Contraception* (1936; repr., New York: Schocken, 1970); Angus McLaren, *Birth Control in Nineteenth-Century England* (London: Croom Helm, 1978); Brian Dolan, ed., *Malthus, Medicine, & Morality: "Malthusianism" after 1798* (London: Brill, 2016).

12 [Francis Place], *To the Married of Both Sexes* ([London]: s.n., n.d.), *To the Married of Both Sexes of the Working People* ([London]: s.n., n.d.), and *To the Married of Both Sexes in Genteel Life* ([London]: s.n., n.d.), SELIGMAN 1823E T55 Green Box, Columbia University Rare Book and Manuscript Library.

13 "What Is Love?" *Republican*, May 6, 1825, 545–569; Richard Carlile, *Every Woman's Book; or, What is Love? Containing Most Important Instructions for the Prudent Regulation of the Principle of Love, and the Number of a Family* (London: R. Carlile, 1826), DRT Digital Store 1578/4474, BL. M. L. Bush, *What Is Love? Richard Carlile's Philosophy of Sex* (London: Verso, 1998) offers a detailed account of *Every Woman's Book*'s creation and publication.

and atheism.[14] As we will see in Chapter 6, some social reformers printed editions of *Moral Physiology* and *Fruits of Philosophy* into the 1870s, selling them in small numbers in their bookshops, by mail order, and through third-party dealers alongside radical classics, like the works of Thomas Paine. By and large, though, support for contraception lost traction in these circles along with hope for revolution.

But the fraught conditions of the 1820s also fostered the birth of the Holywell Street trade, which brought *Every Woman's Book*, *Moral Physiology*, and *Fruits of Philosophy* into conversation with a very different kind of reading material. As they faced a shrinking audience for incendiary political literature, Dugdale, Benbow, Cannon, and a few other radical pressmen identified a growing market for sexual entertainment, and pivoted to serve it.[15] Many of these men continued to attend political meetings and sell political material. In addition to issuing works by the likes of Voltaire and Paine, Dugdale wrote and published fiery pamphlets against the Poor Laws and the Corn Laws in the 1840s, and issued *Bell's Penny Dispatch* (1841–2), a short-lived periodical that railed against slavery, child labour, and worker exploitation.[16] However, these kinds of publications played an increasingly marginal role in their businesses. By the end of the 1830s, they had developed trade in sexually themed publications into a specialized line of work, one that was attracting new players, in league with an array of other urban suppliers of information and entertainment, and chiefly associated with London's Holywell Street.

Inventing a specialized trade in sexual material took time, effort, and willingness to experiment. The libertine dialogues that these publishers had issued at the beginning of the 1820s had an obvious appeal to audiences in search of sexual entertainment. To develop a concentrated trade in sexual material, however, they needed to expand their lists. Practically, there were four routes that publishers could take to get their hands on new content: (1) they could acquire new works by purchasing or commissioning publications, (2) they could write them themselves, (3) they could reprint old publications, or (4) they could rework old publications to create new ones.

From the middle of the 1820s, Cannon, Dugdale, and Benbow distinguished themselves from other publishers by issuing new, straightforwardly erotic novels and prints with niche (usually wealthy) audiences in mind. Some, such as *The Spirit of Flagellation* (1827), a whipping fantasy purporting to be the "Memoirs of Mrs. Hinton, who kept a school many years at Kensington,"

[14] McLaren, *Birth Control*, 85–87. [15] McCalman, *Radical Underworld*, 205–215.

[16] "Works Publishing by W. Dugdale," *Northern Star and Leeds General Advertiser*, April 20, 1844, 2; Marcus [pseud.], *The Book of Murder! A Vade-Mecum for the Commissioners and Guardians of the New Poor Law throughout Great Britain and Ireland* ([London]: William Dugdale, 1839), 1390.g.48, BL; *Bell's Penny Dispatch and Sunday Chronicle*, no. 66–97, BLL01013904216, BL.

were engineered to appeal to the sexual tastes of former public school pupils. Others, such as *The Seducing Cardinal's Amours* (1830), which portrays a group of sex-trafficking monks, and *The Lustful Turk* (1828), which recounts the abduction and sale of an English woman to Ali, the Dey of Algiers, were inspired by anti-Catholic libertine literature and orientalist travel narratives. These works were prized by collectors. However, they were too expensive (early editions of *The Lustful Turk* cost more than four pounds), too labour-intensive to produce, and probably too graphic to sustain a dedicated business.[17] At a time when copyright laws were not as expansive as they are today, and old books were easy to acquire, these publishers also made use of a faster, cheaper method to expand their lists of sexual material and make them attractive to a wider range of readers: they recycled existing publications.

In many cases, Holywell Street publishers expanded their catalogues by renovating old works, bringing their focus to sexual acts by rearranging, deleting, and rewriting portions of the text and appending it with explicit images. Dugdale transformed the eighteenth-century novel *The History of the Human Heart* (1749) into the much racier *Memoirs of a Man of Pleasure* (1827), for instance, by cutting away swaths of material that did not focus on sexual acts and adding steamy illustrations.[18] They also pirated each other's publications and reprinted a motley assortment of old productions that seemed likely to appeal to audiences interested in sex, from classic works of erotic fiction, such as John Cleland's novel *Memoirs of a Woman of Pleasure* (1748), popularly known as *Fanny Hill*, to translations of Ovid's *Art of Love* (2 CE). By mixing new and classic works of erotic fiction and poetry with revised or reframed works from other genres, Holywell Street publishers established an economical product makeup, one that enabled them to tap the cheaper end of the market for sexual entertainment while serving readers who wanted to consume sexual material for other, or additional, reasons. Although the products would change over time, these production principles remained a fixture of the pornography trade through the rest of the century.

Medical works began to trickle into Holywell Street publishers' lists in the 1830s. Works on generation and gynaecology had been framed as books of "secrets" – containers of private knowledge that was normally hidden from view – since the late medieval period, and became the focus of increasing concern about inappropriate engagement after print's introduction in Europe.[19] By the seventeenth century, as

17 See listing in [Edward Duncombe?], *Catalogue of Select Works, Funny, Flash, and Facetious, of the Best Description, Richly Embellished with Plates* ([London]: s.n., c. 1840), DA 676, box 1, item 53, MSCE.

18 Lubey, *What Pornography Knows*, 123–172.

19 Monica Helen Green, "'Diseases of Women' to 'Secrets of Women': The Transformation of Gynecological Literature in the Later Middle Ages." *The Journal of Medieval and Renaissance Studies* 30, no. 1 (2000): 5–40.

Sarah Toulalan has argued, it was taken for granted that "reading about and discussing sexual matters, even in a medical context, was likely to be sexually arousing," and that medical works that addressed such matters needed to be presented to "the right kind of reader who would approach the text with the 'right' attitude."[20] Medical writers often sought to diffuse concerns that they catered to prurience by asserting that the sexual content in their books was necessary and intended only for readers with the appropriate mindset. However, this could have the undesirable effect of highlighting their works' prurient appeal. Disreputable booksellers understood this, and exploited it by producing exaggerated versions of the defences these writers employed: they drew attention to sexual content in works on generation, midwifery, venereal disease, and masturbation by appending them with facetious apologies and warnings. These devices encouraged understandings of sexual knowledge as "secret" in a second sense: voyeuristic, exclusive, and desirable partly because it was dangerous.[21]

The activities of John Joseph Stockdale (c. 1776–1847) illustrate that techniques employed to exploit medical eroticism had not changed much when Holywell Street publishers arrived on the scene. The son of a Republican bookseller, Stockdale acquired his own bookshop in Pall Mall in 1806.[22] From these premises, he issued a wide range of works, from an attack on the M.P. William Cobbett using quotations from his own work, *Cobbett Against Himself* (1807), to a science encyclopedia for schoolchildren.[23] In 1811, more by accident than design, Stockdale began to publish the work of John Roberton. A Scottish specialist in venereal disease, Roberton occupied an awkward place in the medical world. He had little formal training as a surgeon, and his first published work, *A Practical Treatise on the Powers of Cantharides* (1806), has been called "little more than a literary personal advertisement."[24] However, he was well-connected in medical circles, and a member of the prestigious Edinburgh Royal Medical Society. Roberton was hungry for influence, and in 1809, he published a more ambitious book, a 700-page *Treatise on Medical*

[20] Sarah Toulalan, "Pornography, Procreation and Pleasure in Early Modern England," in *The Cambridge Companion to Erotic Literature*, ed. Bradford K. Mudge (Cambridge: Cambridge University Press, 2017), 107, 109.

[21] Harry Newman, "'[P]rophane fidlers': Medical Paratexts and Indecent Readers in Early Modern England," in *Medical Paratexts from Medieval to Modern: Dissecting the Page*, ed. Hannah C. Tweed and Diane G. Scott (Cham: Palgrave Macmillan, 2018), 15–42; Peakman, *Mighty Lewd Books*, 48.

[22] Hannah Barker, "Stockdale, John (c.1749–1814)," in *Oxford Dictionary of National Biography* (Oxford: Oxford University Press, 2004; online ed. 2011), https://doi.org/10.1093/ref:odnb/26541.

[23] John Joseph Stockdale, *Encyclopaedia for Youth; or, An Abridgement of all of the Sciences, for the Use of Schools of Both Sexes* (London: J. J. Stockdale, 1807); William Cobbett, *Cobbett against Himself* (London: John Joseph Stockdale, 1807).

[24] Brenda M. White, "Medical Police. Politics and Police: The Fate of John Roberton," *Medical History* 27, no. 4 (1983): 413.

Police. His ambitions were dashed the following year, when he was expelled from the Medical Society following allegations that he had written "obscene epithets" on ballot papers for its presidential election.[25] Roberton moved to London, where he arrived with the manuscript for a third book, *On the Generative System*, which he hoped would ingratiate him to the city's medical elite.

Plans for the book to be published by Richard Phillips, a Republican and publisher of the *Medical and Physical Journal* (1799–1814), fell through, and Stockdale issued *Generative System* in 1811.[26] To Roberton's horror, Stockdale's advertising for the book emphasized its sexual content, announcing that its twelve illustrations of the reproductive organs "Laid Open" the "Secrets of Nature."[27] Defending sexual content in a medical book was respectable; promoting it in newspapers was not. Roberton frantically published notices in the *Morning Post*, assuring readers that his work afforded "no foundation whatever for the very indecorous Advertisement which, contrary to agreement with the Publisher, has, even subsequent to my remonstrances, been repeated by him."[28] The surgeon wished to gain the patronage of Matthew Baillie, the King's physician, and worried that Stockdale's advertisements would undermine his attempt to flatter Baillie by dedicating *Generative System* to him.

Roberton's bid to win Baillie over was a disaster. Baillie hated the book. He was also so suspicious of Roberton's claims to medical expertise, and so disgusted with Stockdale's advertising, that he published his own letters rebuking Roberton for affixing his name to "an obscene book."[29] Commercially, however, *Generative System* was a success. In the end, Roberton capitulated. He not only permitted Stockdale to issue a new edition but also agreed that Stockdale would become the "sole Proprietor of [his] valuable publications."[30] The partnership produced several editions of *Cantharides*, *Generative System*, and *Medical Police*, and several new compilations on sexual health.

Stockdale continued to frame Roberton's medical publications as entrées to the secrets of the body in advertising material throughout the 1810s. In the 1820s, he set about exploiting the market for sexual material in a more concerted fashion. Fearing for his business's survival after a series of setbacks, including a fire that razed his Pall Mall shop, Stockdale instigated numerous legal battles over his copyrights, and expanded his production of sexually

[25] White, "Medical Police," 415–416.

[26] Roberta McGrath, *Seeing Her Sex: Medical Archives and the Female Body* (Manchester: Manchester University Press, 2002), 43.

[27] "Secrets of Nature Laid Open," *Morning Chronicle*, January 15, 1811, 2.

[28] "I think It Necessary to Inform the Public," *Morning Post*, February 1, 1811, 1.

[29] White, "Medical Police," 416–417.

[30] See the unpaginated Advertisement in John Roberton, *A Practical Essay on the More Important Complaints Peculiar to the Female* (London: Printed for J. J. Stockdale, 1813).

detailed works to pay the bills.[31] Most famously, in 1825, he issued *The Memoirs of Harriet Wilson*, a tell-all that he and Wilson, a courtesan to aristocrats, used to blackmail those connected with its anecdotes before it was issued, which reportedly attracted a crowd of buyers "ten deep" to his shop afterwards.[32] Less well known are Stockdale's quasi-medical productions, starting with *Kalogynomia, or The Laws of Female Beauty* (1821). The book, published under the pseudonym Dr. T. Bell, is sometimes attributed to Roberton, but if Roberton was connected with its composition, he wrote relatively little of it himself. *Kalogynomia*, which details a "Complete system of that Science" of female beauty, is a composite text, constructed by copying from older publications on aesthetics, history, geography, anatomy, physiology, and venereal disease, including Roberton's *Generative System*, and filling in the gaps with original writing.[33]

The result, Roberta McGrath has argued, is a jarring hybrid of medical instruction and erotic narrative, one that purports to teach male readers how to judge female beauty by furnishing them with mixture of anatomical, aesthetic, and sensual descriptions of women's bodies.[34] The section "On Sexual Intercourse," for example, instructs readers on the anatomical structure of the reproductive organs. Where "the [prostate] gland ceases to surround the urethra, and where the caput gallinaginus or verumontanum is found," the book states, borrowing from *Generative System*, "the urethra assumes the name of THE MEMBEROUS PORTION OF THE URETHRA."[35] The tone of the prose shifts when describing the signs of arousal:

> The voluptuous woman, who surrenders herself to the passion, is at first warm, blushing, yielding, and free from constraint; – successive and gradually increasing chills soon take the place of the flush.... At the crisis of passion in both sexes, the motions of the body are vivid and violent; – the whole frame trembles convulsively; – the heart beats against

31 "From the London Gazette: Bankrupts," *Caledonian Mercury*, November 28, 1822, n.p.; John Joseph Stockdale to the Royal Literary Fund, February 5, 1827, ADD MS 589.18.1, BL.

32 Barker, "Stockdale, John (c.1749–1814)."

33 For instance, compare T. Bell [pseud.], *Kalogynomia, or the Laws of Female Beauty: Being the Elementary Principles of that Science* (London: Printed for J. J. Stockdale, 1821), 7–52, with Alexander Walker, "An Attempt to Systematize Anatomy, Physiology, and Pathology," *Annals of Philosophy, or, Magazine of Chemistry, Mineralogy, Mechanics, Natural History, Agriculture, and the Arts* (London: Baldwin, Cradock, and Joy, 1815), 283–292; *Kalogynomia*, 68, with Mr. de Pauw, "On the State of the Fine Arts in Athens," in *The Literary and Biographical Magazine and British Review*, February 1794, 108; *Kalogynomia*, 100–109, with Anthelme Richerand, *The Elements of Physiology*, trans. Robert Kerrison (London: John Murray, 1803), 437–439; *Kalogynomia*, 131 with Robert Heron, *A Collection of Late Voyages and Travels, Chiefly Translated and Arranged from the French and Other Foreign Publications of Neibuhr, Mariti, Beauchamp, &c* [...]. ([London?]: Watson and Co., 1797), 281.

34 McGrath, *Seeing Her Sex*, 48.

35 Compare Bell, *Kalogynomia*, 155 and John Roberton, *On the Generative System: Being an Anatomical and Physiological Sketch on the Parts of Generation, and a Treatise on Their Diseases*, 4th ed. (London: J.J. Stockdale, 1817), 33.

the breast; – in a moment the muscles yield under the weight of pleasure; even intelligence seems extinct. . . .[36]

Kalogynomia's twenty-four plates mirror its composite textual makeup: the images are a jumble of illustrations recycled from other publications, including sketches of the interior and exterior details of the reproductive organs, interior depictions of sexual intercourse, and etchings of nude female statuary.

Ideas about what counts as science change over time and vary between communities.[37] Although it is difficult to do so today, some readers (including Richard Carlile, who alluded to it in *Every Woman's Book*) viewed *Kalogynomia* and similar works as serious scientific interventions.[38] However, as McGrath has emphasized, the book's editorial material leaves little doubt that Stockdale thought its major value lay in its prurient appeal. Stockdale inserted a *nota bene* into the book that emphasizes the plates' eroticism, for instance, by exploiting assumptions that women and youths were especially vulnerable to the influences of print:

Plates 10, 17, 18, 19, 20, 21, 22, 23 and 24 should not be carelessly exposed either to Ladies or to Young Persons. These Plates are therefore stitched up separately. As the work is a scientific one, and calculated both by its mode of construction and its price for the higher and more reflecting class of readers, and as the Plates above enumerated are also entirely scientific and anatomical, the Publisher might have dispensed with this precaution; but he is anxious that these readers should have it in their power to obviate the possibility of the careless exposure of such anatomical Plates: they are therefore detached from the Work and may be locked up separately.[39]

This *nota bene* reworks defences of sexual detail common in medical works to promote *Kalogynomia*'s eroticism. It suggests that the reader is "a discriminating viewer . . . [engaging] in scientific observation rather than sexual voyeurism," even as he invokes the images' stimulating nature by counselling him to lock them away from those who *will* be affected.[40] Stockdale used paratext in this way to construct a readership for *Kalogynomia* that would be complimented by his appeal to their moral prowess even as they were titillated by the dangers he said it represented.

Kalogynomia repeated *Generative System*'s success. After it was published, Stockdale began to fuse material from Roberton's books with new

[36] Bell, *Kalogynomia*, 191–192.

[37] For work on this subject specifically related to publications on sexual matters that later readers have found difficult to take seriously as scientific works, see Kate Fisher and Rebecca Langlands, eds., *Sex, Knowledge, and Receptions of the Past* (Oxford: Oxford University Press, 2015), 20–21; James A. Secord, "Talking Origins," in *Reproduction: Antiquity to the Present*, ed. Nick Hopwood, Rebecca Fleming, and Lauren Kassell (Cambridge: Cambridge University Press, 2018), 375–389.

[38] Bush, *What Is Love?* 35–36. See Chapter 3 for details about the reception of works inspired by *Kalogynomia*.

[39] Bell, *Kalogynomia*, v.

[40] McGrath, *Seeing Her Sex*, 48.

plates and extracts from various sources, fashioning a series of books that he marketed as based on, or related to, *Kalogynomia*.[41] He advertised these works openly for years. None attracted opposition until 1836, when government inspectors discovered an 1824 edition of *Generative System* in Newgate Gaol.[42] Its plates, which were mostly taken from *Kalogynomia*, shocked the inspectors, who urged city officials to prosecute Stockdale for distributing obscene material. The officials refused, noting Roberton's profession as a surgeon and (ironically) the book's dedication to Matthew Baillie. *Generative System*'s scientific status was debated in court anyway, thanks to an audacious libel suit that Stockdale brought against Hansard, the publishers of Parliamentary reports, for printing the inspectors' opinion of the book. Opinions as to whether their assessment was correct varied, but after enjoying three years of free publicity from newspaper reports on the suit, Stockdale won on the basis that Hansard did not enjoy Parliamentary privilege.

As Stockdale's exploits suggests, agents of the book trade were using a variety of techniques to take advantage of medical eroticism at the dawn of the Victorian period. They sometimes sutured texts and images into new combinations to create works for audiences interested in reading about bodies and desires. More often, they simply drew attention existing publications' prurient appeal through paratextual devices such as advertisements, prefaces, and notes. Holywell Street publishers adapted these techniques as they developed a specialized trade in sexual material; but "adapted" is the key word here. Like many booksellers before them, Holywell Street publishers encouraged their customers to read medical works for pleasure. However, they also used these techniques to encourage another kind of engagement with medical works, one inspired by radical arguments for sex education, reproductive autonomy, and female pleasure: they encouraged readers to see these works as containers of a kind of knowledge that could enable them to live out safe, free, and pleasurable sex lives of their own.

41 See Thomas Little [pseud.], *The Beauty, Marriage Ceremonies and Intercourse in the Sexes of All Nations; To Which Is Added the New Art of Love (Grounded in Kalogynomia)* (London: J. J. Stockdale, 1824); Thomas Little [pseud.], *An Introduction to a Natural System of Anatomy, Pathology and Medicine, to Which Is Added a General View of Natural History* (London: J. J. Stockdale, 1825); and Thomas Little [pseud.], *Systems of the Physiology of Camper* (London: J. J. Stockdale, 1825), which are all attributed to the author of *Kalogynomia* but (strangely) published under a different pseudonym. For more on the series, see McGrath, *Seeing Her Sex*, 47.

42 White, "Medical Police," 417. See McGrath, *Seeing Her Sex*, 54–61, for further details about the Newgate and Hansard episodes.

Opening the Catalogue

By 1837, nearly sixty bookshops known for dealing in sexual material operated in London. Many were clustered along a series of thoroughfares stretching out from under the shadow of St. Mary-le-Strand, the Anglican church to the west of the city. Prone to crowding by day and littered with the waste of evening revelry in the West End's theatres, restaurants, and gin palaces, Holywell Street, Wych Street, and Russell Court suited businesses that traded on desire for "secret" knowledge. Standing between the bright, middle-class bustle of the Strand and the poverty-stricken slums of Drury Lane, Holywell Street publishers' shops promised to bring the best of both worlds to readers in print: books, pamphlets, and periodicals that would enable them to indulge in unruly urban pleasures without having to come into contact with hunger, poverty, or shame. A reader who slipped into one of these shops could find the latest in novels about adventure, crime, and vice, bawdy song and joke books, salacious periodicals, guides to London's night life, and, increasingly, medical works on display. Books and prints of a more "curious" nature ("curious" was a common euphemism for sexually explicit content) were available on request. Should readers wish to consider purchases from the comfort of their homes, they could leave with a catalogue of items for sale.[43]

The sheer number of booksellers associated with the trade suggests a healthy market for sexual material. Cannon, Benbow, and Dugdale's friends and family members joined the business, including Dugdale's brothers Thomas and John; the printer John Duncombe and his brother, Edward; and Richard Carlile's son, Thomas Paine Carlile, who operated under his wife's surname, Ward.[44] Over time, new players without evident connections to radical politics entered the trade, including at least one woman, Mary Elliot.[45] The market was large

[43] For more on the number and geography of these shops, see Sigel, *Governing Pleasures*, 21; Lynda Nead, *Victorian Babylon: People, Streets, and Images in Nineteenth-Century London* (New Haven, CT: Yale University Press, 2000), 182; George Frederick Pardon, *The Popular Guide to London and Its Suburbs: Comprising Descriptions of All Its Points of Interest: with Historical, Literary, Statistical and Useful Information* (London: Routledge, Warne, and Routledge, 1862), 80.

[44] See Sigel, *Governing Pleasures* and Straight, "William Dugdale: A Biographical Sketch of an Erotica Publisher, Bookseller and Printer," *The Erotica Bibliophile* for more information about these figures, except Thomas Paine Carlile. Under the name Thomas Ward, Carlile sold sexual material out of a "Parisian Repository" at 103 Strand from 1844 and out of several other addresses after February 1849. For the major details, see John Adcock, "T. Paine of Holywell Street," *Yesterdays Papers* Blog, last modified November 28, 2014, https://john-adcock.blogspot.com/2014/11/t-paine-of-holywell-street_28.html. Advertisements in *The Fly: A Literary and Pictorial Miscellany for 1839* (London: Glover Water Lane, Fleet Street, 1839) suggest that Carlile got started in the business as one of Dugdale's distributors. William Ward, publisher of *Ward's New Catalogue of Parisian Novelties* (Strand: W. Ward, c. 1850), DA 676, box 8, item 22, MSCE, is likely another alias of Carlile's.

[45] Jamie Stoops, "Class and Gender Dynamics of the Pornography Trade in Late Nineteenth-Century Britain," *The Historical Journal* 58, no. 1 (2015): 137–156.

enough to support a number of players because they did not limit their audience to wealthy readers. They aimed to serve a broad, largely male audience that included students, shop-boys, clerks, and tradesmen as well as professionals and aristocrats. To cultivate this audience, the most successful Holywell Street publishers hammered out advertising partnerships and publishing deals with charismatic impresarios like Renton Nicholson, owner of the Garrick's Head and Town Hotel in Covent Garden, a famous destination for bawdy sing-alongs and performances featuring scantily clad women. They also sold a range of inexpensive products, including medical works. The median price for the medical works was two shillings and sixpence, and some could be had for sixpence. At these prices, they were considered "cheap" in the book business: easily within reach of middle-class readers, and feasible purchases for some working-class readers.[46]

Because Holywell Street publishers constantly pirated, traded, and inherited stock from each other, their lists were practically interchangeable. Around thirty-five medical titles circulated through the trade between the late 1830s and the early 1860s, appearing in one catalogue after another.[47] As a collective, these works make up an incredibly diverse body of publications, one that mixes traditional knowledge about procreation with up-to-date information about anatomy; radical writing about the necessity of sexual freedom for both sexes with forbidding lectures on the dangers of masturbation and promiscuity; and practical instruction on how to practise contraception with philosophical discussions about the nature of desire. However, they can be grouped into a few rough categories.

The smallest comprises two allegedly ancient works on procreation. One was *The Secrets of Nature Revealed*, which was derived from parts of the early modern manual *Aristotle's Masterpiece* (1684) and a translation of Nicholas Venette's *La génération de l'homme* (1675), probably *Conjugal Love; or, The Pleasures of the Marriage Bed* (c. 1750).[48] The other was *Aristotle's*

[46] To determine median prices and whether they changed over time (they did not), I analyzed prices in the catalogues listed in Appendix A and newspaper advertisements published in the following newspapers in the years 1842, 1847, 1852, 1857, 1862, and 1867, using Gale's *British Library Newspapers 1800–1900* and *19th Century UK Periodicals* databases: *Aberdeen Journal*, *Bell's Life in London and Sporting Chronicle*, *Berkshire Chronicle*, *Cheshire Observer and General Advertiser*, *Daily Post* (Liverpool), *Derbyshire Times and Chesterfield Herald*, *The Era*, *Freeman's Journal and Daily Commercial Advertiser*, *Liverpool Mercury*, *John Bull and Britannia*, *Morning Chronicle*, *Preston Guardian*, *Reynolds's Newspaper*, and *The Standard*. See Simon Eliot, "Some Patterns and Trends in British Book Production, 1800–1919," *Occasional Papers of the Bibliographical Society* 8 (1994): 59–77 for further information on book pricing during this period.

[47] My discussion draws on advertisements in newspapers in *British Library Newspapers 1800–1900*, *19th Century UK Periodicals*, and *British Newspaper Archive*, and the sales catalogues listed in Appendix A.

[48] See n. 1.

Masterpiece itself. *Aristotle*, which has no connection to the philosopher, was probably Holywell Street publishers' best seller. Sold continuously throughout the nineteenth century, it was enormously popular among readers of all classes and genders: the kind of work that women passed down from generation to generation, and young men passed around with their friends.[49] Holywell Street publishers often advertised multiple differently priced editions for sale, some with coloured plates and some without. Just a single copy of an edition issued by John Duncombe has survived.[50] The dearth of extant Holywell Street editions raises the possibility that these publishers did not issue all or even most of the *Aristotles* they sold, preferring to source them from suppliers who churned them out for many booksellers under a well-known false imprint.[51] High demand for *Aristotle* explains the creation of *Secrets of Nature*: incorporating parts of the famous manual, it was presented as a similar publication by another ancient scholar.

Itself a compilation, *Aristotle* evolved over time. Duncombe's edition is an abridged version popular in the late eighteenth and early nineteenth centuries that provided information about the generative organs, the mechanics of conception, pregnancy, and delivery, and "monstrous births," as well as advice about how to treat various ailments. However, customers of other Holywell Street publishers may have encountered a somewhat different work. Around the mid-nineteenth century, references to sexual intercourse were edited out of many editions of *Aristotle*.[52] An essay on the pleasures and duties of marriage and information about venereal disease were added, and the chapter on monstrous births was expanded to include material on living "eccentricities of nature," such as the conjoined twins Chang and Eng Bunker (1811–74).[53] Some of these changes may have been made to tone down the work during a period in which debate about the limits of publicly acceptable expression intensified: *Aristotle* had a longstanding reputation as a bawdy book.[54]

[49] Jonathan Rose, *The Intellectual Life of the British Working Classes*, 2nd ed. (New Haven, CT: Yale University Press, 2010), 207.

[50] Aristotle [pseud.], *Aristotle's Master-Piece; or, Every Woman's Book! Displaying All the Secrets of Nature, as Exhibited in the Creation of Man!* (London: Printed for James Duncombe, c. 1830), WZ 290 A718 1800, Osler Library of the History of Medicine, McGill University. Although "James Duncombe" is named on the imprint, this edition was printed at John Duncombe's address in Little Queen Street.

[51] The following editions held in the British Library are sometimes attributed to Holywell Street publishers. However, their paper, typefaces, illustrations, and bindings are all very different from those of works cited in this chapter, and they share a common imprint, "J. Smith, High Holborn," which was not associated with anyone in the Holywell Street trade: DE.24.07306; RB.23.a.29207; 1578.3759; 07326.ee.18; 1578.3735; CUP.365.aa.54; and C.194.a.487.

[52] Roy Porter and Lesley Hall, *The Facts of Life: The Creation of Sexual Knowledge in Britain, 1650–1950* (New Haven, CT: Yale University Press, 1995), 128.

[53] Aristotle [pseud.], *Revised Edition of the Works of Aristotle, the Famous Philosopher* [...]. (London: Published by J. Smith, 193, High Holborn, [1857]), 56, 07306.de.24, BL.

[54] See Chapter 4 for an account of possible revisions for this purpose.

However, they mainly seem to have been oriented around bringing the manual into conversation with the present. When they read updated editions of *Aristotle*, Victorian readers experienced the thrill of accessing timeless secrets about generation. However, these secrets were now presented in dialogue with contemporary fascination with congenital variation, concern about venereal disease, and hope for marital fulfilment.

Holywell Street publishers dealt in a wider variety of works on venereal disease, fertility problems, and sexual dysfunction. Many were reprints or translations of bestselling eighteenth-century century works about the dangers of masturbation, including the anonymous pamphlet *Onania: or, The Heinous Sin of Self-Pollution* (c. 1712), Samuel-Auguste Tissot's *L'Onanisme* (1760), and M. D. T. de Bienville's *La nymphomanie* (1771). Others, including James Graham's *Lecture on the Generation, Increase, and Improvement of the Human Species* (c. 1783) and newer productions like R. J. Swaine & Co's *Geneseology, or, the Physiology of Woman* (1850) and R. and L. Perry & Co's *The Silent Friend* (1841), focused on the causes and treatment of infertility, impotence, and venereal disease.[55] Issued by living medical practitioners, works like *The Silent Friend* offered up-to-date information about the body, drawn from the modern science of anatomy. However, they had the same flavour as the older material, issuing stern warnings about the dangers of masturbation and extra-marital sex. During the 1840s and 1850s, Holywell Street publishers hawked these works on behalf of their authors, acting as retailers.[56] By the 1860s, they may have shifted to trading in piracies: these titles were listed at significantly higher prices in their advertisements than they were in advertisements placed by such works' own authors.

The third category, sex and marriage manuals, is even more varied. Some of these works, such as Venette's *Conjugal Love*, were reprints of seventeenth- and eighteenth-century productions that offered a potpourri of advice and anecdotes about fertility, marriage, sexual technique, and desire.[57] Others,

[55] For a Holywell Street edition of one of Graham's publications, see James Jraham [*sic*] [James Graham], *On Impotence and Sterility, or, Private Advice to Those Married Ladies Who Have Been Unable, but Are Eagerly Desirous to Have Children* (London: H. Smith, printer [William Dugdale], n.d.), MC. HQ734.E87 1807F, ML.

[56] This is indicated in the lists of booksellers that appear on the title pages of these works, or in their advertisements. For instance, the title page of Horace Goss, *Woman: Her Physiology and Functions* (London: Published by the Authors, 1853) indicates that it was sold by "Winn, Holywell-street, Strand," while "Just Published … The Silent Friend," *Railway Chronicle*, August 3, 1844, 383 indicates that "Ward, 103 Strand" sold *The Silent Friend*.

[57] Although it was advertised, I have not seen an edition of *Conjugal Love* issued by a Holywell Street publisher apart from *Secrets of Nature*, which excerpts it. T. Graham, *Conjugal Love; or, The Mysteries of Hymen Unveiled* (London: H. Smith [William Dugdale], n.d.), MC. HQ734. E87 1807D, ML is not an edition of Venette's work but a reprint of G. A. Douglas, *The Nature and Causes of Impotence in Men, and Barrenness in Woman, Explained*, 3rd ed. (London: Printed for J. Brett, 1758), EPB/B/20800, WL.

such as *The Philosophy of Kissing* (c. 1840), a rambling paean to the delights of kissing and the insights of the science of phrenology, were original.[58] Few of the latter have survived, but like *Kalogynomia* they appear to have been compiled from a variety of medical, scientific, aesthetic, historical, and legal works. Most of the text of Dugdale's *Marriage, Historically, Philosophically, Legally, Physiologically and Pathologically Examined* (c. 1842), attributed to Henry Horne, M.D., was taken from *The Philosophy of Marriage* (1837), a book by Michael Ryan, a London-based obstetrician and medical lecturer, which Dugdale also sold intact.[59] To create his *Marriage*, Dugdale excised parts of Ryan's work, including most of its religious references, and combined it with a chapter from Robert Dale Owen's contraception manual *Moral Physiology*. These editorial manoeuvres transformed the text. Ryan's *Marriage* is a sprawling survey of reproductive functions, problems, and arrangements that condemns contraception on the grounds that it would break down restraints on female sexuality. Horne's *Marriage* is a shorter cross-cultural exploration of reproductive arrangements that endorses contraception on the grounds that people of both sexes should not suffer for gratifying their desires.

Horne's *Marriage* provides a bridge to the final and perhaps most compelling category, works on contraception. This category is a reminder of the Holywell Street trade's roots in radical publishing: Carlile's *Every Woman's Book*, Owen's *Moral Physiology*, and Knowlton's *Fruits of Philosophy* were all staples of Holywell Street publishers' catalogues.[60] Two of Dugdale's editions of Knowlton's pamphlet have survived.[61] The main text is identical to contemporary editions issued by social reformers, but Dugdale's are furnished with two new anatomical plates (Figure 1.2). Printed on a single fold-out sheet appended to the pamphlet's title page, these images illustrate Knowlton's descriptions of the female reproductive organs. One is an engraving of the

58 *The Philosophy of Kissing, Anatomically and Physiologically Explained* (London: H. Smith, [William Dugdale] c. 1840), EPB/P/41132, WL. The section on phrenology appears to be loosely adapted from lectures by George Combe, whose materialist *Constitution of Man* (1828) was popular in radical circles.

59 Henry Horne, M. D. [pseud.], *Marriage, Historically, Philosophically, Legally, Physiologically, and Pathologically Examined* (London: H. Smith [William Dugdale], c. 1842). There are two extant copies of this publication: 1) MC. HQ734.E87 1807B, ML and 2) 162.3 H81m, KIL. Compare the text with Michael Ryan, *The Philosophy of Marriage in Its Social, Physical, and Moral Relations* (London: John Churchill, 1837) and Robert Dale Owen, *Moral Physiology: Or, a Brief and Plain Treatise on the Population Question* (London: James Watson, 1842).

60 It is possible that Thomas Paine Carlile supplied the trade with *Every Woman's Book*. His brother Alfred published an edition in 1838 (Tab.603.a.27, BL), which he distributed. See *Fly*, 60.

61 Charles Knowlton, *Fruits of Philosophy, or, The Private Companion of Young Married People* (London: Dugdale, Russell Court, Drury Lane, 1838), EPB/A/61972, WL; Charles Knowlton, *Fruits of Philosophy, or, The Private Companion of Young Married People* (London: Printed and Published by H. Smith [William Dugdale], c. 1845), MC. HQ734. E87 1807E, ML.

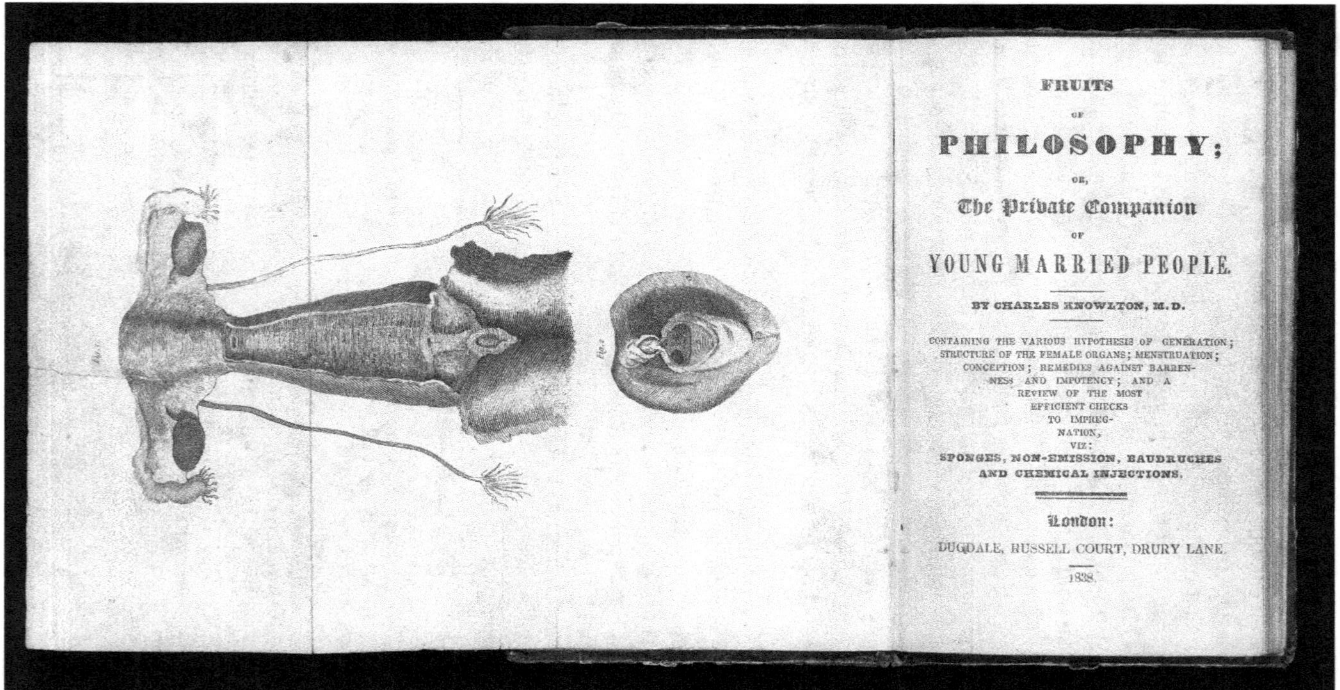

Figure 1.2 Fold-out illustration and title page of Charles Knowlton, *Fruits of Philosophy, or, The Private Companion of Young Married People* (London: Dugdale, Russell Court, Drury Lane, 1838), EPB/A/61972, WL. Wellcome Collection, CC BY-NC 4.0.

reproductive system, spanning from the ovaries to the opening of the vagina. The other depicts a spread vulva, drawing attention to the locations of the clitoris, clitoral hood, labia, and hymen. If readers flipped to the back of the pamphlet, they would find a numbered key that names each anatomical element, and a letter allegedly written by a physician named Athanasius Griskin, who takes credit for the plates and key. Positioning Griskin as an expert in contraceptive techniques, the letter focuses almost exclusively on the benefits of the baudruche, or "condem" (condom). The device is superior to contraception methods advocated by Knowlton or Owen, Griskin argues, because it is more effective at preventing pregnancy, stops the spread of venereal disease, and can even help "the man who goes off like wild fire" satisfy women by enabling him to "keep himself back" during intercourse.[62]

Additionally, Holywell Street publishers sold at least two original pamphlets on contraception.[63] One, *On the Use of Night Caps; or, Seven Years' Experience on the Practicability of Limiting the Number of a Family*, is attributed to "a Married Man with Six Children!"[64] Dugdale published the only extant copy, probably in 1844. Its style and verbatim overlaps with Griskin's letter suggest that Dugdale was its author. *Night Caps* was clearly influenced by Carlile's work. Like *Every Woman's Book*, it defends the right of couples to "be the best judges of their own situation," ridicules religious authorities, and emphasizes women's right to enjoy sex, freed from the mortal risks of pregnancy and the emotional devastation of miscarriage.[65] However, its tone is markedly different from *Every Woman's Book*, which anxiously defends itself against imputations of impropriety, insisting that "all subjects may be philosophically discussed, when they are discussed with a view to the acquisition or communication of knowledge."[66] Written as a direct address to a mixed-gender readership, *Night Caps* has the flavour of a sales pitch delivered

[62] Knowlton, *Fruits* (Dugdale, 1838), 58–59.

[63] William Dugdale additionally advertised a two-penny pamphlet called *A Private Hint to Young Married People*, attributed to Charles Combe, M. A., which reportedly instructed people "how to prevent an increase in their families." See "Advertisement: Now Publishing," *Paul Pry*, October 11, 1856, 8. It is likely that *Bride's Own Book; or, Chaste Counsel for the Wedding Day*, a 6*d* pamphlet advertised in many Holywell Street catalogues, also contained information about contraception or abortion. Although Holywell Street publishers' descriptions of the work are vague, they often include the quotation from *Cain* discussed below.

[64] *On the Use of Night Caps, or, Seven Years' Experience on the Practicality of Limiting the Number of a Family, by the Best Known Methods, Including Some Valuable and Novel Information, Never before Published, by a Married Man with Six Children!* (London: J. Turner [William Dugdale], [1844?]), P.C. 30.a.33, BL. The first known advertisement for *Night Caps* appears in "Works Published by H. Smith," *Satirist; or, The Censor of the Times*, February 4, 1844, 8. The pamphlet's instructions for postal orders further suggest a publication date around this time. However, the addresses printed on the title page and on page 24, which are crossed out, suggest that *Night Caps* could have been first published as early as 1832.

[65] *Night Caps*, 3.

[66] Carlile, *Every Woman's Book*, iv.

by a skilled showman, careening between thundering invective, bawdy humour, and gentle cajoling. Its narrator goes out of his way to create an atmosphere of bar-room intimacy: he litters the text with double entendres, often refers to his own sexual experiences, and makes naughty asides. "Ladies and gentlemen," he exclaims at one point, "I hope you are all married. If you are not, the omission cannot be attributed to *me*."[67]

Although *Night Caps* describes several contraceptive techniques, most of the text is devoted to addressing reservations that readers might have about its recommended method, the "night cap," or "French letter" (condom). *Night Caps'* narrator concedes that the device dulls sexual sensation for men. However, he suggests strategies for improving it and appeals to readers' sense of manly virtue, opining that a husband's first duty is not to his own pleasure but to his wife's well-being. Women must be protected from the ravages of childbearing, and if their partners are willing to experiment with using the night cap, they will be rewarded for their efforts:

> Let the gentleman only procure one, and he may be quite certain to be rewarded by a hearty laugh from his wife at its singularity . . . Let it be tried *on*, and the experiment would be found not complete without it being *tried in*. At one of the numerous contacts most married people enjoy, this experiment would be interesting from its novelty.[68]

Night Caps anticipates and diffuses other objections, too: about condoms' reputation as filthy devices used by prostitutes, about the expense of using them, about the risk of breakage, and even about judgement from friends. "Pshaw! madame," the narrator retorts. "It is no affair of theirs whether you lie in lawn, linen, or calico, or whether your husband does, or does not, cover his head with a night cap."[69] Eventually, it becomes clear that *Night Caps* was meant to function, at least partly, as an advertisement: the pamphlet winds up with an appeal to readers to purchase night caps from the publisher.

The other pamphlet, *The Connubial Guide; or, Married People's Best Friend*, draws on radical writing about contraception in a very different way. The only extant copy was issued by Edward Duncombe under the name John Wilson in the early 1840s and published under the pseudonym "Intercidona."[70] Although the title and pseudonym, the name of a Roman goddess of protection for labouring women, suggest a sex manual or midwifery book, the front cover offers a clue to the pamphlet's contents by quoting lines from George Gordon, Lord Byron's drama *Cain* (1821):

67 *Night Caps*, 19. 68 *Night Caps*, 11. 69 *Night Caps*, 21.

70 Intercidona [pseud.], *The Connubial Guide; or, Married People's Best Friend* (London: John Wilson [Edward Duncombe], c. 1843), NZ Z492, Beinecke Library. *The Connubial Guide* was likely first published in 1840. The first known advertisement for the pamphlet was issued by William Dugdale under the name H. Smith in "Just Published," *Satirist; or, the Censor of the Times*, June 21, 1840, 2.

To give birth to those
Who can but suffer many years, and die
Methinks is merely propagating death
And multiplying murder

The Connubial Guide is essentially a digest: the twelve-page pamphlet streamlines material from radical works on contraception, cutting away almost all of their philosophical content to offer a focused survey of contraceptive techniques. Stating their object "to diffuse . . . necessary knowledge amongst all ranks," Intercidona only briefly defends contraception from what they consider the sole plausible objection to it: that it is "unnatural, seeing that no part of the bodily organization is adapted for the purpose."[71] Reminding readers that overpopulation gives rise to poverty and hunger, and that humans "interfere with the intentions of nature" every day, Intercidonia reasons, "Is it not better for us, being, as we are, in an artificial state, to adopt artificial means to prevent an artificial increase in our numbers?"[72]

The rest of the pamphlet describes a variety of methods of controlling reproduction, citing Owen, Knowlton, and Carlile's pamphlets and the wisdom of several unnamed individuals. However, it rejects all but one. In Intercidonia's opinion, withdrawal is too difficult for men to follow through with. Vaginal sponges are unreliable. French letters are "likely to tear," and also "filthy," and it is "impracticable" for female partners to take exercise immediately after intercourse. Unusually for birth control pamphlets, *The Connubial Guide* provides a recipe for an abortifacient containing sulphate of potass or soda, though it claims that the recipe is also useless, producing only "a violent action on the bowels."[73] Ultimately, Intercidona advocates vaginal douching with an alkaline solution after intercourse, noting that the method is proposed in Knowlton's *Fruits of Philosophy.* Conveniently, a Dr. M. sells such a preparation through Wilson's shop. The final paragraph, which describes the symptoms of pregnancy, obliquely suggests that Wilson's customers can also arrange abortions with Dr. M.[74]

Just on its own, this motley collection of publications highlights some important features of sexual knowledge's circulation during the first decades of the Victorian period. First, it emphasizes that old ways of thinking about the body and sexuality continued to circulate in print beyond exchanges of

[71] Intercidona, *Connubial Guide*, 4, 6.

[72] Intercidona, *Connubial Guide*, 6–7. Intercidona may be taking their argument from Knowlton's fourth edition of *Fruits of Philosophy*. See Robert Jütte, *Contraception: A History* (Cambridge: Polity, 2008), 108.

[73] Intercidona, *Connubial Guide*, 10.

[74] "Dr. M." may have worked with several Holywell Street publishers: *Hints to Men about Town, or, Waterfordiania* [. . .]. (London: Henry Smith [William Dugdale], c. 1841), 30 reports that readers can procure treatments for venereal disease from a Dr. M. through Dugdale's shop.

Aristotle's Masterpiece, though *Aristotle* was undoubtedly the most popular early modern work on procreation. Holywell Street editions of early modern medical works and descriptions of them in sales catalogues also suggest that readers would not necessarily have perceived the ideas that they communicated as "old": while publishers highlighted and even fabricated the "ancient" status of some productions, such as *Secrets of Nature*, other seventeenth- and eighteenth-century works, such as *Onania: or, The Heinous Sin of Self-Pollution*, were reprinted and sold alongside newer works like *The Silent Friend* without a word about their origins. While scholars have long recognized that medical perspectives from earlier periods lived on in oral tradition, these catalogues underscore just how much currency older models of the body and sexuality had in cheap print during the first decades of the Victorian period.

This material also emphasizes that trade in birth control literature was far more active than previously thought. Historians often assume that works describing contraceptive techniques circulated in low numbers between the mid-1830s and the mid-1870s, and that their sole sellers were social reformers who inherited Knowlton's and Owen's pamphlets.[75] Yet, other players clearly sold these pamphlets and Carlile's *Every Woman's Book*; wrote, published, and sold other works inspired by them; and sometimes inserted extracts from them into other kinds of publications, as in Dugdale's made-over edition of Michael Ryan's *Philosophy of Marriage*. It is also clear that these pamphlets, and reworkings and elaborations on them, were used to promote products (and possibly, *The Connubial Guide* suggests, services) that theoretically enabled people to prevent or end pregnancy, protect themselves or their partners from venereal disease, and have more satisfying sex lives. As well as promoting condoms, contraception pamphlets sometimes served as resources for copy for stand-alone advertisements for the devices, where their utility as a prophylactics for venereal disease was often highlighted alongside, or instead of, their utility for preventing pregnancy.[76] Prices for the pamphlets ranged from two pence to two shillings and sixpence, but the condoms, which were made by hand out of treated animal gut, were quite expensive, priced between six and twenty-one shillings per dozen. Nevertheless, they had buyers. One customer annotated a sales catalogue with a note indicating the price for William Dugdale's "best quality" condoms (Figure 1.3).

[75] This idea seems to have originated in Himes's *Medical History of Contraception*, 231, and been elaborated in subsequent scholarship on Victorian contraception. For instance, see McLaren, *Birth Control*, 90; Hera Cook, *The Long Sexual Revolution: English Woman, Sex, and Contraception, 1800–1975* (Oxford: Oxford University Press, 2004), 76–77. See Chapter 6 for an argument as to why this narrative arose and persisted through the twentieth century.

[76] For example, see the unpaginated advertisement for French letters in Wm. Ward [Thomas Paine Carlile?], *The Man of Pleasure's Illustrated Pocket-Book for 1850* (London: Wm. Ward's Bachelor's Repository of Arts, 1850), DA 679.M285, MSCE, which derives most of its text from Knowlton's *Fruits of Philosophy*.

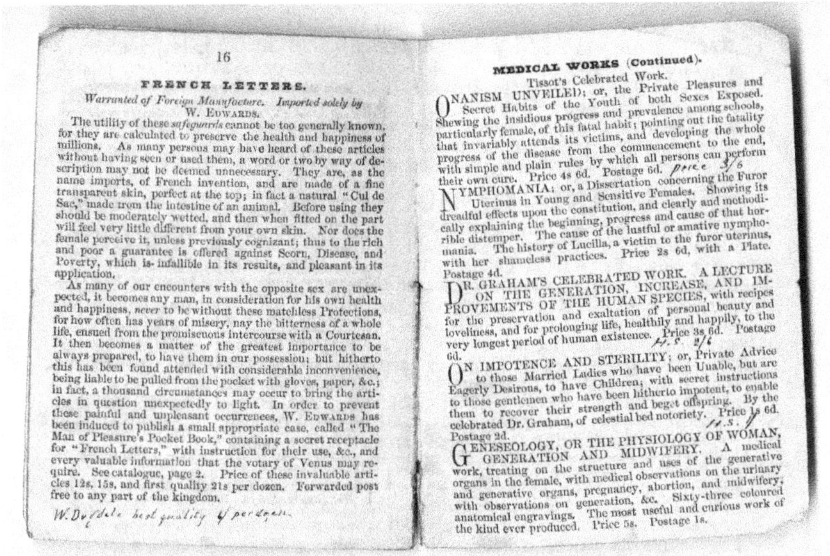

16

FRENCH LETTERS.

Warranted of Foreign Manufacture. Imported solely by W. EDWARDS.

The utility of these *safeguards* cannot be too generally known, for they are calculated to preserve the health and happiness of millions. As many persons may have heard of these articles without having seen or used them, a word or two by way of description may not be deemed unnecessary. They are, as the name imports, of French invention, and are made of a fine transparent skin, perfect at the top; in fact a natural "Cul de Sac," made from the intestine of an animal. Before using they should be moderately wetted, and then when fitted on the part will feel very little different from your own skin. Nor does the female perceive it, unless previously cognizant; thus to the rich and poor a guarantee is offered against Scorn, Disease, and Poverty, which is infallible in its results, and pleasant in its application.

As many of our encounters with the opposite sex are unexpected, it becomes any man, in consideration for his own health and happiness, *never* to be without these matchless Protections, for how often has years of misery, nay the bitterness of a whole life, ensued from the promiscuous intercourse with a Courtesan. It then becomes a matter of the greatest importance to be always prepared, to have them in our possession; but hitherto this has been found attended with considerable inconvenience, being liable to be pulled from the pocket with gloves, paper, &c.; in fact, a thousand circumstances may occur to bring the articles in question unexpectedly to light. In order to prevent these painful and unpleasant occurrences, W. EDWARDS has been induced to publish a small appropriate case, called "The Man of Pleasure's Pocket Book," containing a secret receptacle for "French Letters," with instruction for their use, &c., and every valuable information that the votary of Venus may require. See catalogue, page 2. Price of these invaluable articles 12s, 15s, and first quality 21s per dozen. Forwarded post free to any part of the kingdom.

MEDICAL WORKS (Continued).

Tissot's Celebrated Work.

ONANISM UNVEILED; or, the Private Pleasures and Secret Habits of the Youth of both Sexes Exposed. Shewing the insidious progress and prevalence among schools, particularly female, of this fatal habit; pointing out the fatality that invariably attends its victims, and developing the whole progress of the disease from the commencement to the end, with simple and plain rules by which all persons can perform their own cure. Price 4s 6d. Postage 6d.

NYMPHOMANIA; or, a Dissertation concerning the Furor Uterinus in Young and Sensitive Females. Showing its dreadful effects upon the constitution, and clearly and methodically explaining the beginning, progress and cause of that horrible distemper. The cause of the lustful or amative nymphomania. The history of Lucilla, a victim to the furor uterinus, with her shameless practices. Price 2s 6d, with a Plate. Postage 4d.

DR. GRAHAM'S CELEBRATED WORK. A LECTURE ON THE GENERATION, INCREASE, AND IMPROVEMENTS OF THE HUMAN SPECIES, with recipes for the preservation and exaltation of personal beauty and loveliness, and for prolonging life, healthily and happily, to the very longest period of human existence. Price 3s 6d. Postage 6d.

ON IMPOTENCE AND STERILITY; or, Private Advice to those Married Ladies who have been Unable, but are Eagerly Desirous, to have Children; with secret instructions to those gentlemen who have been hitherto impotent, to enable them to recover their strength and beget offspring. By the celebrated Dr. Graham, of celestial bed notoriety. Price 1s 6d. Postage 2d.

GENESEOLOGY, OR THE PHYSIOLOGY OF WOMAN, GENERATION AND MIDWIFERY. A medical work, treating on the structure and uses of the generative organs in the female, with medical observations on the urinary and generative organs, pregnancy, abortion, and midwifery, with observations on generation, &c. Sixty-three coloured anatomical engravings. The most useful and curious work of the kind ever produced. Price 5s. Postage 1s.

Figure 1.3 Advertisements for French letters and medical works. *Ward's New Catalogue of Parisian Novelties* (Strand: W. Ward, c. 1850), page 16 and inner back cover, DA 676, box 8, item 22, MSCE. Courtesy Lilly Library, Indiana University, Bloomington, Indiana.

Access to these materials was not confined to people living in London. The mid-nineteenth century was a period of unprecedented expansion for the press, and it quickly became the primary mechanism through which Holywell Street publishers connected with readers. Over time, it enabled them to expand their advertising out of London and across the country, penetrating even the smallest provincial towns. During the 1830s and early 1840s, Holywell Street publishers advertised in a handful of papers that targeted urban male readers. Favoured venues included *Bell's Life in London*, which published news on sports, politics, foreign events, entertainment, and crime; the Tory weekly *The Age*, whose readers were thought "fast gentlemen"; and the *Poor Man's Guardian*, a radical penny weekly.[77] Over the course of the 1840s, however, they steadily advertised in more and more urban venues. Some Holywell Street publishers dabbled in periodical publishing, and advertised medical works in their own productions. Dugdale promoted them in every issue of *Bell's Penny Dispatch*, and later in his salacious penny periodical *Peeping Tom* (1850), which targeted an

[77] "*Age* (1825–1843)," in *Dictionary of Nineteenth-Century Journalism in Great Britain and Northern Ireland*, ed. Laurel Brake and Marysa Demoor (London: Academia, 2009), 8.

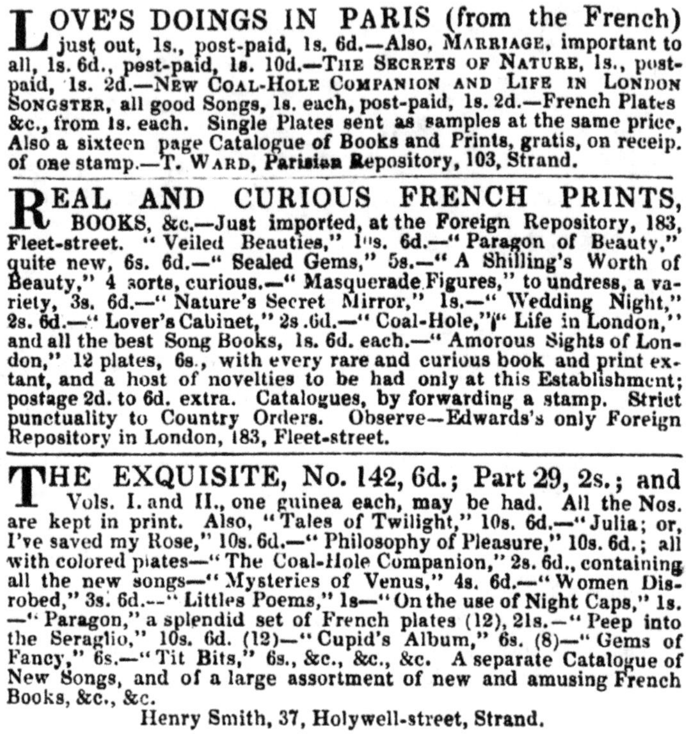

LOVE'S DOINGS IN PARIS (from the French) just out, 1s., post-paid, 1s. 6d.—Also, MARRIAGE, important to all, 1s. 6d., post-paid, 1s. 10d.—THE SECRETS OF NATURE, 1s., post-paid, 1s. 2d.—NEW COAL-HOLE COMPANION AND LIFE IN LONDON SONGSTER, all good Songs, 1s. each, post-paid, 1s. 2d.—French Plates &c., from 1s. each. Single Plates sent as samples at the same price, Also a sixteen page Catalogue of Books and Prints, gratis, on receip. of one stamp.—T. WARD, Parisian Repository, 103, Strand.

REAL AND CURIOUS FRENCH PRINTS, BOOKS, &c.—Just imported, at the Foreign Repository, 183, Fleet-street. "Veiled Beauties," 1''s. 6d.—"Paragon of Beauty," quite new, 6s. 6d.—"Sealed Gems," 5s.—"A Shilling's Worth of Beauty," 4 sorts, curious.—"Masquerade Figures," to undress, a variety, 3s. 6d.—"Nature's Secret Mirror," 1s.—"Wedding Night," 2s. 6d.—"Lover's Cabinet," 2s. 6d.—"Coal-Hole," "Life in London," and all the best Song Books, 1s. 6d. each.—"Amorous Sights of London," 12 plates, 6s., with every rare and curious book and print extant, and a host of novelties to be had only at this Establishment; postage 2d. to 6d. extra. Catalogues, by forwarding a stamp. Strict punctuality to Country Orders. Observe—Edwards's only Foreign Repository in London, 183, Fleet-street.

THE EXQUISITE, No. 142, 6d.; Part 29, 2s.; and Vols. I. and II., one guinea each, may be had. All the Nos. are kept in print. Also, "Tales of Twilight," 10s. 6d.—"Julia; or, I've saved my Rose," 10s. 6d.—"Philosophy of Pleasure," 10s. 6d.; all with colored plates—"The Coal-Hole Companion," 2s. 6d., containing all the new songs—"Mysteries of Venus," 4s. 6d.—"Women Disrobed," 3s. 6d.—"Littles Poems," 1s—"On the use of Night Caps," 1s. —"Paragon," a splendid set of French plates (12), 21s.—"Peep into the Seraglio," 10s. 6d. (12)—"Cupid's Album," 6s. (8)—"Gems of Fancy," 6s.—"Tit Bits," 6s., &c., &c., &c. A separate Catalogue of New Songs, and of a large assortment of new and amusing French Books, &c., &c.

Henry Smith, 37, Holywell-street, Strand.

Figure 1.4 Holywell Street publishers' advertisements. *The Era*, June 2, 1844, 2. Content provided by The British Library Board, with thanks to The British Newspaper Archive.

overlapping audience to *Bell's Life*. He also advertised medical works in his 4*d* weekly *The Exquisite* (1842–4) and 3*d* weekly *Gems for Gentlemen* (c. 1850), which serialized erotic stories and were aimed at a slightly more upmarket audience (Figure 1.4).[78]

The late 1840s and early 1850s marked enormous expansions in Holywell Street advertising, thanks to new opportunities opened up by the abolition of most "taxes on knowledge": duties on newspapers that had been introduced in

[78] *Peeping Tom: Wit, Fun, and Facetia* [*sic*] (London: H. Smith [William Dugdale], [1850]). Nos. 1–52, bound, in *London Low Life: Street Culture, Social Reform, and the Victorian Underworld* (Adam Matthew Digital, 2011-), https://www.amdigital.co.uk/collection/london-low-life; *The Exquisite: A Collection of Tales, Histories and Essays, Funny, Fanciful, and Facetious* [. . .]. (London: H. Smith [William Dugdale], [1842–44]), vol. I–IV, bound, P.C.20.B.1, BL; *Gems for Gentlemen: A Collection of Amatory Tales and Adventures* (London: William Johns, c. 1850), Nos. 1–24, bound, RB.23.b.5321, BL.

the eighteenth and early nineteenth centuries with the aim of suppressing dissent.[79] The ending of taxes on newspaper advertising in 1853 seems to have been especially significant. The tax represented such a huge expense to publishers that one industry commentator claimed its effect was "the virtual suppression of pamphlets and low-priced books."[80] While massive increases in the production of cheap print during the 1840s emphasize that this assessment was exaggerated, the abolition of the tax cut the costs of advertising in newspapers in half.[81] Publishers like William Dugdale and Edward Duncombe put their savings to work and promoted their wares across the country in a plethora of provincial newspapers, such as the *North Wales Chronicle*, and periodicals for bored travellers, like *Herapath's Railway Journal*. Advertising in these venues may not have changed their audience much in terms of its demographics: although women and working-class men did read them, these periodicals' largest audience was middle-class men.[82] It did mean, however, that Holywell Street publishers now reached prospective readers across the country.

Advertising so widely would have been pointless without the postal service, whose dramatic expansion in the 1830s, and introduction of the penny stamp in 1840, enabled Holywell Street publishers to communicate with readers in remote locations and transport their wares to them cheaply and easily.[83] Readers living virtually anywhere in the United Kingdom could send away for the medical publications that they advertised in newspapers, or for their sales catalogues, which described them alongside explicit fiction and images. In doing so, Holywell Street publishers claimed, readers could rest assured that their transactions were private. Orders could be placed under pseudonyms, paid for with postage stamps enclosed with the order, and picked up at "any Post-office in the United Kingdom" in a sealed envelope. "If [the reader's] name be Ramsbottom, or Cockburn, or any other name," Dugdale advised winkingly, "he may write … under the signature of Harrison, Jackson, Williamson, or plain A.B.C., Post-office, — to be left till called for."[84] In reality, readers could not be assured of

79 Martin Hewitt, *The Dawn of the Cheap Press in Victorian Britain: The End of 'Taxes on Knowledge,' 1849–1869* (London: Bloomsbury, 2013), 24.

80 John Chapman, *Cheap Books and How to Get Them* (London: Chapman, 1852), 7.

81 It is worth noting that advertising campaigns were still quite expensive after 1853. Based on the number of advertisements they published and posted costs, Dugdale and Duncombe would each have spent £13 3*s* 6*d* on advertising under the names Henry Smith and John Wilson in *Bell's Life in London* alone in 1855, for instance. The extent to which Holywell Street publishers advertised during this period offers further evidence that they were doing very good business.

82 Andrew Hobbs, *A Fleet Street in Every Town: The Provincial Press in England, 1855–1900* (Cambridge: Open Book, 2018), 54–62.

83 For further information, see Catherine J. Golden, *Posting It: The Victorian Revolution in Letter-Writing* (Gainesville: University Press of Florida, 2009).

84 *Night Caps*, 23–24. Postage stamps could be exchanged for money at post offices for a fee of 2.5 percent, and were routinely used to purchase books. See *First Report of the Postmaster General on the Post Office: Presented to both Houses of Parliament by Command of Her Majesty* (London: George E. Eyre and William Spottiswoode, 1855), 13.

discretion. Letters and packages were sometimes opened. However, in Britain, pornographers' mails were not subject to concerted attempts at interception until end of the century. Readers could reasonably expect privacy, though not quite to the degree that Holywell Street publishers claimed.[85]

Marginalia in sales catalogues further emphasizes the material accessibility of these works, showing that readers could compare prices and choose among suppliers. One reader annotated a number of entries in *Ward's New Catalogue of Parisian Novelties* (c. 1850) with different prices. At top of the catalogue's opening page, he wrote, "The prices written here are the ones charged by H.S. Smith 37 Holywell St Strand, or W. Johns 35 Holywell St also sent Thos Ward 2 St Martin's Ct St Martin's Lane + T Hicks 34 Holywell St. H.S. Stands for Henry Smith [William Dugdale] who is decidedly the cheapest of the lot."[86] Other marginalia emphasizes that Holywell Street publishers did not uniformly serve a well-educated audience, though it also draws attention to the fact that some readers would have had difficulty interpreting their wares. One reader of a catalogue called *A Select Catalogue of Books; Facetious and Amorous* (c. 1845) had to look up, or ask someone to translate, unfamiliar terms.[87] On the first page of the catalogue, words in a blurb for a work of erotic fiction are numbered "1" and "2" and clarified at the bottom of the page: "1 lanugo – soft hairs, 2 labia – <u>cunt</u>." On the second page, this reader attempted to decipher a riot of terms in a section advertising French prints for sale, writing "Chastity" alongside "La Pudeur"; "maiden-head" alongside "Le Pucelage"; "favours" alongside "Bien fait." As if delighted with his discoveries, he appended a translation of a banner reading "Petite Bibliotheque [*sic*] Joyeuse" with an exclamation: "THE JOLLY LITTLE LIBRARY O! HO!"

The Jolly Little Library

How did Holywell Street publishers want readers to engage with the medical works that they sold? In amplifying radical views about the necessities of sexual freedom and equal pleasure, works like *Night Caps*, *The Connubial Guide*, and Horne's *Marriage* suggest that some shared Carlile, Owen, and Knowlton's beliefs that medical knowledge could help people live better, more egalitarian lives, freed from shame about their bodies and desires, and the burden of children they could not afford to feed. When he transformed Michael

85 For more on postal privacy, see Kate Thomas, *Postal Pleasures: Sex, Scandal, and Victorian Letters* (Oxford: Oxford University Press, 2011); Colette Colligan, *A Publisher's Paradise: Expatriate Literary Culture in Paris, 1890–1960* (Amherst: University of Massachusetts Press, 2014), 145–147, and Chapter 7.

86 *Ward's New Catalogue*, 1.

87 *A Select Catalogue of Books; Facetious and Amorous* ([London]: s.n., n.d.), DA 676, box 6, item 51, MCSE.

Ryan's *Philosophy of Marriage* into a godless marriage-guide-cum-contraception-manual, perhaps Dugdale still saw himself as a soldier in a war against blinkered sexual ideologies. Yet, this literature's function as advertising material raises questions about his and other Holywell Street publishers' aims in spreading these views. Additionally, only a handful of the medical works that Holywell Street publishers sold are obvious contributions to a progressive political project. Even in their updated forms, manuals like *Aristotle* were incredibly old-fashioned, and hasty compilations like *The Philosophy of Kissing* were incredibly vapid. Works like *The Silent Friend* and *Onania: or, The Heinous Sin of Self-Pollution*, with their dire warnings about the dangers of masturbation and promiscuity, are even more awkward companions to the contraception literature.

At the same time, many of these works are not obvious companions to the pornographic fiction and images that made Holywell Street publishers notorious. Some do have a clear prurient appeal. Venette's *Conjugal Love* describes the mechanics of copulation in lyric detail, while Ryan's *Marriage* reproduces titillating excerpts from travel narratives that inspired novels like *The Lustful Turk.*[88] Yet, critics of *The Silent Friend* claimed that its descriptions of venereal disease and sexual debility were engineered to elicit horror and anxiety in readers, and readers of *Aristotle's Masterpiece* often expressed disappointment on discovering that its main focus is the development of the foetus and not, as its reputation implied, sexual acts. Richard Carlile grumbled that *Aristotle* was a bestseller solely because it was known "as a smuggled book."[89]

Even thematically, Holywell Street publishers' medical and pornographic output is an awkward fit. Much of the latter, for instance, depicts queer sex. Sex scenes between women are common, and many novels feature gender-bending scenes involving cross-dressing, ejaculating dildoes, and other props. Holywell Street publishers were clearly conscious of a market for material on queer sex and gender presentation outside fiction. Several sold reprints of old pamphlets about the lives of cross-dressers and "hermaphrodites."[90] Dugdale issued an original work that provided men seeking male sex partners with a guide to cruising: under the guise of telling readers how to avoid "*Margeries, Poofs,*

88 For example, see Ryan, *Philosophy of Marriage*, 99.

89 Richard Carlile, "To Old William Wilberforce, Saint and Self-Styled Suppressor of Vice," *Republican*, March 18, 1825, 322. For further details about critics' opinions of *The Silent Friend* and similar works, see Chapter 2.

90 Holywell Street publishers often advertised an illustrated pamphlet called *Bigenio, an Hermaphrodite*. An incomplete edition issued by Dugdale survives. See *The Life and Surprising Adtentures* [*sic*] *of Bigenio, an Hermaphrodite, or Man-Woman, and Woman-Man* ([London]: Printed by H. Smith [William Dugdale], c. 1842), EPB/P/68210, WL. *Cohen*, 1836, Old Bailey Proceedings Online (t18361024-2351) suggests that some of these publisher-booksellers also sold Henry Fielding's *The Female Husband* (1746). See Jen Manion, *Female Husbands: A Trans History* (Cambridge: Cambridge University Press, 2020) for details about such pamphlets and their popularity.

&c" on forays around London, his *Yokel's Preceptor* (c. 1844) spells out exactly where such men gathered, how readers could identify them, and how they signalled sexual interest.[91] Yet, medical descriptions of queer bodies, acts, and desires were rare in the Holywell Street trade. A handful of the medical works briefly discuss conditions that disturb gender binaries, such as "hermaphrodism" (*Aristotle's Masterpiece*) and eunuchism (Ryan's *Marriage*). Medical discussions of same-sex sex did not appear in the pornography trade until 1881, however, in essays appended to the novel *The Sins of the Cities of the Plain*.[92]

The medical material's overwhelming focus on white bodies is also conspicuous when set against nineteenth-century pornography, which often luxuriates in describing racialized bodies and supposedly foreign sexual practices. *The Lustful Turk*, for instance, unremittingly exoticizes the Dey's body, those of his eunuchs, and those of the members of his multiethnic harem, and ends with a triumphant imperial twist: finally freed, the Dey's "white slave" carries his severed penis and testes back to Britain in a jar, where they are put on display as specimens in a girls' school.[93] References to racialized bodies and allegedly foreign sexual practices appear in a number of the medical works. However, they are never the main focus of the text, and usually very brief. Only Ryan's *Marriage* breaks with this trend by including lengthy discussions of polygamy and sexual development among the inhabitants of "warm countries." Dugdale clearly thought this material would compel readers: he not only retained them in the text of Horne's *Marriage* but highlighted them on the title page. Yet, neither he nor his competitors adapted other medico-scientific material with this focus.

To make sense of Holywell Street publishers' hopes for their medical works, it is less helpful to try to find commonalities across their wares than it is to consider how they were framed. These publisher-booksellers' lists were not painstakingly curated affairs. They were thrown together on an ad hoc basis, shaped by a combination of opportunity, perceptions about what would sell, book-trade traditions, and, in my estimation, political beliefs. Diverse as they were, though, each publication contributed to something larger: a catalogue of sexually themed products – a "jolly little library," if you will – that could serve a wide range of needs, tastes, and budgets. It was the catalogue itself that brought these works into coherence, presenting them as materials that, in different ways, supported the enactment of a hazy, pleasure-centred fantasy of sexual autonomy that complemented the convictions of revolutionary

91 *The Yokel's Preceptor: or, More Sprees in London! Being a Regular and Curious Show-Up of All the Rigs and Doings of the Flash Cribs in this Great Metropolis* (London: H. Smith [William Dugdale], c. 1844), 5–7, Cup.364.ee.14, BL.

92 See "A Short Essay on Sodomy" and "Tribadism" in Jack Saul, *The Sins of the Cities of the Plain; or, The Recollections of a Mary Ann* (1881; repr., Olympia, WA: Olympia, 2006), 115–120.

93 *The Lustful Turk* (1828; repr., Olympia, WA: Olympia, 2006), 120–121. For further details on these tropes in nineteenth-century pornography, see Colligan, *Traffic*, 45–55.

libertines like Dugdale and was also very good for business. By placing individual works within this larger context and further steering interpretation through strategic editing and paratextual devices, Holywell Street publishers encouraged readers to "yield to the dictates of love and perform its joyous rites" by performing multiple readings and consuming multiple products.

Holywell Street publishers marketed a number of medical works as titillating reading material. This was especially true of seventeenth- and eighteenth-century works on masturbation, fertility, and generation, which already had a history of being framed as containers of secret knowledge in the book trade and depicted bodies and desires in ways that may have felt racier than modern productions, which often had a more technical focus on anatomy and physiology. Holywell Street publishers often used elements of the language they employed to market pornographic novels to describe these works. Sales catalogues allude to the "Extraordinary and Curious" nature of these publications, the "remarkable," "unexpurgated" detail of the cases they recount, and sometimes warn readers of the moral danger that the "Secrets of Nature" they unveil might present to "youth and unmarried females."[94] Sometimes, titles would be altered to suggest "secret" content. Edward Dyer framed a translation of Tissot's forbidding *L'Onanisme* in voyeuristic terms by titling it *Onanism Unveiled; or, The Private Pleasures and Secret Habits of the Youth of Both Sexes Exposed*, while William Dugdale swapped the prosaic title of one eighteenth-century fertility pamphlet, *The Nature and Causes of Impotence in Men, and Barrenness in Woman, Explained*, for a title that heralded revelation: *Conjugal Love; or, The Mysteries of Hymen Unveiled.*[95]

Carlile's comment about *Aristotle*'s undeserved reputation suggests that some readers considered this framing fraudulent. However, others probably found medical works exciting sexually. Francis Place reported feeling "a near-erotic thrill" as a teenager when he rummaged through anatomy textbooks in second-hand bookshops.[96] *Aristotle* reportedly acted as an equivalent for less well-off readers, providing, as Mary Fissell has pointed out, "the most easily accessible pictures of a naked woman in cheap print."[97] Walter, the narrator of the anonymous autobiography *My Secret Life* (1888), paints a vivid picture of these reading experiences, describing how he devoured *Aristotle* with a friend

94 These quotations are from H. G. Brook, *Catalogue of Fast and Funny Literature* (London: H. G. Brook, n.d.), DA 676, box 1, item 52, MSCE.

95 Edward Dyer, *A Catalogue of Facetious and Humorous Books* (London: Edward Dyer, n.d.), 6. DA 676, box 1, item 51, MSCE. See n. 57 for information about *Conjugal Love*, whose title was probably meant to recall Nicholas Venette's work.

96 Francis Place, *The Autobiography of Francis Place: 1771–1854*, ed. Marty Thale (Cambridge: Cambridge University Press, 1972), 46–47.

97 Mary Fissell, "Making a Masterpiece: The *Aristotle* Texts in Vernacular Medical Culture," in *Right Living: An Anglo-American Tradition of Self-Help Medicine*, ed. Charles E. Rosenberg (Baltimore, MD: Johns Hopkins University Press, 2003), 61.

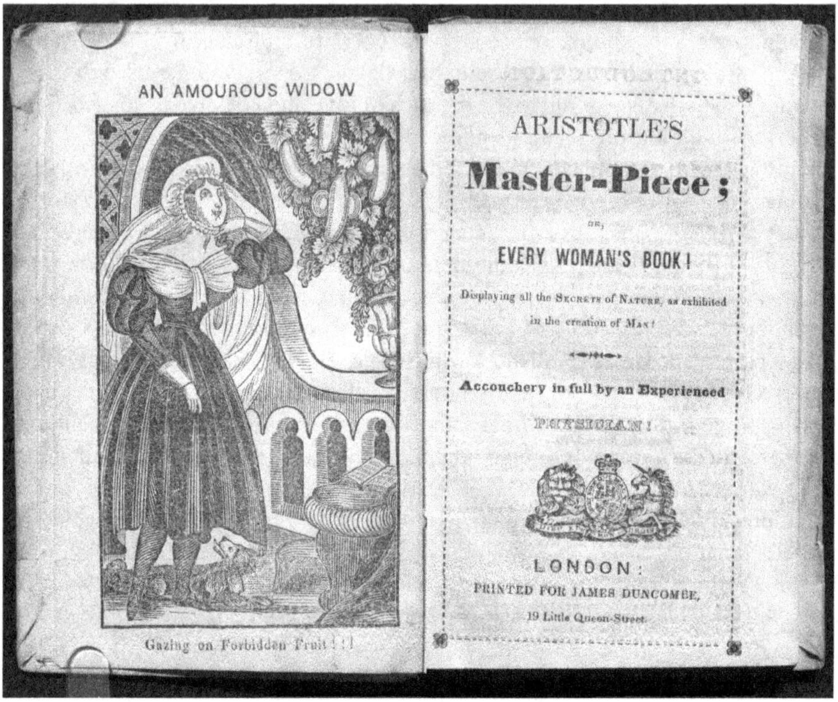

Figure 1.5 Frontispiece and title page, *Aristotle's Master-Piece; or, Every Woman's Book! Displaying All the Secrets of Nature, as Exhibited in the Creation of Man!* (London: Printed for James Duncombe, c. 1830), WZ 290 A718 1800, Osler Library of the History of Medicine, McGill University. By courtesy of McGill University Libraries.

in his youth, then lent it to a servant in hopes of seducing her.[98] Holywell Street publishers sometimes added material to medical works to enhance their prurient appeal. John Duncombe met readers' expectations of a book with a bawdy reputation by furnishing his edition of *Aristotle* with a bawdy frontispiece (Figure 1.5). "AN AMOUROUS WIDOW Gazing on Forbidden Fruit!!!" its caption exclaims. The frontispiece depicting a nude woman in *Secrets of Nature* performs a similar kind of work, adding an erotic element to the book and setting a tone that could make its descriptions of procreation more exciting. The frontispiece to Horne's *Marriage*, which depicts one woman undressing another while a third peeps through the door, functions in a similar way.[99] The

[98] *My Secret Life* (Amsterdam: Privately Printed for Subscribers, 1888), chapter 3.

[99] This frontispiece appears in the Kinsey Institute's copy of Horne's *Marriage*, but not in the Morris Library's copy.

image of the vulva that Dugdale appended to Knowlton's *Fruits of Philosophy* could be interpreted as another device in this tradition.

Night Caps offers a more elaborate example of an addition that turned a notably bawdy medical work into a means of entertainment. The pamphlet is appended with a short fictional vignette, "A Case Worth Knowing By All Females," which tells the story of a physician who diagnoses an unmarried young woman with "unsatisfied … sexual sensations."[100] At her mother's request, he treats her anxiety, depression, and menstrual problems by having sex with her. This narrative is allegedly appended to the pamphlet to demonstrate the benefits of the "night cap," which the doctor employs to ensure that he does not get his patient pregnant or pass on a venereal disease. The vignette is not sexually explicit, and arguably more medical than fictional: most of the text is given over to the doctor's explanation of the mechanics of conception and contraception, which reprises information covered in *Night Caps*' main text. Nevertheless, it's a titillating device for reinforcing the pamphlet's message, one that turns the whole manual into a kind of erotic story by association.

Although they can be interpreted as erotic, it is important to recognize that the vignette appended to *Night Caps* and the illustration of the vulva in Dugdale's editions of *Fruits of Philosophy* are also didactic. Both communicate information about the human body – the mechanics of conception and the location of the clitoris – covered in the main text, offering instruction in alternative ways that readers might consider more interesting or accessible. The degree to which Holywell Street publishers emphasized the utility of medical information on sexual matters is what set them apart from previous disreputable publishers, who capitalized on medical eroticism by winking and nudging at "secret" content. While they did their own winking and nudging, Holywell Street publishers always apprised readers of their medical works' practical use-value. One of the bookseller Edward Dyer's catalogues, for instance, emphasizes that *Secrets of Nature* relays "safe and certain methods" of curing impotence and fertility; that a work on venereal disease called *Tabes Dorsalis* offers "an explanation of the symptoms and precautions, and the method of cure"; and that *Fruits of Philosophy* provides "a review of the most efficient checks of impregnation."[101] Moreover, Holywell Street publishers wove medical knowledge together with fantasy in ways that demonstrated how readers could apply it to enjoy the kinds of sex lives they aspired to. *Night Caps*' vignette offers perhaps the most direct example of this technique. However, Holywell Street publishers also did so more subtly by evoking idealized unions in which couples enjoyed frequent, mutually pleasurable,

[100] *Night Caps*, 24. [101] Dyer, *Catalogue of Facetious*, 10–11.

non-reproductive sex in contraception literature, and, in works aimed at single young men, an aspirational figure from low urban culture: the fast man.

The latter is best illustrated by Holywell Street publishers' insertion of medical material into two ephemeral genres: night guides and flash periodicals. Flash periodicals, which sported suggestive titles like *Sam Sly*, *The Fast Man*, and *Peeping Tom*, were extremely popular during the 1840s and 1850s.[102] They usually cost a penny and were not sexually explicit. However, they skirted the bounds of propriety, offering up lurid stories about love, vice, and crime; biographies of courtesans; bawdy jokes and sketches; theatrical reviews; and local gossip. Taken together, this material painted a glamourous picture of fast life in London and other urban centres engineered to appeal to young male readers. Dugdale's *Peeping Tom* routinely reprinted extracts on venereal disease, reproductive physiology, and contraceptive techniques from *Dr. Graham's Lectures*, *The Silent Friend*, *Night Caps*, and other medical works that he listed for sale in the periodical's advertising section.[103] With the exception of the excerpt from *Night Caps*, which urges readers to purchase night caps from *Peeping Tom*'s publisher, these extracts were presented without any direct contextualization. However, while their placement in a bawdy periodical could be taken to suggest that medical information was titillating, it also relayed a different message: that readers who wanted to live like fast men needed medical knowledge.

Night guides made what was implicit in flash periodicals explicit. This genre of guidebook is best known for providing addresses and reviews of brothels in major cities.[104] However, night guides also functioned as a combination of conduct manual and escapist reading: they evoked the fantasy of a sexually sophisticated, self-assured man about town and purported to teach readers how to be one. Most night guides contain "flash dictionaries," which induct readers into the mysterious wordplay of cockney slang. Some include pages of advice about how to dress, speak, drink, gamble, fight, and pay sex workers. And some provide advice on how to avoid the most undesirable outcome of a night in a brothel: venereal disease. The medical advice that these works proffered was, again, not original. It was mostly excerpted from works that Holywell Street publishers advertised in the back pages of the guides alongside bawdy songbooks, erotic prints, and so on. For the

[102] On flash periodicals in Britain, see Donald J. Gray, "Early Victorian Scandalous Journalism: Renton Nicholson's *The Town* (1837–42)," *The Victorian Periodical Press: Samplings and Soundings*, ed. Joanne Shattock and Michael Wolff (Toronto: University of Toronto Press, 1982), 317–348. On the American context, see Patricia Cline Cohen, Timothy J. Gilfoyle, and Helen Lefkowitz Horowitz, *The Flash Press: Sporting Male Weeklies in 1840s New York* (Chicago: University of Chicago Press, 2008).

[103] See *Peeping Tom*, "Sequel to Dr. Graham's Lectures," 18–19; "On Checks to Impregnation," 58; "The Silent Friend," 83–84, 88; "An Extract from Dr. Graham's Lecture," 120; "On the Present State of Prostitution in Paris," 151; "Prostitution in London," 31, 34.

[104] Phillip Howell, "Sex and the City of Bachelors: Sporting Guidebooks and Urban Knowledge in Nineteenth-Century Britain and America," *Ecumene* 8, no. 1 (2001): 20–50.

shop-boys, clerks, and students who were these guides' target audience, however, it is doubtful that originality mattered. What mattered was access to useful advice.

Hints to Men About Town; or, Waterfordania (c. 1841), a guide attributed to "a Sporting Surgeon," provides such readers with three detailed chapters on the functions of the reproductive organs, the symptoms of gonorrhoea and syphilis, and how these infections can be prevented or, should efforts at prevention fail or be forgotten, treated. Most of this material appears to have been copied from Michael Ryan's *Philosophy of Marriage* or his later book *Prostitution in London* (1839).[105] However, the spirit in which it is presented in *Hints* is very different. Going even further than *Night Caps*, which depicts sexual desire as a healthy, normal condition in both sexes, *Hints* frames promiscuity in young men as natural and venereal disease as a preventable risk of living life to the fullest. At one point, it sneers at the work it excerpts:

> "Avoid," says he, "chambermaids and servant girls, avoid courtezans – avoid milliners, dress makers, bonnet makers, stay makers, the ladies to be met with at Vauxhall, Tea Gardens, Concert Rooms, &c. &c. &c." Why, what a thrice double ass is this same book maker – if these rules be attended to, there would be no danger of infection, no necessity for laying down rules for its prevention. And besides, how is it to be expected that such wise saws or aphorisms are even to be retained at these moments when passion or lust takes possession of the breast, and when prudence and wisdom flee from it? No, this is utterly impossible. It is when better judgment has been overcome by the impulse of the moment, that he requires the aid of art to ward off the danger he may have incurred.[106]

Hints encourages readers to educate themselves about venereal disease so they can enjoy sex with many people while mitigating the consequences. More broadly, it encourages readers to look beyond language about sexual sin seared into many medical works on the topic to get to useful advice, an against-the-grain mode of reading that framing works like *Onania* as arousing also encouraged. Notably, Holywell Street publishers also encouraged this mode of reading by other means, such as creating in-jokes by retaining content that railed against vice in their renovated works. Horne's *Marriage*, for example, retains a rant quoted in Ryan's *Philosophy of Marriage* against the "open exhibition of disgustingly indecent books and pictures" in London. Having purchased Horne's *Marriage* from one of the "miscreants" who, the author complains, "insult females by exhibiting and selling, with absolute impunity, horrible and indecent representations," readers knew that they were not to read moralizing passages straight.[107]

[105] Major, verbatim text overlaps suggest that Dugdale derived most of the content for these chapters from one of these books. However, it is difficult to determine which one because, as Chapter 3 discusses, Ryan habitually reused his own work as well as that of others. For instance, compare *Hints*, 17 with Ryan, *Philosophy of Marriage*, 352 and Michael Ryan, *Prostitution in London: With a Comparative View of that of Paris and New York* (Paris: Baillière, 1839), 412.

[106] *Hints to Men*, 14.

[107] Compare Horne, *Marriage*, 12 and Ryan, *Philosophy of Marriage*, 15.

Holywell Street publishers' trade in cheap medical works made good business sense. It supported a robust trade in condoms and occasionally other medical products and services. More broadly, marketing medical works not just as racy reading material but also as useful companions to sexual entertainment enabled Holywell Street publishers to source content quickly and cheaply, and encouraged readers to purchase multiple products in ways that a narrower trade in erotic fiction or images would not. Indeed, they actively fostered this kind of consumer behaviour by habitually cross-advertising medical, bawdy, and pornographic publications. In addition to advertising them in the same catalogues and newspaper advertisements, as the back cover of *Secrets of Nature* suggests, they often inserted advertisements for pornographic and bawdy productions into their medical works, and vice versa. With these resources, customers could choose from various genres according to their needs again and again: first a night guide or a flash paper, then a manual on venereal disease and a packet of French letters, then a pornographic novel or an erotic plate – or the other way around. Holywell Street publishers' shops were destinations for sexual discovery that were accessible to middle- and probably some working-class readers across the nation by the early 1850s. The price of entry could be as low as a day-old newspaper, an envelope, and a penny stamp.

Some scholars have characterized the Holywell Street trade as a sorry departure from its roots in revolutionary politics: "too hollow and fantastic, too parasitic on the genres it tried to burlesque, too commercially expedient, to be a subversive cultural force," Iain McCalman memorably concludes.[108] Holywell Street publishers clearly aspired to profit from public appetite for sexual information and entertainment. Yet, as the next chapter emphasizes, this was a period in which desire was frequently presented in cheap print as virtually absent in women and as a weakness in men. In this context, they performed a kind of radical work through their noisy, bawdy affirmation of Victorian men's and women's sexual curiosity, appetites for pleasure, and desire to take control of their reproductive lives. The ways Holywell Street publishers transformed different elements of medical and radical print cultures into a glittering commercial enterprise that promoted sexual pleasure and bodily autonomy laughed at medical authority, embarrassed more conservative social reformers, and, as we will see, dragged medical works into obscenity trials in the 1850s. However, the emergent pornography trade's traffic in medical works escaped significant opposition for a long time, partly because it was eclipsed by businesses that presented different and more direct challenges to medical authority. Such businesses are the subject of the next chapter.

[108] McCalman, *Radical Underworld*, 235.

2 Stereotyped Knowledge

Branwell Brontë, brother of the novelists Charlotte, Emily, and Anne, noted the title of a work that interested him in a battered notebook. "manhood. the causes of its premature decline," he scribbled, "by J. L. Curtis & Co, London."[1] It was 1841. Brontë was living in Luddenden Foot, a tiny village in West Yorkshire, and trying to forget that he was a failure. He aspired to be a painter and a poet. Yet, his portraits had not sold, his poems had been refused by publishers, and his letters to influential authors and artists had gone unanswered.[2] He had been relieved to find employment as a tutor for the sons of a retired country magistrate, only to be sacked less than a year into the job. Rumour had it that one of the servants was pregnant with his child.[3] Brontë was now working as a clerk on the new Leeds and Manchester railway line. Luddenden Foot's rail station was little more than a shack, and trains did not come through it often. Brontë wiled the days away by doodling in his ledgers and, reportedly, matched the alcoholic station-master pint for pint.[4] How could J. L. Curtis's *Manhood: The Causes of Its Premature Decline with Directions for Its Perfect Restoration* (1840) not attract the eye of a man who, at only twenty-four, believed that he had failed to live up to his potential? The title must have seemed to speak to Brontë personally, to promise an explanation for his struggles, and a guide to setting things right.

Manhood was not made for Branwell Brontë, but it was created for, and found an international audience in, young men like him. In 1841, the work was being advertised all over the British Isles. A decade later, it had been translated into four European languages and was being promoted all over the world. By 1855, readers from Lima to Madrid, Calcutta to Adelaide would have been familiar with *Manhood*'s title, if not the work itself. Advertisements for it appeared everywhere: in the classified sections of local newspapers, in the back pages of

1 Patrick Branwell Brontë, "Brearley Hill," with doodles and notes, 1841, BC MS 19c Bronte/B3/14/c, University of Leeds Digital Library, http://digital.library.leeds.ac.uk/id/eprint/6950.
2 Daphne DuMaurier, *The Infernal World of Branwell Brontë* (Garden City, NY: Doubleday, 1961), 127.
3 Juliet Barker, *The Brontës* (London: Weidenfeld and Nicholson, 1994), 334.
4 DuMaurier, *Infernal World*, 154.

travel guides and how-to books, on the walls of military barracks and back alleys, and above public urinals. Issued under a pseudonym by a medical practitioner named Joseph Lambert, or possibly Joseph La'Mert, *Manhood*'s longevity is as striking today as its globe-spanning circulation. Lambert sold various editions out of his premises in Albemarle Street, West London, into the 1870s, and others hawked it under a variety of titles and attributions into the early 1900s. Yet, *Manhood* was not an extraordinary publication. It was merely one of the more successful of a panoply of cheap manuals on venereal disease and sexual debility that began to deluge the print marketplace in the 1840s. People who framed themselves as experts in the treatment of sexual problems made, published, and sold these works at the local, national, and sometimes international levels, supported by a finely tuned advertising machine that far surpassed Holywell Street publishers' in the sheer volume of its output.

The author-publishers of these manuals usually called themselves "consulting surgeons," adopting a term from hospital practice, and that is the term I will use to refer to them here – not because they were the only practitioners to use the title but because the only other term closely identified with these figures was a pejorative: "quack."[5] Deriving from the Dutch *kwakzalver*, a term for "a person who cures with home remedies," "quack" often implied a doctor who exaggerated his expertise or claimed to effect miracle cures.[6] However, in medical circles it was also volleyed at practitioners who made a more benign error: "those who tell the truth in their advertisements, but, doing so [i.e. advertising], adopt a course not countenanced by the profession."[7] Self-promotion was considered uncouth in the class-conscious medical world. Medical men were supposed to develop reputations sufficient to support a career by patiently cultivating – or being born with – social networks.[8] Quacks embraced a lower-rent way of attracting patients, one that, in the eyes of other doctors, aligned medicine with the low social status and

5 As with my use of "pornography" and "pornographer" in discussions of pre-1880s contexts, I recognize that my use of this term needs some qualification. "Consulting surgeon" was a title used by other kinds of practitioners, and not all practitioners working in Lambert's style adopted it (though most did). Given that they play a major role in this book's narrative, I desired a term that could be used to refer to this specific kind of medical practitioner. Previously, I used "commercial medical dealer," but colleagues found it awkward and not sufficiently specific. "Irregular" also seemed too broad: there were irregular practitioners of many kinds. In referring to these figures by using the most common term they used to describe themselves, I ultimately chose to follow Maritha Burmeister, whose work on public anatomical museums informs this chapter.

6 *Oxford English Dictionary Online*, s.v. "quacksalver, n," accessed October 2, 2020, www.oed.com/view/Entry/155643.

7 Quoted in Maritha Burmeister, "Popular Anatomical Museums in Nineteenth-Century England" (PhD diss., Rutgers University, 2000), 83.

8 For more on the ways doctors traditionally cultivated trust through social networks and a study of how the expansion of the print marketplace challenged this tradition in a slightly earlier period, see Hannah Barker, "Medical Advertising and Trust in Late Georgian England," *Urban History* 36, no. 3 (2009): 379–398.

moral quagmires of trade: they spoke to prospective patients directly through public lectures, demonstrations, and, now most of all, through print.

Many consulting surgeons would have qualified as quacks under both definitions of the term. All of them qualified under the latter. They not only made massive investments in print advertising but also exploited the multifunctionality of the book to advance their interests. The cheap manuals that they created by compiling excerpts from existing publications offered Victorian readers a cornucopia of information about reproduction and sexual health. At the same time, the manuals acted as instruments that consulting surgeons used to cultivate trust in their expertise and facilitate the sale of other products and services. The techniques that consulting surgeons used to make and sell these works were similar to Holywell Street publishers'. However, this chapter argues that their effects on the market for sexual knowledge were quite different. The incestuous nature of the copying involved in creating consulting surgeons' manuals and the sheer scale of their circulation meant that they blanketed the Victorian world with a standardized model of sexuality that soldered desire with male weakness. Ubiquitous in foreign and especially colonial territories, trade in these manuals can be thought of as an element of cultural imperialism, one that displaced indigenous knowledges in India, Australasia, the Caribbean, and North and South America with a mass-produced model of sexuality imported from Europe.

At first glance, these manuals and their makers are unlikely characters in a book that explores debate about medical works' potential to deprave and corrupt. Consulting surgeons' manuals were not known as bawdy books, nor did they invite such a reputation. Their representations of sex and the body imported from their sources a highly technical focus on anatomy and physiology, and they displayed images of disease and disability that readers typically framed as the opposite of erotic. Nor did these manuals obviously encourage sexual rebellion: one of their most notable features is their extreme, conservative moralism. Even so, these manuals entered the story this book tells because their makers exploited an ambiguity that, as we will see, aroused greater anxiety among regular practitioners during this period than the blurry boundary between the medical and erotic: the uncertain line between information and advertisement. By exploiting that ambiguity, consulting surgeons threatened regular medicine economically and existentially. Their self-identification as medical experts and their use of print as a vehicle for self-promotion attracted patients in droves and associated a profession anxious to assure the public that it was learned and trustworthy with the low status of trade and the exaggerations of advertising.[9] Moreover, their manuals seemed to undermine the

[9] For more on advertising's associations with exaggeration during this period, see Anat Rosenberg, *The Rise of Mass Advertising: Law, Enchantment, and the Cultural Boundaries of Modernity* (Oxford: Oxford University Press, 2022), 308.

credibility of all medical literature. These cut-and-paste productions raised the question of whether it was possible to distinguish between published evidence of expertise and a hollow performance aimed at extracting profit.

Paper Museums

The brashly commercial brand of medicine that consulting surgeons engaged in had existed since the seventeenth century.[10] Almost immediately after the printing press was introduced to Britain in 1476, medical practitioners had seized the opportunity to spread word about their remedies through print.[11] The ending of government licensing for printing and publishing in 1695 gave them freer rein to experiment with the medium, and set off a boom in the production of vernacular works aimed at readers who were not medical experts.[12] As Mary Fissell has shown, informational and promotional print forms quickly became entangled in this context. Medical guides and pamphlets coexisted with handbills advertising medical practice in early modern print culture, with practitioners often using each form to present themselves in a different way. However, these forms also merged into a hybrid genre that functioned simultaneously as instructive reading material and as advertisements for medical products and services, a genre demonstrated by some of the contraception pamphlets examined in the previous chapter.

By the late eighteenth and early nineteenth centuries, this hybrid genre – "the most commercial and market-like [aspect] of medical print," Fissell notes – had become especially associated with trade in remedies for impotence, infertility, and venereal disease.[13] James Graham's *Lecture on the Generation, Increase, and Improvement of the Human Species* (c. 1783), hawked by Holywell Street publishers decades after Graham's death, offers a great deal of information about procreation. It also suggests a variety of means through which readers could preserve or enhance their fertility,

10 Mary Fissell, "The Marketplace of Print," in *Medicine and the Market in England and Its Colonies, c. 1450–c. 1850*, ed. Mark S. R. Jenner and Patrick Wallis (Basingstoke: Palgrave Macmillan, 2007), 108–132; W. F. Bynum and Roy Porter, eds., *Medical Fringe and Medical Orthodoxy, 1750–1850* (London: Croom Helm, 1987); Roy Porter, *Health for Sale: Quackery in England, 1660–1850* (Manchester: Manchester University Press, 1989); Alan Mackintosh, *The Patent Medicines Industry in Georgian England: Constructing the Market by the Potency of Print* (Basingstoke: Palgrave Macmillan, 2018); David Boyd Haycock and Patrick Wallis, "Quackery and Commerce in Seventeenth-Century London: The Proprietary Medicine Business of Anthony Daffy," *Medical History* 25 (2005): 1–36.

11 Mary Fissell, "Popular Medical Writing" in *The Book in the Renaissance*, ed. Andrew Pettegree (New Haven, CT: Yale University Press, 2010), 297–318.

12 Fissell, "Marketplace of Print," 114.

13 Fissell, "Marketplace of Print," 126. For more on irregular Georgian-era advertising and distribution practices, see John Strachan, *Advertising and Satirical Culture in the Romantic Period* (Cambridge: Cambridge University Press, 2011), 15, 53; Mackintosh, *The Patent Medicines Industry*, 18, 119–152; and Porter, *Health for Sale.*

including by seeking out customized advice from Graham "at the very moderate price of ONE GUINEA."[14] Other examples include Samuel Solomon's three-shilling *Guide to Health, or, Advice to Both Sexes* (1782) and William Brodum's two-volume, five-shilling *Guide to Old Age, or Cure for the Indiscretions of Youth* (1795), which warned readers against masturbation on the grounds that it would harm them physically, mentally, and morally, and promoted their authors' cures for the damage.[15]

Trade in these kinds of manuals skyrocketed around 1840. Over the next twenty years, it only increased even as prices plummeted from a median three shillings in 1840 to below one shilling in 1860.[16] Like Georgian irregulars before them, consulting surgeons advertised their manuals in a wide range of venues and sold them directly to customers and through networks of newspaper offices, bookshops, stationers, and apothecaries. However, they took advantage of expanding transport infrastructures to sell them across much wider geographic distances. As with Holywell Street productions, Britons could order consulting surgeons' manuals directly from addresses listed in advertisements, pay for them with postage stamps, and have them delivered in a sealed envelope for a fee of one or two pence. By the late 1840s, readers in the British colonies had relatively easy access to many of these manuals, which were advertised in newspapers and almanacs in Canada, Australia, New Zealand, and India.[17] Colonial readers could pick up copies from local booksellers, or order them directly from London for a six-penny fee.

[14] James Graham, *A Lecture on the Generation, Increase, and Improvement of the Human Species* ([London]: Typis excusum Jac. Graemaei, c. 1783), 51. EPB/A/25278, WL. See Porter, *Health for Sale*, 161–163 for more on Graham's career.

[15] Samuel Solomon, *A Guide to Health, or, Advice to Both Sexes in a Variety of Complaints* [. . .]. (London: Printed for the author, c. 1797), WZ 260 S691g 1797, NLM; William Brodum, *A Guide to Old Age, or Cure for the Indiscretions of Youth*. 2 vols. (London: J. W. Meyers, 1797), WZ 260 B866g 1797, NLM. For pricing, see "A Guide to Health," *Hereford Journal*, March 21, 1798, 4; "Brodum's Guide to Old Age," *Hampshire Chronicle*, June 10, 1797, 3.

[16] To determine median prices and changing patterns in pricing over time, I compiled prices from advertisements published in the following newspapers in the years 1842, 1847, 1852, 1857, 1862, and 1867 using Gale's *British Library Newspapers 1800-1900* and *19th Century UK Periodicals* databases: *Aberdeen Journal*; *Bell's Life in London and Sporting Chronicle*; *Berkshire Chronicle*; *Cheshire Observer and General Advertiser*; *Daily Post (Liverpool)*; *Derbyshire Times and Chesterfield Herald*; *The Era*; *Freeman's Journal and Daily Commercial Advertiser*; *Liverpool Mercury*; *John Bull and Britannia*; *Morning Chronicle*; *Preston Guardian*; *Reynolds's Newspaper*; and *The Standard*. See Fissell, "Marketplace of Print," 111–114 for an analysis of prices for seventeenth- and eighteenth-century manuals of this type.

[17] For examples of colonial advertisements, see "St. Andrew's Library, Calcutta," *The Friend of India*, June 3, 1847, 352; "Curtis on Manhood," *The Bombay Almanack and Book of Direction for 1858* (Bombay: Bombay Gazette Press, 1858), n.p.; "Manhood: The Causes of Its Premature Decline," *The Courier*, December 15, 1849, 1; "The Silent Friend," *Portland Guardian and Norman by General Advertiser*, July 12, 1858, 4; "On Nervous and Generative Diseases," *Haszard's Gazette*, October 26, 1852, cover sheet.

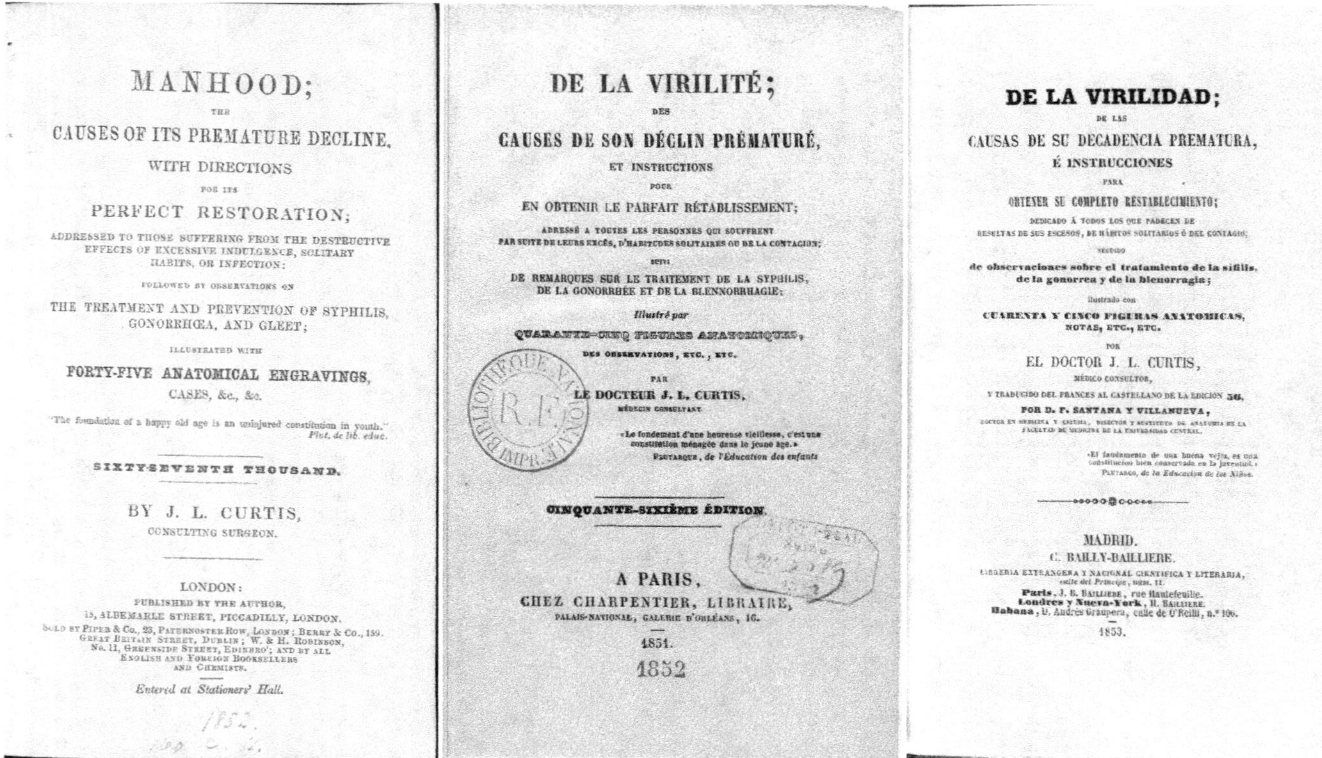

MANHOOD;
THE
CAUSES OF ITS PREMATURE DECLINE,
WITH DIRECTIONS
FOR ITS
PERFECT RESTORATION;
ADDRESSED TO THOSE SUFFERING FROM THE DESTRUCTIVE EFFECTS OF EXCESSIVE INDULGENCE, SOLITARY HABITS, OR INFECTION:
FOLLOWED BY OBSERVATIONS ON
THE TREATMENT AND PREVENTION OF SYPHILIS, GONORRHŒA, AND GLEET;
ILLUSTRATED WITH
FORTY-FIVE ANATOMICAL ENGRAVINGS,
CASES, &c., &c.

"The foundation of a happy old age is an uninjured constitution in youth."
Plut. de lib. educ.

SIXTY-SEVENTH THOUSAND.

BY J. L. CURTIS,
CONSULTING SURGEON.

LONDON:
PUBLISHED BY THE AUTHOR,
15, ALBEMARLE STREET, PICCADILLY, LONDON.
SOLD BY PIPER & CO., 23, PATERNOSTER ROW, LONDON; BERRY & CO., 159, GREAT BRITAIN STREET, DUBLIN; W. & H. ROBINSON, NO. 11, GREENSIDE STREET, EDINBRO'; AND BY ALL ENGLISH AND FOREIGN BOOKSELLERS AND CHEMISTS.

Entered at Stationers' Hall.

DE LA VIRILITÉ;
DES
CAUSES DE SON DÉCLIN PRÉMATURÉ,
ET INSTRUCTIONS
POUR
EN OBTENIR LE PARFAIT RÉTABLISSEMENT;
ADRESSÉ A TOUTES LES PERSONNES QUI SOUFFRENT PAR SUITE DE LEURS EXCÈS, D'HABITUDES SOLITAIRES OU DE LA CONTAGION;
SUIVI
DE REMARQUES SUR LE TRAITEMENT DE LA SYPHILIS, DE LA GONORRHÉE ET DE LA BLENNORRHAGIE;
Illustré par
QUARANTE-CINQ FIGURES ANATOMIQUES,
DES OBSERVATIONS, ETC., ETC.
PAR
LE DOCTEUR J. L. CURTIS,
MÉDECIN CONSULTANT

« Le fondement d'une heureuse vieillesse, c'est une constitution ménagée dans le jeune âge. »
PLUTARQUE, *de l'Éducation des enfants*

CINQUANTE-SIXIÈME ÉDITION.

A PARIS,
CHEZ CHARPENTIER, LIBRAIRE,
PALAIS-NATIONAL, GALERIE D'ORLÉANS, 16.
1851.
1852

DE LA VIRILIDAD;
DE LAS
CAUSAS DE SU DECADENCIA PREMATURA,
É INSTRUCCIONES
PARA
OBTENER SU COMPLETO RESTABLECIMIENTO;
DEDICADO Á TODOS LOS QUE PADECEN DE RESULTAS DE SUS ESCESOS, DE HÁBITOS SOLITARIOS Ó DEL CONTAGIO;
SEGUIDO
de observaciones sobre el tratamiento de la sifilis, de la gonorrea y de la blenorragia;
Ilustrado con
CUARENTA Y CINCO FIGURAS ANATOMICAS,
NOTAS, ETC., ETC.
POR
EL DOCTOR J. L. CURTIS,
MÉDICO CONSULTOR,
Y TRADUCIDO DEL FRANCES AL CASTELLANO DE LA EDICION 56,
POR D. F. SANTANA Y VILLANUEVA,
DOCTOR EN MEDICINA Y CIRUJIA, DISECTOR Y SUSTITUTO DE ANATOMIA EN LA FACULTAD DE MEDICINA DE LA UNIVERSIDAD CENTRAL.

« El fundamento de una buena vejez, es una constitucion bien conservada en la juventud. »
PLUTARCO, *de la Educacion de los Niños.*

MADRID.
C. BAILLY-BAILLIERE.
LIBRERIA ESTRANGERA Y NACIONAL CIENTIFICA Y LITERARIA, calle del Príncipe, núm. 11.
Paris, J. B. BAILLIERE, rue Hautefeuille.
Londres y Nueva-York, H. BAILLIERE.
Habana, D. Andres Graupera, calle de O'Reilli, n.° 106.
1853.

Figure 2.1 Title pages of three editions of J. L. Curtis, *Manhood. Manhood: The Causes of Its Premature Decline* [. . .]. (London: Published by the Authors, [1852]), *De la virilité; des causes de son déclin prématuré* [. . .]. (Paris: Charpentier, 1851), and *De la virilidad, de las causas de su decadencia prematura* [. . .]. (Madrid: C. Bailly-Bailliere,1853). Courtesy of The Bodleian Libraries, University of Oxford, (OC) 160 c.11, CC-BY-NC 4.0, The Bibliothèque Nationale de France, 617.463 (23e éd.), and the author's private collection.

A few consulting surgeons gained a truly global audience from the late 1840s by having their manuals translated into other languages (Figure 2.1).[18] Joseph Lambert's *Manhood* was translated into German, French, Spanish, Dutch, Danish, and Polish and issued in a variety of foreign countries by local publishers. Although the Danish and Polish translations appear to have been unauthorized, the rest were commissioned by Lambert himself. The Jordan family, owners of Perry & Co, the medical firm that issued one of *Manhood*'s chief competitors, *The Silent Friend* (1841), had the work translated into Italian and French and printed abroad under similar arrangements. Samuel La'Mert, Lambert's brother, had perhaps the widest international reach: he issued his manual *Self-Preservation* (1841) in German, Russian, French, Dutch, Italian, Spanish, and Portuguese.[19] Notices for these translations were extremely common in Europe, Latin America, and the Caribbean throughout the mid-nineteenth century. Readers in Barcelona, Rotterdam, Paris, and Torino, Rio de Janeiro, Lima, Caracas, and Havana saw advertisements for J. L. Curtis's *De la virilidad* and *Manbaarheid*, Perry & Co's *L'ami discret* and *L'amico discreto*, and Samuel La'Mert's *A preservação pessoal* in cheap books and local newspapers among notices for estate sales and employment announcements.[20] As in Britain and its colonies, foreign-language readers were instructed to purchase the manuals in person from local booksellers or to write to purchase them by post.

When they received their orders, what readers would have found in their hands was a small, slender book, usually bound in cheap cloth or paper boards, whose design strongly emphasized its intended audience: people with no medical education. Along with the binding, size, and weight of the volumes, the title pages of consulting surgeons' manuals set them apart from solid octavo tomes intended for medical practitioners. Hearkening to older print traditions, they featured lengthy subtitles that spelled out, in shifting sizes and styles of type, details about what was contained within that would now, in a book written for medical men, be left to the table of contents. Readers did not have to rely on bibliographical clues, however, to know that they were these manuals' target audience. They could simply scan the

[18] As with the English versions, these translations were published in many editions. For examples, see Appendix B.

[19] An unauthorized version of *Self-Preservation* was also issued in Danish in 1866. See Samuel La'Mert, *Fat Mod!*, in Appendix B.

[20] For examples of advertisements for translations, see "Manbaarheid," *Onze Tolk: Letterkundig Nieuwsblad*, August 20, 1872, 230; "L'ami discret," *La Patrie*, January 22, 1855, 4; "La Préservation Personnelle," *Jornal do Commercio*, March 21, 1861, 3; "Nova Edicio em Portuguez," *Jornal do Commercio*, October 10, 1862, 3; "De La Virilidad," *Comercio*, June 28, 1853, 1 ; "De La Virilidad," *Pasatiempo*, July 6, 1853, 8; "De La Verilidad," *Diario de la Marina*, August 10, 1853, 1; "La Preservación Personal," *Mercurio de Valparaiso*, August 1, 1872, 4; "Preservacion Personal," *Diario de Avisos, y Semanario de las Provincias*, October 24, 1855, 1.

subtitle. J. Jordan & Co's *Human Frailty* (1842) describes itself as "a popular medical work." I. A. Jacques & Co's *The Secret Preceptor* (1852) brands itself "a popular treatise." La'Mert's *Self-Preservation* calls itself "a popular inquiry."[21] This presentation was not meant to suggest a watered-down summary of medical facts but to imply democratized knowledge: that these manuals, as the introduction to Horace Goss's *Woman: Her Physiology and Functions* (1853) proclaims, enabled "readers who may be ignorant of the structure of the human body, to arrive at a clear and proper knowledge of the wonderful mechanism of man."[22]

Most of these manuals delivered on their promise to provide the uninitiated with a real medical education. The first fifty pages of *The Silent Friend* present readers with detailed information about how the parts of the body operate in tandem, like "that complex and delicate piece of machinery, a watch."[23] A series of engravings, furnished with labels identifying anatomical features, accompany the work's review of anatomy and physiology, which sets up two longer sections devoted to "derangement and impairment of [the] function and structure" of the human body: "Onanism and Its Consequences" and "Venereal and Syphilitic Diseases." The latter describes in detail how gonorrhoea and syphilis are contracted, what their symptoms are, and how they should be treated. Like the section on anatomy and physiology, this section is furnished with engravings. One brings together five images of the penis and testes, swollen, leaking, and marred with syphilitic sores. Another depicts chancres on the inner thighs and abdomen. Although many people probably perused these manuals out of sheer curiosity, marginalia suggests that they were used as a means of self-diagnosis: some readers customized them by annotating them with recipes for medicines to treat issues described in the text.[24]

Consulting surgeons' manuals thus offered people a means of understanding their bodies in modern, "scientific" ways, grounded in the study of anatomy,

[21] J. Jordan & Co, *Human Frailty: A Popular Work on the Awful Results Produced by the Dangerous Effects of an Inordinate Indulgence of the Passions, Youthful Imprudence and Infection* [. . .]. (London: Published by the Authors, 1842); I. A. Jacques & Co, *The Secret Preceptor; or, The Grandeur & Vigour of Man, Physically, Mentally, and Morally Vindicated, Illustrated & Displayed* [. . .]. (London: Published by the Authors, [1852]); Samuel La'Mert, *Self-Preservation: A Medical Treatise on the Secret Infirmities and Disorders of the Generative Organs, Resulting from Solitary Habits, Youthful Excess, or Infection* [. . .]. (London: Published by the Author, 1852).

[22] Horace Goss, *Woman: Her Physiology and Functions* [. . .]. (London: Published by the Author, 1853), v.

[23] R. and L. Perry & Co, *The Silent Friend: A Medical Work Treating of the Anatomy and Physiology of the Organs of Generation and Their Diseases* [. . .]. (London: R. and L. Perry & Co., 1847), 7.

[24] For instance, a recipe for a medicine containing copaiba balsam, an extract from a South American tree used to treat gonorrhoea, is dashed out on the last page of J. L. Curtis, *Mannheit: die Ursachen ihrer vorzeitigen Abnahme und Belehrungen über ihre vollständige Wiederherstellung* [. . .]. (Leipzig: Orthaus, 1851), Author's private collection.

that older popular works, such as *Aristotle's Masterpiece*, did not.[25] It is important to recognize, though, that these manuals enabled some people to understand their bodies better than they did others. Although it does cover female anatomy, physiology, and experiences of venereal disease, the focus of *The Silent Friend* is overwhelmingly male experience. Not one of its engravings depicts a female body. This was typical of the genre, which, like some of the works examined in the previous chapter, primarily addressed young men like Branwell Brontë: unmarried, equipped with a small amount of disposable income, and desperately in search of self-knowledge. At least two manuals for women were issued in Britain, however, and they provided comparably detailed information tailored to female concerns: R. J. Swaine & Co's *Geneseology, or, The Physiology of Woman* (1850) and Goss's richly illustrated *Woman*, which circulated in Britain for at least twenty-five years.[26] Each offers a compendium of information about the anatomy and physiology of the female body, pregnancy, miscarriage, labour and delivery, menstruation, venereal disease, injuries from childbirth, and fertility.

Like *The Silent Friend*, *Woman* invites readers to gaze in wonder at the marvellous mechanisms of the human body even as it tacitly acknowledges a range of practical reasons that a woman would seek out a book on reproductive health. Unlike male-oriented manuals, which tend to have few but lengthy chapters, *Woman* is organized as a reference book, with a series of short sections indicated in the table of contents. A reader who was trying to conceive could consult the manual's introductory "Observations on Generation," which describe the mechanics of coition and conception, and causes of infertility. A reader preparing for the birth her first child could thumb through to a series of engravings that illustrate the delivery of a baby and the placenta (Figure 2.2). A reader who had suffered a miscarriage – or was hoping to induce an abortion – could refer to a series of tables that describe the appearance of embryonic tissue at various stages of development. A reader who suspected that she had contracted a venereal disease could compare her own vulva with illustrations depicting the vulvas of diseased patients.

In addition to providing readers with medical information, consulting surgeons' manuals offered a moral lesson, one that was, again, mostly aimed at men.

[25] Burmeister, "Popular Anatomical," 135 makes a similar point about public anatomical museums, discussed below.

[26] R. J. Swaine & Co, *Geneseology, or, the Physiology of Woman: A Medical Work, Treating on the Structure and Uses of the Generative Organs in the Female* [. . .]. (London: Published and sold by the authors, 1850). Jah 03294, Thomas Fisher Rare Book Library, University of Toronto. A similar manual, whose title positioned it as a companion to *Manhood*, was published in the United States. See A. G. Hall, *Womanhood: Causes of Its Premature Decline, Respectfully Illustrated: Being a Review of the Changes and Derangements of the Female Constitution* [. . .]. (Rochester, NY: E. Shepard, 1845). 24.a.248, Frances A. Countway Library of Medicine, Harvard University.

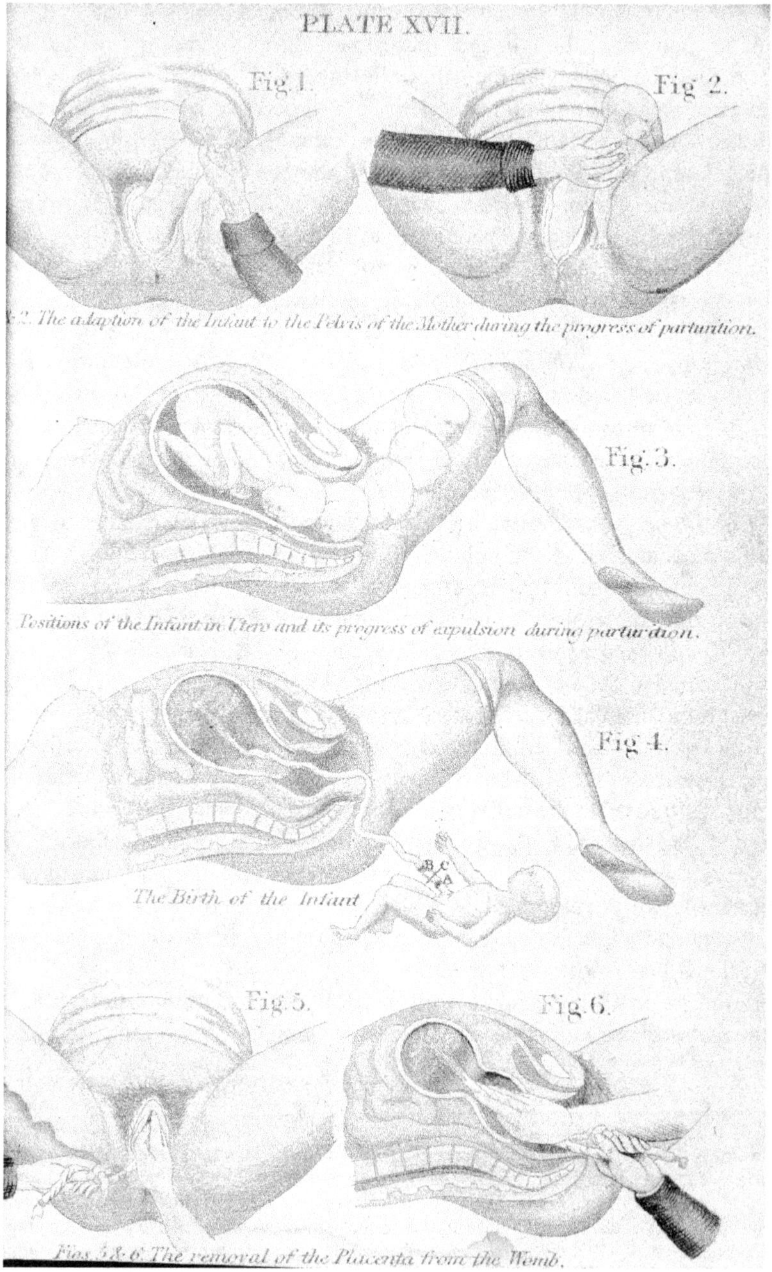

Figure 2.2 Plate 10, illustrating childbirth, in Horace Goss, *Woman: Her Physiology and Functions* (London: Published by the Authors, 1853), (OC) 160 c.66, Weston Library, Oxford. Courtesy of The Bodleian Libraries, University of Oxford, CC-BY-NC 4.0.

Women's sexual health problems are portrayed as beyond their control in manuals for both genders: their origins lie in the capricious nature the female body and the actions of careless, faithless men.[27] In men, the same health problems are depicted as the consequences of abject failures of self-control. Readers may have found *The Silent Friend*'s descriptions of anatomy and the symptoms of gonorrhoea and syphilis enlightening. If they read the work from cover to cover, however, they would have had to pass over lengthy descriptions of the suffering of men who failed to master their sexual urges, and lectures that decried the selfishness of those who brought venereal disease to the marriage bed:

> How degraded and utterly lost . . . must that man be, who, knowing himself to be tainted by disease, or so debilitated by early and guilty excesses, that it is next to impossible that he should give life to any but tainted and doomed progeny – doomed in the mother's womb! who yet dares to offer his polluted and shattered frame at the pure shrine of female love.[28]

While sex is framed as a self-affirming activity in many Holywell Street productions, in consulting surgeons' manuals sexual desire is collapsed with male weakness. Desire, as Ellen Rosenman has observed, produces flaccid, leaking male bodies; disordered, incontinent minds; disease-ravaged wives; deformed offspring; broken relationships; and shattered ambitions. In order preserve their manhood in every one of its senses, men must become masters of their desires, denying themselves pleasure even to the point of rationing marital intercourse.[29]

Medical journalists often deemed these works' descriptions of the perils of sexual indulgence "disgusting, demoralizing, [and] deceptive."[30] Yet, as historians have often pointed out, they trafficked the same ideas as works written for medical specialists. French treatises like Léopold Deslandes's *De l'onanisme et des autres abus veneriens* (1835) and Claude François Lallemand's *Des pertes séminales involontaires* (1836–44), and the English medical works that they inspired, alleged that even behaviour that did not spread venereal disease, such as masturbation, damaged men, feminizing them by weakening their bodies and reducing the "penis, symbol and site of virility . . . to a vulnerable, flaccid body part."[31] In fact, the relationship between these works and consulting surgeons' manuals was even more concrete. Consulting

27 Sally Shuttleworth observes the same representation of female health in advertisements for menstrual drugs in "Female Circulation: Medical Discourse and Popular Advertising in the Mid-Victorian Era," *Body/Politics: Women and the Discourses of Science*, ed. Mary Jacobus, Evelyn Fox Keller, and Sally Shuttleworth (New York: Routledge, 1989), 47–68.

28 *Silent Friend*, 1847, vii.

29 Ellen Bayuk Rosenman, *Unauthorized Pleasures: Accounts of Victorian Erotic Experience* (Ithaca, NY: Cornell University Press, 2003), 20, 18–27, 41–8.

30 "The Anatomy of Quackery," *Medical Circular and General Medical Advertiser*, October 12, 1853, 283.

31 Rosenman, *Unauthorized Pleasures*, 27. For more on these ideas in regular and irregular medical works, see Lesley A. Hall, "Forbidden by God, Despised by Men: Masturbation,

surgeons did not simply take ideas from other publications. They took their words. Works like *Manhood*, *The Silent Friend*, and *Woman* were not written so much as they were assembled. While Holywell Street publishers tended to revise and reframe existing works for new audiences, consulting surgeons habitually generated content out of them, tearing passages, paragraphs, and occasionally whole chapters out of multiple books, pamphlets, and articles to create productions of their own.

It can be difficult to determine exactly which sources the authors of these manuals used to create them because compilation was such a common method of composition at the time. The American practitioner Seth Pancoast's *Porneio-Kalogynomia-Pathology: Boyhood's Perils and Manhood's Curse* (1858) appears to borrow from *Kalogynomia, or The Laws of Female Beauty* (1821), the hybrid of medical description and erotic narrative examined in the previous chapter, for example, but it could theoretically have borrowed from some of *Kalogynomia*'s sources instead.[32] That said, much of the text in these manuals matches verbatim with writing in standard textbooks on anatomy, physiology, and surgery, such as Sir Astley Cooper's *Lectures on the Principles and Practice of Surgery* (1825). Books on sexual debility and venereal disease, including John Bacot's *A Treatise on Syphilis* (1829) and John Roberton's *On the Diseases of the Generative System* (1811), or translations of foreign works on these topics, including Deslandes's and Lallemand's treatises, also appear to have been common sources. Others include midwifery textbooks, anti-masturbation pamphlets like *Onania: or, The Heinous Sin of Self-Pollution* (c. 1712), works on the history and philosophy of marriage, including Michael Ryan's *Philosophy of Marriage* (1837), and works that had inspired the consulting surgeon's manual as a genre, such as Simeon Solomon's *Guide to Health*. Chunks of text in *Manhood*, ranging from paragraphs to pages, match material in most of the works I have named.[33] *Woman*'s content seems to have been derived from

Medical Warnings, Moral Panic, and Manhood in Great Britain, 1850–1950," *Journal of the History of Sexuality* 2, no. 3 (1992): 365–387; Elizabeth Stephens, "Pathologizing Leaky Male Bodies: Spermatorrhea in Nineteenth-Century British Medicine and Popular Anatomy Museums," *Journal of the History of Sexuality* 17, no. 3 (2008): 421–438; Shuttleworth, "Female Circulation," 51–64.

32 S. Pancoast, *Porneio-Kalogynomia-Pathology: Boyhood's Perils and Manhood's Curse* [. . .]. (Philadelphia: s.n., 1858), WJA P188o 1858, NLM.

33 Compare J. L. Curtis, *Manhood: The Causes of Its Premature Decline, with Directions for Its Perfect Restoration* [. . .]. (London: Published by the Author, 1852), 8–10 with *Onania: or, The Heinous Sin of Self Pollution*, 4th ed. (London: Printed for the Author, 1725), 10, 13, 186, 5, 8; *Manhood*, 37–39 with T. M. Caton, *A Practical Treatise on the Prevention and Cure of the Venereal Disease* (London: Samuel Highley, 1809), 114–117; *Manhood*, 11, with John Roberton, *On the Generative System*, 4th ed. (London: J. J. Stockdale, 1817), 77; *Manhood*, 86–87, with John Bacot, "A Treatise on Syphilis," reprinted in William Atkinson, *Popery Unmasked and Her Supporters Exposed* (Leeds: T. Inchbold, 1829), 123–125; *Manhood*, 25–26 with Astley Cooper, *Lectures on the Principles and Practice of Surgery*,

textbooks for medical students and encyclopedia entries on midwifery, embryology, and anatomy.[34]

That these works are compilations would not necessarily be obvious to a casual reader. Consulting surgeons combined parts of other publications skilfully. They often expanded excerpted text with writing of their own, modernized the language of excerpts from old books and pamphlets, made excerpts from specialized textbooks and treatises more accessible by omitting, paraphrasing, or explaining technical terms, and changed the implied audience where necessary. For instance, while Sir William Lawrence instructs surgeons how to relieve painful symptoms of gonorrhoea in his *Lectures on Surgery* (1830):

> In the first place, you may get a basin of cold water, and let the patient, with a sponge or piece of lint, bathe the part so as to cool it as much as possible. Then you press gently upon the swollen glans with the thumb, or thumb and finger of one hand, while you gradually draw over it the contracted orifice of the prepuce with the thumb and finger of the other hand. If you proceed slowly, squeezing out the blood from the glans as well as you can, so as to reduce its size, then managing to push it gradually into the opening of the orifice, at the same time that you draw the prepuce gently forward, you will usually succeed in replacing the parts, and thus relieve the patient from a state which to him is one of considerable alarm and apprehension, besides being very painful.[35]

Manhood explains the procedure to prospective patients:

> What we would advise in this case is, to get a basin of cold water, and let the patient, with a spunge or piece of lint, bathe the part so as to cool it. Then the surgeon is to press gently with the thumb the swollen glans, or with the thumb and finger of one hand, whilst he gradually draws over it the contracted orifice of the prepuce with the thumb and finger of the other. He is to proceed slowly, squeezing out the blood from the glans, as well as he

2nd ed. (London: F. C. Westley, 1830), 469–470; *Manhood*, 78–83, with William Lawrence, *Lectures on Surgery, Medical and Operative* [. . .]. (London: F. C. Westly, 1830), 365–370; *Manhood*, 25–26 with Wooster Beach, *The American Practice of Medicine*, 2nd ed. (New York: Kelley & La Tourette, 1836), 374; *Manhood*, 8, 11, 37 with Michael Ryan, *The Philosophy of Marriage* (London: John Churchill, 1837), 64, 18, 26; *Manhood*, 53, with Francis Burdett Courtenay, *Practical Essays on the Debilities of the Generative System* (London: T. Hill, 1839), 43; *Manhood*, 77, 85, 89–91 with Langston Parker, *The Modern Treatment of Syphilitic Diseases* (London: John Churchill, 1839), 32, 51, 52–55; *Manhood*, 54, 61–62, 73 with François Lallemand, *A Practical Treatise on the Causes, Symptoms and Treatment of Spermatorrhœa*, 2nd ed., trans. Henry J. McDougall (London: John Churchill, 1851), 344, 354–355, xiii; and *Manhood*, 21, 45–51, with Richard Dawson, *An Essay on Marriage; Being a Microscopic Investigation into Its Physiological and Physical Relations* [. . .]. (London: Hugh Hughes, 1848), 39, 5–6 and 58–63.

[34] For examples, compare Goss, *Woman*, 1 with John Mason Good, *The Study of Medicine*, 3rd rev. ed., vol. 4. (London: Thomas and George Underwood, 1829), 3; *Woman*, 8, 14, 29 with Andrew Fyfe, *A Compendium of the Anatomy of the Human Body: Intended Principally for the Use of Students*, vol. II (Edinburgh: Pillan and Sons, 1810), 189, 281, 293; *Woman*, 34 with "Abortion," *Encyclopædia Brittanica: or, A Dictionary of Arts, Sciences, and Miscellaneous Literature*, 5th ed. (Edinburgh: Printed at the Encyclopaedical Press, 1817), 37.

[35] Lawrence, *Lectures on Surgery*, 370.

can, so as to reduce its size, then managing to push it gradually into the opening of the orifice, at the same time that he draws the prepuce gently forward, and he will then succeed in replacing the parts, and in relieving the patient from a very distressing and painful situation.[36]

Even so, it is possible to read consulting surgeons' manuals less as original productions than as showcases: their authors gathered information and perspectives from a variety of works and framed them so that they spoke in new ways to new audiences.[37]

Indeed, the consulting surgeon's manual arguably functioned as the paper equivalent of the public anatomical museum, another popular Victorian source of sexual knowledge.[38] Emerging in Europe in the eighteenth century, these urban attractions were inspired by collections of models and specimens used for training in medical schools. Entry to medical school collections was usually restricted to students, lecturers, and governors. However, anyone could enter a public anatomical museum for a shilling during daytime hours, or half a shilling between five and ten o'clock in the evening, a convention introduced in the 1830s to encourage working-class attendance.[39] Just as consulting surgeons did in the first pages of their manuals, the owners of Victorian public anatomical museums drew on the rhetoric of public education and working-class uplift to frame them as venues that provided ordinary people with vital knowledge, grounded in the science of anatomy, that enabled them to understand their bodies in revelatory ways. "Know Thyself!" was a constant refrain in advertising material for these destinations.[40]

The kinds of knowledge that people gleaned from the manuals and the museums roughly matched up too. Just as readers of *The Silent Friend* were treated to a detailed lesson in anatomy, visitors to Rackstrow's Museum in London, one of the city's first public anatomical museums, were urged to gaze at specimens of skulls and brains, wax models of the nervous and respiratory systems, and a full-body "anatomical Venus" outfitted with glass vessels filled

[36] *Manhood* (1852), 84.

[37] My phrasing is inspired by Mary Thomas Crane, *Framing Authority: Sayings, Self, and Society in Sixteenth-Century England* (Princeton, NJ: Princeton University Press, 1993), 92, which describes an early modern conception of writing centred on "gathering and framing" traditional materials.

[38] The comparison I make here builds on Burmeister's observations in "Popular Anatomical," 179–208. For further information about public anatomical museums in Britain, see Samuel Alberti, *Morbid Curiosities: Medical Museums in Nineteenth-Century Britain* (Oxford: Oxford University Press, 2011); Carin Berkowitz, "The Beauty of Anatomy: Visual Displays and Surgical Education in Early-Nineteenth-Century London," *Bulletin of the History of Medicine* 85, no. 2 (2011): 248–278; Elizabeth Hallam, *The Anatomy Museum: Death and the Body Displayed* (London: Reaktion, 2008); Elizabeth Stephens, *Anatomy as Spectacle: Public Exhibitions of the Body from 1700 to the Present* (Liverpool: Liverpool University Press, 2011).

[39] Burmeister, "Popular Anatomical," 106.

[40] Burmeister, "Popular Anatomical," 93–120.

with a fluid that looked like blood.[41] But getting to know oneself also entailed getting to know the reproductive self in isolation. Displays of embryos in various stages of development, models of pregnant women, and exhibits devoted to illustrating the effects of venereal disease were routine features of these museums. Some historians have argued that like illustrations in consulting surgeons' manuals, these exhibits taught visitors how to check their bodies for signs of disease, though museum owners (again, like consulting surgeons) typically framed them as lessons in the benefits of chastity.[42]

Public anatomical museums and consulting surgeons' manuals were also alike in that they both repurposed tools initially created for medical students. As glass jars containing preparations multiplied in medical school collections, duplicates were deaccessioned and sold off at auction, where they were bought up by museum owners and put on public display. After the passage of the 1832 Anatomy Act made cadavers easier for medical schools to come by, wax and plaster models previously used for instruction were also sold off in large numbers. While it is sometimes suggested that museum owners displayed models depicting venereal disease solely to titillate or horrify, Maritha Burmeister has theorized that they initially became common in public anatomical museums because they were plentiful in the second-hand market.[43] Rendered in wax, models of venereal disease were considered excellent teaching tools: evidence of disease on the skin could be observed in models in ways that were impossible when working with illustrations and even with patients.[44] Old models regularly made their way to auction as more up-to-date models were introduced.

Education went hand in hand with entertainment more explicitly in public anatomical museums, however, than it did in consulting surgeons' manuals. Early nineteenth-century public anatomical museums had more in common with *Wunderkammers* than teaching collections: they displayed models and specimens of human body parts alongside replicas of Greek statues, stuffed exotic animals, and Egyptian mummies.[45] From the 1830s, as they aligned themselves with public education movements, they became more self-consciously "scientific." Victorian anatomical museum owners often declared that their displays sought "not to gratify a prurient curiosity, but to present the scientific observer with a general and correct view of the perfect and wonderful structure of the body."[46] Even so, they catered to fascination with sexual and racial difference. Joseph Kahn's Anatomical and Pathological Museum in

[41] Rackstrow's Museum, *A Brief Description of Those Curious and Excellent Figures of the Human Anatomy in Wax* (London: s.n., c. 1790), DRT Digital Store 7423.cc.6, BL; Alberti, *Morbid Curiosities*, 148.

[42] Alberti, *Morbid Curiosities*, 199.

[43] Burmeister, "Popular Anatomical," 78.

[44] Alberti, *Morbid Curiosities*, 152.

[45] Burmeister, "Popular Anatomical," 36.

[46] Quoted in Burmeister, "Popular Anatomical," 60.

London, one of the largest in the metropolis, exploited Britons' lingering memories of Saartjie Baartman, the Khoikhoi woman known for her buttocks and genitals who had been displayed in London in 1810 under the name Hottentot Venus. Kahn displayed Baartman's likeness in an ethnological exhibit called the Gallery of All Nations alongside wax models of various racial "types" and exhibited the "enormous" labia of other Khoikhoi women in glass jars alongside the preserved genitals of European men and women, bringing the unsavoury conclusion of *The Lustful Turk* to life.[47]

In some cases, museum owners created displays that straddled the line between fact and fiction in the interest of attracting visitors. One of Kahn's displays, introduced in 1855, depicted the "Niam-Niams of Central Africa," a people supposedly burdened with an "elongation of the vertebral column" which resembled a tail. An image of the wax display in a pamphlet issued to promote it depicts a nude family. The father and child expose their buttocks, revealing a short, tail-like appendage. The mother reclines. Her hand covers her vulva, but her chest is thrust towards the viewer, displaying her breasts. Extrapolating on common colonialist depictions of indigenous Africans as "wild" and "savage," the text accompanying the image portrays all of the family members as "lower animals" with primitive instincts and base appetites.[48] Of course, such creatures did not exist. Indeed, Kahn's pamphlet includes extracts from the *Lancet* that dismiss reports on which the display was based as "Oriental fantasy."[49] Despite his claim that his displays were not "exaggerated in the slightest degree," however, Kahn promoted the myth on the basis that it was possible that men with tails existed. In Kahn's telling, this justified displaying models of fictive people alongside real wonders of the human body, blending medical fact and imperialist fantasy.[50]

Until the mid-1850s, regular medical practitioners also treated consulting surgeons' manuals and public anatomical museums very differently. Prominent organs of the medical profession attacked the former as "disgusting" and "deceptive" even as they spoke of the latter approvingly, opining that making the science of anatomy known to members of the public could only increase their confidence in medical expertise. The *Lancet* praised Kahn's Museum when it opened in 1851, deeming its anatomical and ethnological models "very beautiful" and its guides well-informed.[51] Public anatomical museums soon became

47 See *Catalogue of Dr. Kahn's Anatomical Museum* ([London]: Printed by J. Golbourn, [1851]), 27. 7305.de.9.(9.), BL and *Catalogue of Dr. Kahn's Anatomical and Pathological Museum* ([London]: Printed by J. Golbourn, [1853]), 26, 49. For an analysis of Baartman's story and its afterlives, see Sadiah Qureshi, "Displaying Sara Baartman, the 'Hottentot Venus,'" *History of Science* 42, no. 2 (2004): 233–257.

48 *Men with Tails: Remarks on the Niam-Niams of Central Africa; Comprising an Introduction, by Dr. Kahn* [. . .]. (London: W. J. Colbourn, 1855), [16], a49361, RCS.

49 *Men with Tails*, 10. 50 *Men with Tails*, 2.

51 "Dr. Kahn's Museum," *Lancet*, August 13, 1853, 156.

subject to medical opposition, however, and the *Lancet* reversed its opinion. This may be partly because some museum owners introduced audacious displays like the Niam-Niam exhibit to attract visitors, representing them as science. However, several historians have argued that rising medical opposition to these museums had more to do with the fact that museum owners were adopting the practices of, or forging partnerships with, consulting surgeons, shifting from being mere displayers of medical knowledge to claimants to practical medical expertise.[52]

According to Burmeister, the history of Kahn's Museum offers a good sense of how and why owners of public anatomical museums and authors of their paper equivalents merged in the 1850s. Although his museum was a critical success, Kahn found it difficult to turn a profit from ticket sales alone. As he sought to make his business more profitable, he not only introduced more sensational displays but also began to offer medical services. In 1855, the same year in which he opened the Niam-Niam exhibit, Kahn began to advertise his availability for private consultations for sexual health problems illustrated in his displays, and hand out museum guides that included extracts from a one-shilling pamphlet on "obstacles to a happy union" called *The Philosophy of Marriage* which promoted him as an expert in their treatment. Unfortunately, no copy of the pamphlet survives today.[53] However, the extracts suggest that *Marriage* was heavily inspired by, and consequently very similar to, most consulting surgeons' manuals, down to the origins of its text in longer, more technical medical and scientific works.[54]

Even as he imitated consulting surgeons, Kahn charged them with pretended expertise. He was an especially vocal critic of Perry & Co, publishers of *The Silent Friend*. The company's owners, the Jordan family, recognized public anatomical museums' potential to attract customers, however, and found a diplomatic solution to their problem. The Jordans purchased anatomical models from Kahn to display in their consulting rooms, and then persuaded him to bring them into his business as silent partners.[55] The museum quickly became a vehicle for promoting the Jordans' business. Attendants began to distribute copies of *The Shaols and Quicksands of Youth* (1856),

52 Alan W. Bates, "Dr Kahn's Museum: Obscene Anatomy in Victorian London." *Journal of the Royal Society of Medicine* 99, no. 12 (2006): 618–624; Burmeister, "Popular Anatomical," 21; Stephens, "Pathologizing," 432–435.

53 The British Library lists a copy of Kahn's *Philosophy of Marriage* in its catalogue, but it is marked as destroyed. According to Kahn, it was translated into four languages by 1860. See "The Philosophy of Marriage," *John Bull*, December 29, 1860, 15. However, I have not been able to locate any foreign editions of Kahn's *Marriage*, or any advertisements for them.

54 For instance, compare "Extracts from the Forty-Seventh Edition of Dr. Kahn's Treatise on the Philosophy of Marriage" in *Handbook of Dr. Kahn's Museum* ([London]: Printed by W. Snell: 1863), M9498, WL, 101 with Gideon Anderson, *Thoughts on Animalcules; or, a Glimpse of the World Revealed by the Microscope* (London: John Murray, 1846), 11.

55 See Burmeister, "Popular Anatomical," 195 for further details about Kahn's partnership with the Jordans.

a version of *The Silent Friend* presented as Kahn's work, to visitors, which directed readers to seek out a range of products and services that the Jordans offered under Kahn's name. The partnership inspired many imitators.[56] Aligned with consulting surgeons and their manuals, public anatomical museums became full-service destinations through which Victorians could acquire sexual knowledge through the actions of viewing, listening, speaking, and reading.

Copies of Copies

Consulting surgeons framed their manuals as democratic productions that made vital knowledge accessible to any literate person. It is crucial to recognize that they functioned in this way for many readers. However, as the fact that Kahn only began to sell them when he had a medical practice to promote emphasizes, their major function for their authors was self-promotion. Exploring how this function shaped the consulting surgeon's manual can expand our understanding of the cultural implications of this strand of the trade in sexual knowledge and unpack its implications for other medics. Here, I wish to make two points. First, the techniques that consulting surgeons used to work up manuals that could persuade readers of their expertise led to a striking sameness in the ways they represented the body and sexuality: they blanketed Britain, and indeed the globe, with uncannily similar portrayals. Second consulting surgeons' treatment of medical knowledge in print undermined its authority in the eyes of other practitioners, and implicated all medical works as potential fronts for self-promotion.

That the consulting surgeon's manual was essentially a form of content marketing was not a secret. All of these manuals draw attention to their authors' availability for consultations to diagnose health problems in person or by letter – sometimes in several different languages – in advertisements appended to the text, within the text itself, in footnotes, or in all of these places at once.[57] Many manuals also recommend, and often incorporate stand-alone advertisements for, proprietary ointments, lotions, pills, balms, and tinctures to prevent or cure the same health problems. Like the manual itself, these products could be purchased by post or in person, at their authors' consulting rooms, through chemists, druggists, booksellers, and newspaper offices scattered across Britain

[56] Richard Daniel Altick, *The Shows of London* (Cambridge, MA: Harvard University Press, 1978), 341–342; Burmeister, "Popular Anatomical," 195–196.

[57] For instance, J. L. Curtis, *De la virilidad: de las causas de su decadencia prematura é instrucciones para obtener su completo restablecimiento* [. . .]. (Madrid: C. Bailly-Baillière, 1853) includes several pages of instructions for purchasing medicines or consultations by letter from London, aimed at Spanish-speaking patients located in France, Belgium, the German lands, Spain, Portugal, India, the West Indies, Mexico, and North and South America.

and, in some cases, at bookshops and newspaper-offices located in other countries.[58] In contrast to the manuals, these products and services were expensive and probably only sought out by a fraction of the manuals' readers. A guinea – the standard fee for a visit from an authoritative physician, a lesson from one of London's better violin teachers, or a year's subscription to a circulating library – was the going rate for a consultation.[59]

A course of medicine could cost far more. The Cordial Balm of Syriacum, a treatment for "weakness, debility, deficiency of natural strength, and relaxation of the vessels" sold by the authors of *The Silent Friend*, cost eleven shillings per bottle.[60] Their Preventive Lotion, which allegedly removed "all danger from [the] indiscriminate sexual intercourse" that they sternly instructed readers to avoid, cost thirty-three shillings per bottle, or five pounds for a case of six.[61] Thankfully, financial ruin appears to have been the worst consequence of using these medicines, something that cannot be said of many regular treatments for venereal disease, which could contain mercury, arsenic, or sulphur.[62] According to one chemical analyst, the Cordial Balm of Syriacum contained "weak spirits, sweetened with moist sugar, and flavoured with aniseed, spearmint, benzoin, and tolu, with the addition, probably, of some tincture of cantharides," blistering extracts from the beetle *Lytta vesicatoria* commonly used to treat venereal disease. The Preventive Lotion was "a solution of zinc, coloured with a vegetable dye."[63]

Other aspects of consulting surgeons' manuals functioned as promotional devices in more subtle ways. From the surgeon's point of view, for instance, a major purpose of manual's main text, tables, and illustrations was to cultivate trust in his expertise, giving the impression of a practitioner with an enormous breadth of learning and experience. Consulting surgeons reinforced this impression by employing paratextual devices that aligned them with elite medicine. Many published under aliases derived from the names of eminent medical practitioners, such as Perry, Cooper, and Brodie.[64] They also claimed

58 For example, see the lengthy list of suppliers at the end of *Silent Friend* (1847).

59 Anne Digby, *Making a Medical Living: Doctors and Patients in the English Market for Medicine, 1720–1911* (Cambridge: Cambridge University Press, 1994), 186; David J. Golby, *Instrumental Teaching in Nineteenth-Century Britain* (London: Routledge, 2017), 97; Simon Eliot, "Books and Their Readers: Part I," in *The Nineteenth-Century Novel: Realisms*, ed. Delia da Sousa Correa (London: Routledge, 2000), 23. Foreign-language editions of consulting surgeons' manuals often list equivalent prices in foreign currency.

60 "The Anatomy of Quackery," *Medical Circular and General Medical Advertiser*, September 14, 1853, 204.

61 *The Silent Friend* (1847), 116, 168.

62 See Anne R. Hanley, *Medicine, Knowledge, and Venereal Diseases in England, 1886–1916* (Basingstoke: Palgrave Macmillan, 2016) for further information about treatments for venereal disease.

63 "The Anatomy of Quackery," *Medical Circular and General Medical Advertiser*, October 12, 1853, 284–285.

64 Courtenay, *Revelations*, 79.

to be members of elite medical institutions, such as the Royal College of Surgeons of England, on the title pages of their manuals, or told readers that they consulted in famous hospitals. Not all of these claims were false. The Jordans merely had to emphasize the genuine qualifications of one of their own, Robert Jacob Jordan, to associate themselves with elite medicine, telling readers of *The Silent Friend* that they had "confided their prescriptions to a Physician of the Royal University of Erlangen, and Member of the Royal College of Surgeons of England."[65]

Other features of these manuals aimed to persuade readers to avail themselves of the expertise that they saw displayed on the page. Medical journalists often suggested that their searing accounts of suffering were engineered to send readers into a frenzy, inspiring panicked purchases of patent medicines or hurried arrangements for consultations. Journalists considered detailed descriptions of spermatorrhoea, a disease thought to result from the excessive discharge of sperm whose symptoms were supposed to include "anxiety, nervousness, lassitude, impotence, and, in its advanced stages, insanity and death," especially effective for this purpose because spermatorrhoea's symptoms were easily brought on by hypochondria.[66] Tales of the devastating effects of scanning these manuals were rife in the medical press. Before perusing a consulting surgeon's manual, one story went, a young man "never had any idea that men were liable to such a malady," but after reading it, "he began to fancy that he might, perhaps, unknowingly, labour under the disease." He visited its author and was informed, of course, that his "urine was loaded with semen." A fee-book for treatment was produced, and the hapless man was persuaded to part with a hundred guineas for a cure he did not require.[67]

The manuals' vivid descriptions of decline may well have had this effect. However, it is doubtful that they would have been effective had consulting surgeons not also worked to demonstrate that they were sympathetic to their readers' problems, and that they recognized the need for delicacy and discretion in treating them. As a rule, consulting surgeons' manuals assure readers that the details of medical consultations, and even the fact that a consultation has taken place, will be kept strictly confidential. "I am enabled to afford relief without even knowing the residences of the parties who receive it at my hands," a typical note on discretion claims. "Inviolable secrecy, and certain relief, are the boons, then, that I offer to suffering humanity."[68] Goss's *Woman* repeatedly addresses concerns about privacy specific to women. For instance, the author

[65] "The Silent Friend," *Elgin Courant, and Morayshire Advertiser*, July 22, 1859, 2.

[66] Rosenman, *Unauthorized Pleasures*, 32.

[67] Francis Burdett Courtenay, *Revelations of Quacks and Quackery: A Series of Letters by "Detector,"* 3rd ed. (London: Baillière, Tindall & Cox, 1865), 88–89.

[68] Samuel La'Mert, *Self-Preservation: A Medical Treatise on the Secret Infirmities and Disorders of the Generative Organs* [. . .]. (London: Published by the Author, 1852), 99–100.

emphasizes that those seeking expert treatment would not have to be examined by, or forced to relay personal details to, a male medical practitioner. Prospective patients could choose to consult Goss's wife, a "Consulting-Accoucheuse" who had the "discretion of a lady" and expertise equal to her husband.[69] Should readers find it difficult to imagine writing or speaking to a consultant of any gender about embarrassing health problems, they could turn to the manual for help. Most manuals offer detailed descriptions of the kind of information that should be included in a letter to the author, and some even tell readers how to structure one. Should readers remain uncertain, they could model their letters on the "cases" that fill the back pages of many consulting surgeons' manuals: anonymized letters or rewritings of letters allegedly posted to the authors from clients which testified to their skills and experience.

While it was framed as – and functioned for many people as – an informational genre, the consulting surgeon's manual was thus overwhelmingly oriented around cultivating trust in a *particular* consulting surgeon or firm of surgeons, and persuading readers to avail themselves of their services. Everything about it aimed to convey a very individualized impression of the author(s) and their expertise. And yet, as the ease with which I am generalizing suggests, these manuals were extraordinarily alike. They were not just put together using the same methods. Nor did they simply hew to a predictable set of generic conventions. They also drew on very similar, and frequently the same, materials. The images of flaccid penises and swollen testes, syphilitic chancres and drooling onanists that appear in these works are interchangeable, and, as the examples in Figure 2.3 suggest, are often different copies of the same illustrations.

The same is true of the manuals' textual content. Although most of the text in consulting surgeons' manuals originated in works in other genres, the manuals share enormous amounts of that text with each other. The 1852 edition of *Manhood* and the 1844 edition of *Brodie's Medical Work on Virility* alone share over 4,000 words of verbatim text, or about ten percent of the text of each manual. The 1852 edition of *Manhood* also shares substantial amounts of verbatim text with *The Silent Friend*, *Self-Preservation*, extracts from Kahn's *Philosophy of Marriage*, C. J. Lucas and Co's *Manly Vigour* (1841), *The Secret Preceptor* (1852), Walter de Roos's *Silent Hints on Certain Subjects* (1852), Henry Smith's *The Warning Voice, or Private Medical Friend* (1860), and L. J. Kahn's *Nervous Exhaustion: Its Cause and Cure* (1870); and these works share substantial amounts of verbatim text with each other that do not appear in *Manhood*. In addition to copying from other sources, consulting surgeons copied from their prior publications and from each other when they created their

[69] Goss, *Woman*, 70.

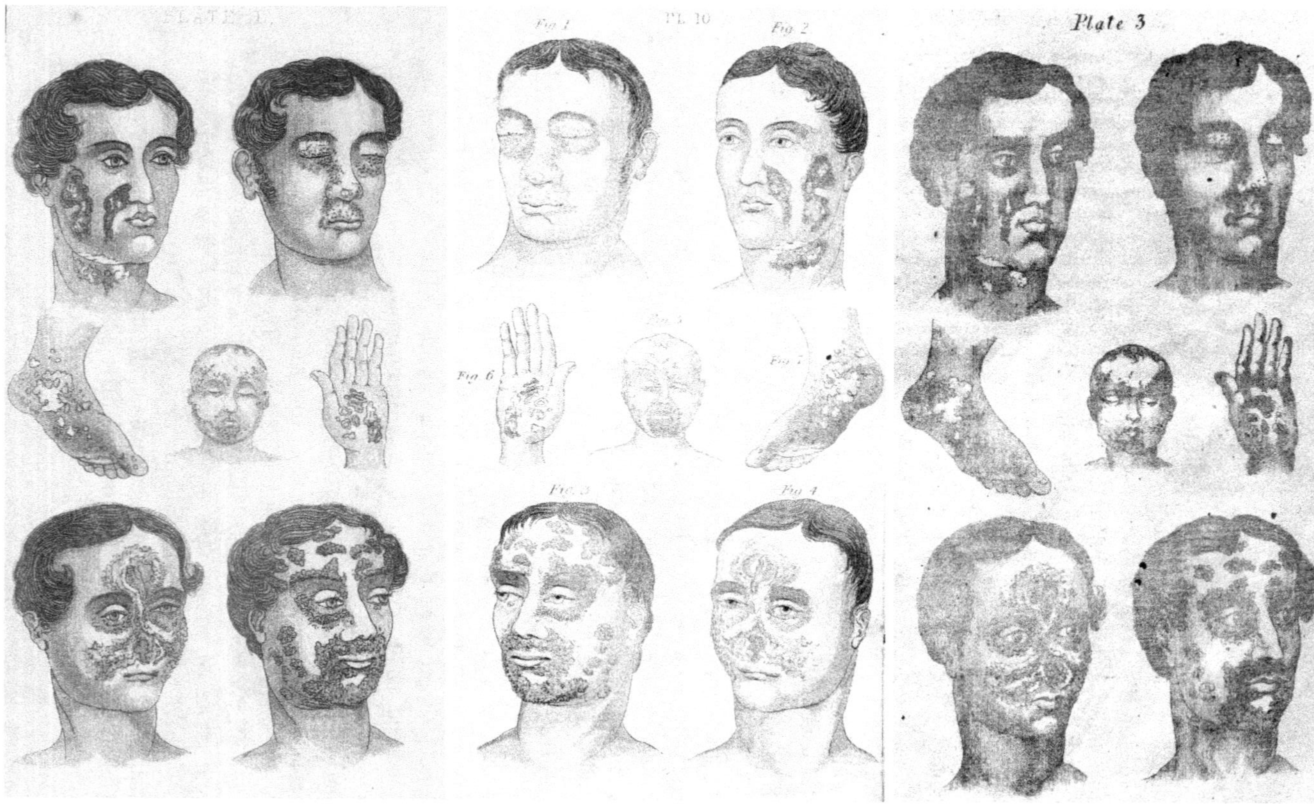

Figure 2.3 Different copies of the same illustration. Plate 1 in I. A. Jacques, *The Secret Preceptor* (Newcastle on Tyne: Published by the Authors, [1852]), Plate 10 in Samuel La'Mert, *Self-Preservation* (London: Published by the Author, 1852), and Plate 3 in John A. Lewis, *Controul of the Passions* ([Liverpool?]: Published by the authors, [1854]). By courtesy of the Bodleian Libraries, University of Oxford, (OC) 160 c.31 and (OC) 160 c.37, and The University of Liverpool Library, SPEC 2017.a.023.

manuals, and also when they issued new, expanded editions.[70] As a result, the descriptions of anatomy, venereal disease, and sexual debility that appear in these works frequently overlap verbatim. So, too, does the text of cases, of advertisements for proprietary medicines, of instructions for how to write to the author, and of anecdotes from medical practice: features of these manuals that were supposed to be specific to the author. The specificity of the consulting surgeon's manual was a total fiction.

That these manuals promoted the same views of the body and sexuality and that they circulated so widely and for so long have some compelling implications for the history of sexual knowledge. Holywell Street publishers' catalogues attest to great variety in the kinds of knowledge available in the Victorian print marketplace. Such publishers' scavenging fostered diverse lists that incorporated models of the body and sexuality from different times, places, and perspectives. Consulting surgeons' manuals demonstrate that roughly the same principles of composition could have the effect of standardizing and amplifying a single perspective. Regardless of whether the author was Perry & Co, Curtis & Co, or Joseph Kahn, these manuals spread the same view of sexuality as inherently white, male, and weak around and around. The same descriptions of drooling onanists and oozing penises filled colonial spaces at a time when indigenous people's literatures on sexuality were being erased; European centres from Stockholm to Madrid; and cities across the United States, where local practitioners copied British manuals and claimed them as their own. Although most of these manuals were first published in the 1840s and 1850s, many reached later generations of readers as a result of continuous repackaging by their creators and by other agents: versions of the most successful consulting surgeons' manuals were advertised around the world into the early twentieth century.[71]

[70] This can be discerned by tracking text overlaps in various editions of consulting surgeons' manuals and how they changed over time. For example, the 1840 edition of *Manhood* contains a paragraph that seems to have originated in *Onania: or, The Heinous Sin of Self-Pollution*. The 1847 edition of *The Silent Friend* contains the exact same paragraph. In *The Silent Friend*, the author followed this paragraph with a paragraph that matches one in John Roberton's *On the Generative System* (1811), which does not appear in the 1840 edition of *Manhood*. The 1852 edition of *Manhood*, however, reproduces the exact same 950-word, two-paragraph block of text containing material from both *Onania* and *Generative System*. Compare *Onania: or, The Heinous Sin of Self-Pollution* (London: C. Corbett, 1752), 186–187; *Manhood* (1840), 5–8; *Silent Friend* (1847), 63–68; Roberton, *Generative System* (1817), 77; *Manhood* (1852), 10–11.

[71] On the sanitization, erasure, and transformation of indigenous sexual knowledges in the British colonies, see Anjali Arondekar, *For the Record: On Sexuality and the Colonial Archive in India* (Durham, NC: Duke University Press, 2009); Deana Heath, *Purifying Empire: Obscenity and the Politics of Moral Regulation in Britain, India and Australia*. (Cambridge: Cambridge University Press, 2010). For examples of foreign English editions and reworkings of British consulting surgeons' manuals, see Léopold Deslandes, *Manhood: The Causes of Its Premature Decline: With Directions for Its Perfect Restoration* (Boston: Otis, Broaders, 1842), S.65,

The scale at which some of these manuals were produced only strengthened this effect. Consulting surgeons' claims about sales – Joseph Kahn bragged that he had sold a million copies of *The Philosophy of Marriage* by 1872, and others reported similar figures – are hard to trust since they appear in advertising material.[72] Court records suggest, however, that the most successful manuals were distributed in the tens and even hundreds of thousands in Britain, giving them a circulation comparable with many hymnals and primers.[73] When the proprietors of Kahn's Museum were prosecuted for distributing obscene material in 1873, an episode covered in Chapter 5, Joseph Smale, a printer working out of Hale Street, Southwark, testified that between 1866 and 1872 alone he issued 43,250 copies of *The Philosophy of Marriage* for Kahn's museum, and 30,000 copies of another work (probably *The Shaols and Quicksands of Youth*) on a similar topic.[74] These numbers reflect local production by a single printer over six years. Editions of *Manhood* and *Self-Preservation* were issued for decades by many agents in a number of different countries, in several different languages.

In these contexts, it does not seem surprising that in the 1920s and 1930s, long after doctors had stopped believing that masturbation ruined men's health, many of the older men who wrote to sex education campaigners like Marie Stopes worried that they had destroyed their bodies by indulging in it.[75] That these views lived on cannot entirely be attributed to manuals like *Manhood*, of course. Old medical ideas enjoyed extended lives, especially in rural and working-class communities where people gained much of their information about sex and reproduction through oral tradition. And, as Holywell Street publishers' mocking of these works suggests, not everyone took their warnings about the dangers of sexual indulgence seriously. That the same portrayals of weakened, feminized men, destroyed by their own desires, circulated around the globe for several generations must have had some effect on people's ideas about sex and gender, health and morality, however. Although knowingly reading old medical knowledge was a common early Victorian experience, for

New York Academy of Medicine Library; Becklard, Eugène and M. Sherman Wharton. *The Physiologist, or, Sexual Physiology Revealed* [. . .]. (s.l.: s.n., 1846), HMD W6 P3 v. 5829, NLM; Lima and Samuel La'Mert, *The Science of Life; or, Self-Preservation* (Melbourne: s.n., 1883), 613.02/L, Mitchell Library Collection, State Library of New South Wales; Samuel La'Mert, *The Silent Friend: Dr. Lamert's Science of Life* [. . .]. (Melbourne: Will Andrade, 1898), SLT 613.042. L18S, State Library of Victoria.

72 "Dr. Kahn's World-Renowned Anatomical Museum," *Leed's Times*, January 27, 1872, 1.

73 Alexis Weedon, *Victorian Publishing: The Economics of Book Production for the Mass Market, 1836–1916* (London: Ashgate, 2003), 92.

74 See *Davidson, Dennison, and Romilly*, 1873. Old Bailey Proceedings Online (t18730203-167).

75 Simon Szreter and Kate Fisher, *Sex before the Sexual Revolution: Intimate Life in England, 1918–1963* (Cambridge: Cambridge University Press, 2010), 107.

later readers so, too, was encountering late Georgian and early Victorian medical perspectives posing as up-to-date information.

The fact that medical journalists often derisively referred to consulting surgeons and their expertise as "stereotyped" helps unpack the implications of their collective standardization of sexual knowledge for other claimants to medical authority. Stereotyping was one of several new printing techniques that facilitated fast, cheap publishing during the mid-nineteenth century. Involving the use of a mould to cast an exact replica of a set block of type, it sped up the process of printing new copies of successful publications. Instead of painstakingly resetting type when a book or pamphlet sold out, printers could simply dust off stereotype "plates" created from the type initially used to print it. It is probably not a coincidence that the growing popularity of stereotyping aligned with falling prices for consulting surgeons' manuals and their growing circulation in colonial and foreign markets. Stereotyping made low-price, high-volume sales strategies more feasible, and facilitated transnational bookselling by enabling publishers to print their works abroad. Sending stereotypes from city to city and country to country was often cheaper than transporting publications themselves, which were heavier and more easily destroyed.[76]

In other words, stereotypes were copies that enabled the production of more copies. They "froze" previously mobile knowledge (or, at least, type) in place and facilitated virtually infinite commercial reproduction. The stereotype was an apt metaphor for consulting surgeons' derivative, "arrested" performance of expertise, and the fact that medical journalists quickly took it on as a descriptor for their output – referring to "stereotype quack pathologies," to consulting surgeons' "stereotyped oration," to the usual "stereotyped subjects of quack treatment" – offers insight into the nature of the anxieties that their practices aroused in other medics.[77] Consulting surgeons packaged information largely produced by and for medical practitioners and used it to sell themselves to the public as experts over and over again. Like the false names and qualifications on some of their manuals' title pages, the knowledge they claimed did not necessarily extend from anything more than copying. The uncanny sameness of consulting surgeons' manuals made this obvious to other practitioners and seemed to offer evidence that their authors were not legitimate experts. The

[76] Stereotyping also seems to have facilitated the reprinting of these manuals under other names: stereotypes of *Manhood*, for instance, were auctioned off to publishers in the United States. See "A. M. Merwin, Auctioneer," *The Literary World*, May 19, 1849, 446. For more detailed information about the stereotype process and its implications for publishing and bookselling, see Aileen Fyfe, *Steam-Powered Knowledge: William Chambers and the Business of Publishing, 1820–1860* (Chicago: University of Chicago Press, 2012), 33–35.

[77] "The Nostrum Trade," *Boston Medical and Surgical Journal*, September 13, 1848, 131; "Quacks and Quackery," *Medical Times and Gazette*, February 28, 1874, 236; "Quacks," *Health: A Weekly Journal of Domestic and Sanitary Science*, January 25, 1883, 259; "Saturday, November 7, 1846," *Medical Times*, November 7, 1846, 113.

manuals' obvious function as a form of content marketing seemed to further expose consulting surgeons as exploiters of expert knowledge for personal gain.

That other practitioners castigated authors of these manuals even in cases where they had formal medical training and were members of elite medical societies – Robert Jacob Jordan and Samuel La'Mert, for instance, both initially belonged to the Royal College of Surgeons – emphasizes that medical opposition to consulting surgeons was not simply rooted in concern about unqualified medical practice, however. It also derived from the feeling that consulting surgeons' practices were a threat to medicine's credibility. Consulting surgeons seemed to undermine medical authority by highlighting the profession's interests in the market, and therefore its vulnerability to degenerating into charlatanism.[78] At the same time, they undermined medical authority by simultaneously under- and over-performing expertise. Their manuals were theatrical, even lurid in their display of medical knowledge, and, yet, depthless, unapologetically derivative. Medical men might have claimed, had the term then existed, that the consulting surgeon's manual looked like a gimmick, a form characterized by a mixture of laboured superfluity and disappointing vacuity that the critic Sianne Ngai has argued is capitalism's most embarrassing aesthetic category.[79] Because of its identification with medical practice, the consulting surgeon's manual threatened to make medicine itself look like a gimmick: all flash for the crowds, and no substance behind it.

Cash in the Quack's Corner

Thus far, I have argued that the challenge that consulting surgeons and, increasingly, owners of public anatomical museums presented for medical authority was essentially reputational. Even in cases where these figures were formally qualified medical experts, their brash commercialization of medical knowledge seemed to undermine medicine's credibility as a trustworthy, scientific profession and the authority of its print culture. As we shall see, this potential effect on the profession greatly worried regular medical practitioners. However, the economic competition that consulting surgeons represented was also a source of serious concern for other medics. Given the global scale of some of the businesses I have described, I think that their concern about economic competition deserves closer attention. Nowhere is this concern more evident than in the ways regular practitioners discussed consulting surgeons' use of direct advertising to promote their manuals. Ongoing features on consulting surgeons' advertisements in medical journals

[78] Rosenberg, *Rise of Mass Advertising*, 308.

[79] Sianne Ngai, *Theory of the Gimmick: Aesthetic Judgement and Capitalist Form* (Cambridge, MA: Harvard University Press, 2020), 2.

chart other doctors' increasing obsession with finding the answer to a single question: How much money did consulting surgeons make?

As I have suggested, consulting surgeons' advertisements were absolutely everywhere during the mid-nineteenth century. Although they advertised their manuals on posters in public places, hired boys to distribute handbills promoting them in the streets, and paid publishers to insert advertisements for them in all manner of books, their advertisements were especially ubiquitous in periodicals. While Holywell Street publishers became wide advertisers in the 1840s and 1850s, they were small-time players compared to consulting surgeons, who advertised so widely and so frequently that many readers could be certain of encountering several notices for their manuals every time they bought a newspaper or magazine. Readers of the *Morning Chronicle* and of *Reynolds's Newspaper*, of the *Farmer's Magazine* and of the *Banker's Magazine*, of *Bell's Life in London* and of the *Railway Record* saw advertisements for *Manhood* and *The Silent Friend* in every issue. Between the late 1830s and the mid-1840s readers encountered a mean four advertisements for consulting surgeons' manuals per issue in newspapers.[80] By the mid-1850s, the mean had jumped to nine.

Women's periodicals are the only secular genre in which advertisements for these manuals were uncommon. The fact that such periodicals carried many advertisements for treatments for fertility and menstrual problems emphasizes that this is not because irregulars ignored female complaints, however, but because they typically addressed men's and women's concerns differently in print. Men were perceived as reluctant to seek out medical advice and in need of persuasion to do so; women were considered either more open to persuasion through direct advertising or less able to spend time or money on manuals. Some of the drugs aimed at women were certainly as successful as some of the manuals aimed at men, and they were advertised and distributed in similar ways, on similar scales.[81] Widow Welch's Female Pills, a drug company established in 1787 by the booksellers Catherine and George Kearsley, employed many of the same sales strategies as the authors of *Manhood* and *The Silent Friend*, selling pills to treat menstrual "obstructions" (phrasing that could be interpreted to suggest abortion or simply menstrual irregularity) by mail order in sealed envelopes across the country and around the world.[82] By the mid-1840s, when Lambert and the Jordans were just getting started on colonial sales, Widow

80 These calculations are based on periodicals collected in the Gale's *British Library Newspapers, 1800-1900* and *19th Century UK Periodicals* historical newspaper databases.

81 As Sally Shuttleworth observes in "Female circulation," 49, as in manuals for men, advertisements for treatments for women's reproductive problems employed alarmist language, though this as focused on "confirm[ing] contemporary beliefs in the peculiar delicacy of the female system and the pernicious impact of [irregular or disturbed] menstruation."

82 For more on the language used in these kinds of advertisements, see Andrea Carnevale, Denise McGuire, and Johanna Kelly, "'Removes All Obstacles': Abortifacients in Nineteenth-Century Toronto and Beyond," *International Journal of Historical Archaeology* 20 (2016): 743–767.

Welch's was already established in Australia. By the early 1870s, its pills were being advertised in Canada, India, and China.[83]

The bottom right-hand corner of a periodical's advertising page was known as the "quack's corner," as this was the place where editors typically published both kinds of advertisements.[84] This convention attuned readers to locating them quickly, a process that irregulars helped along by making their advertisements visually distinctive. Advertisements for books issued by literary publishing houses favoured the elegant aesthetics of white space: such publishers paid newspaper proprietors handsomely to spread out letters and words. Holywell Street publishers' advertisements prized economy: they typically ran no more than eight lines, comprising a header, a list of short titles and prices, and an address. Advertisements for consulting surgeons' manuals stood out because they were thick with description, creating a rectangle of text sometimes twenty times the size of adjacent advertisements. They were often the manuals in microcosm, offering chapter descriptions; details about their authors' qualifications, addresses, and the times when they were available for consultations; snippets from endorsements and reviews; and, in some cases, promotional language for proprietary medicines (Figure 2.4).[85]

These advertisements aroused a variety of responses. Many readers found them compelling and wanted to believe their claims. As Anat Rosenberg has demonstrated, some readers collapsed the ubiquity of an advertisement with its trustworthiness: "I believed the statement contained in that advertisement for the reason," one reported, "that I saw it, or a similar advertisement, a number of times."[86] Other readers considered consulting surgeons' advertisements a nuisance. Just as the religious tracts that evangelicals issued by the ton from the 1830s came to be seen as junk mail, unasked for and unwelcome, readers often framed irregular advertisements as a kind of spam that clogged up textual space.[87] The subject matter could make advertisements for consulting surgeons' manuals especially irritating: when readers complained about them,

83 See "Widow Welch's Female Pills," *South Australian Register*, October 23, 1847, 4; "To Parents and Guardians," *The Times of India*, October 25, 1865, 4; "To Parents and Guardians," *The North-China Herald and Supreme Court & Consular Gazette*, October 4, 1870, 253; "Harbor Grace Medical Hall," *The Star and Conception Bay Semi-Weekly Advertiser*, June 7, 1872, n.p.

84 William Acton, *The Functions and Disorders of the Reproductive System in Childhood, Youth, Age, and Advanced Life: Considered in Their Physiological, Social, and Moral Relations*, 2nd ed. (London: John Churchill, 1858), 91.

85 Courtenay, *Revelations*, 9; "The Indecent Advertising Quacks," *Medical Press and Circular*, February 27, 1867, 192–193. "Medical Quacks," *Edinburgh Christian Magazine*, April 1853, 25; Percy Pickford, *On True and False Spermatorrhoea* (London: H. Baillière, 1852), 18.

86 Quoted in Rosenberg, *Rise of Mass Advertising*, 83. See also Burmeister, "Public Anatomical," 191–193.

87 Leah Price, *How To Do Things with Books in Victorian Britain* (Princeton, NJ: Princeton University Press, 2012), 139–174.

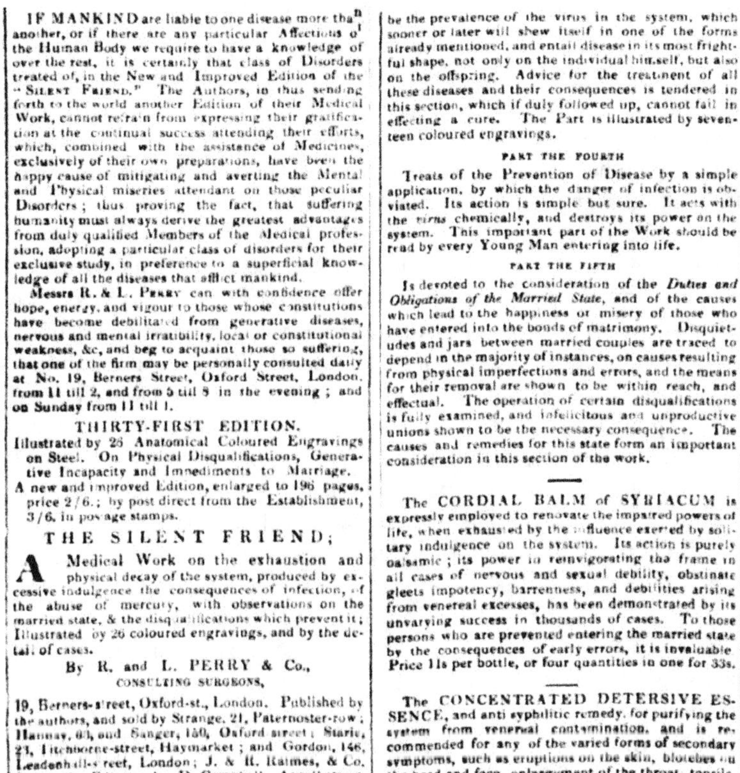

IF MANKIND are liable to one disease more than another, or if there are any particular Affections of the Human Body we require to have a knowledge of over the rest, it is certainly that class of Disorders treated of, in the New and Improved Edition of the "SILENT FRIEND." The Authors, in thus sending forth to the world another Edition of their Medical Work, cannot refrain from expressing their gratification at the continual success attending their efforts, which, combined with the assistance of Medicines, exclusively of their own preparations, have been the happy cause of mitigating and averting the Mental and Physical miseries attendant on those peculiar Disorders; thus proving the fact, that suffering humanity must always derive the greatest advantages from duly qualified Members of the Medical profession, adopting a particular class of disorders for their exclusive study, in preference to a superficial knowledge of all the diseases that afflict mankind.

Messrs R. & L. PERRY can with confidence offer hope, energy, and vigour to those whose constitutions have become debilitated from generative diseases, nervous and mental irratibility, local or constitutional weakness, &c, and beg to acquaint those so suffering, that one of the firm may be personally consulted daily at No. 19, Berners Street, Oxford Street, London, from 11 till 2, and from 5 till 8 in the evening; and on Sunday from 11 till 1.

THIRTY-FIRST EDITION.

Illustrated by 26 Anatomical Coloured Engravings on Steel. On Physical Disqualifications, Generative Incapacity and Impediments to Marriage.

A new and improved Edition, enlarged to 196 pages, price 2/6.; by post direct from the Establishment, 3/6. in postage stamps.

THE SILENT FRIEND;

A Medical Work on the exhaustion and physical decay of the system, produced by excessive indulgence the consequences of infection, of the abuse of mercury, with observations on the married state, & the disqualifications which prevent it; Illustrated by 26 coloured engravings, and by the detail of cases.

By R. and L. PERRY & Co.,
CONSULTING SURGEONS,

19, Berners-street, Oxford-st., London. Published by the authors, and sold by Strange, 21, Paternoster-row; Hannay, 63, and Sanger, 150, Oxford street; Starie, 23, Titchborne-street, Haymarket; and Gordon, 146, Leadenhall-street, London; J. & R. Raimes, & Co. Leith-walk, Edinburgh; D. Campbell, Argyll-street, Glasgow; J. Priestley, Lord-street, and T. Newton, Church-street, Liverpool; R. H. Ingham, Market-place, Manchester.

PART THE FIRST

Is dedicated to the consideration of the *Anatomy* and *physiology* of the organs which are directly or indirectly engaged in the process of reproduction. It is illustrated by six coloured engravings.

PART THE SECOND

Treats of the infirmities and decay of the system produced by over indulgence of the passions, and by the practice of solitary gratification. It shews clearly the manner in which the baneful consequences of this indulgence operate on the economy in the impairment and destruction of the social and vital powers. The existence of nervous and sexual debility and incapacity with their accompanying train of symptoms and disorders, are traced by the chain of connecting results to their cause. This section concludes with an explicit detail of the means by which these effects may be remedied, and full and ample directions for their use It is illustrated by three coloured engravings, which fully display the effects of physical decay.

PART THE THIRD

Contains an accurate description of the diseases caused by infection, and by the abuse of mercury; primary and secondary symptoms, eruptions of the skin, sore throat, inflamation of the eyes, disease of bones, gonorrhœa, gleet, stricture, &c., are shown to depend on this cause. Their treatment is fully described in this section. The effects of neglect, either in the recognition of disease or in the treatment, are shewn to be the prevalence of the virus in the system, which sooner or later will shew itself in one of the forms already mentioned, and entail disease in its most frightful shape, not only on the individual himself, but also on the offspring. Advice for the treatment of all these diseases and their consequences is tendered in this section, which if duly followed up, cannot fail in effecting a cure. The Part is illustrated by seventeen coloured engravings.

PART THE FOURTH

Treats of the Prevention of Disease by a simple application, by which the danger of infection is obviated. Its action is simple but sure. It acts with the *virus* chemically, and destroys its power on the system. This important part of the Work should be read by every Young Man entering into life.

PART THE FIFTH

Is devoted to the consideration of the *Duties and Obligations of the Married State*, and of the causes which lead to the happiness or misery of those who have entered into the bonds of matrimony. Disquietudes and jars between married couples are traced to depend in the majority of instances, on causes resulting from physical imperfections and errors, and the means for their removal are shown to be within reach, and effectual. The operation of certain disqualifications is fully examined, and infelicitous and unproductive unions shown to be the necessary consequence. The causes and remedies for this state form an important consideration in this section of the work.

The CORDIAL BALM of SYRIACUM is expressly employed to renovate the impaired powers of life, when exhausted by the influence exerted by solitary indulgence on the system. Its action is purely balsamic; its power in reinvigorating tha frame in all cases of nervous and sexual debility, obstinate gleets impotency, barrenness, and debilities arising from venereal excesses, has been demonstrated by its unvarying success in thousands of cases. To those persons who are prevented entering the married state by the consequences of early errors, it is invaluable Price 11s per bottle, or four quantities in one for 33s.

The CONCENTRATED DETERSIVE ESSENCE, and anti syphilitic remedy, for purifying the system from venereal contamination, and is recommended for any of the varied forms of secondary symptoms, such as eruptions on the skin, blotches on the head and face, enlargement of the throat, tonsils, and uvula; threatened destruction of the nose, palate, &c. Its action is purely detersive, and its beneficial influence on the system is undeniable. Price 11s and 33s per bottle.

The 5*l* cases of Syriacum or Concentrated Detersive Essence can only be had at 19, Berners street, Oxford street, London; whereby there is a saving of 1*l* 12s, and the patient is entitled to receive advice without a fee, which advantage is applicable only to those who remit 5*l* for a packet.

PERRY'S PURIFYING SPECIFIC PILLS constitute an effectual remedy in all cases of gonorrhœa, gleet, stricture, and diseases of the urinary organs. Price 2s 9d, 4s 6d, and 11s per box.

Consultation fee, if by letter 1*l*. Patients are requested to be as minute as possible in th edescription of their cases.

Attendance daily at 19, Berners street, Oxford street, London, from 11 to 2, and from 5 to 8; on Sundays from 11 to 1.

Sold by Messrs WATTON, CHRONICLE office, Shrewsbury; Allbut and Son, booksellers, Market place, Hanley; R and W Wright, druggists, Stafford; Mander, Weaver, and Co. druggists, Wolverhampton; W Parke, bookseller, High street, Wolverhampton; Pennell and Mark, booksellers, High street, Kidderminster; Deighton, Journal office, Worcester; James Chillcott, bookseller, Broad street, Leominster; Draper, chemist, Broad street, Hereford; John Moore, chemist, Broad street, Newtown, Wm. Edwards, chemist, Denbigh; and John Beale, chemist, High street, Wrexham, of all of whom may be had the Silent Friend.

Figure 2.4 Advertisement for Perry & Co's *The Silent Friend*. *Shrewsbury Chronicle*, September 7, 1849, 1. Content provided by The British Library Board, with thanks to The British Newspaper Archive.

they invariably recalled the embarrassment of seeing sexual health problems aired at the family breakfast table.

For medical journalists, these advertisements were a source of data: it was thought that they could enable estimates of the size of consulting surgeons' businesses – and potentially the size of their income. In 1845, a writer for the *Lancet* searched seven daily papers, nearly a hundred weekly papers, and an unspecified number of "magazines, monthlies, and quarterlies . . . miscellaneous publications, and . . . country newspapers" for advertisements placed by five consulting surgeons.[88] Collectively, these sources published 626 advertisements on behalf of the surgeons each week. By the *Lancet*'s reckoning, this added up to 32,650 advertisements a year. Since most consulting surgeons' notices were lengthy, it estimated that they cost at least ten shillings apiece. This meant that five consulting surgeons alone probably spent more than 16,000 pounds a year on periodical advertising, two-thirds the amount that Richard Bentley, one of Britain's largest literary publishers, spent on book advertising annually.[89] Medical journalists used the same method to estimate consulting surgeons' collective annual spending during the 1850s and 1860s. The figures they arrived at ranged between 50,000 and 65,000 pounds.[90]

As the authors of these studies often pointed out, however, these estimates did not cover a variety of advertising-related expenditures. They excluded the costs of paper, printing, and distribution for posters and handbills, and payments for placing advertisements in guides and almanacs. They also excluded the cost of puffs: allegedly independent writing about a consulting surgeon's manual whose praise had been paid for.[91] Some puffs, as one journalist explained, were framed "as news . . . to draw attention to the advertisement" that the surgeon had placed elsewhere in a periodical.[92] Others masqueraded as independent reviews, which consulting surgeons often quoted in their advertisements, framing them as unasked-for endorsements.[93] Given the nature of the manuals' subject matter, puffs were sometimes evasive as to what they were actually about. One 1856 "review" of *Manhood* in the *Mark Lane Express* employs vague language about self-improvement to describe the manual, for

[88] Review of *Brodie's Secret Companion, Lancet*, November 22, 1845, 563–565. For an earlier example of this kind of accounting, see Charles Cowan, *The Danger, Irrationality, and Evils of Medical Quackery* (London: Sherwood, 1839), 24–25. For a later example, see "Vicious Advertisements," *Lancet*, March 21, 1851, 262–263.

[89] "The Commerce of Literature," *Westminster Review*, April 1852, 276.

[90] See Courtenay, *Revelations*, 11 and J. Teevan, *An Exposure of the Most Nefarious and Heartless System of Swindling Ever Tolerated in Any Civilized Community* (London: S. J. Cuckow, 1851), 7.

[91] For example, see "Quack Advertisements," *Chambers's Edinburgh Journal*, January 23, 1847, 62.

[92] J. D. Burn, *The Language of the Walls: And A Voice from the Shop Windows; or, The Mirror of Commercial Roguery. By One Who Thinks Aloud* (Manchester: Abel Heywood, 1855), 91.

[93] "Quacks and Quack Medicines," *Penny Magazine*, December 29, 1838, 500.

instance, praising its commitment to addressing the "duty of all men to study the laws of their body no less than of the mind."[94]

Medical journalists' calculations also excluded international advertising costs, which would have significantly added to consulting surgeons' overhead. Possibly to save money as well as time, consulting surgeons put little effort into adapting their advertisements for new geographic contexts. The advertisements that Joseph Lambert, the Jordans, and Samuel La'Mert placed in colonial periodicals are identical to the advertisements they placed in periodicals at home, save for the names and addresses of suppliers. Advertisements placed in foreign-language newspapers were often translated from British versions line for line.[95] It is important to keep in mind, however, that identical advertising copy would have been interpreted differently in foreign and colonial contexts than it would have been in Britain. As Peter Yeandle has argued, for instance, advertising addressing concerns about "manly vigour" in the British colonies spoke to anxieties about white health and Western imperial strength in ways that it did not in Britain.[96]

Finally, bespoke advertising arrangements complicated attempts to calculate consulting surgeons' advertising expenditures. Some newspaper proprietors reportedly charged irregulars 300 or 400 percent more than they did other customers, figuring that they could afford it.[97] Apparently, this was especially true of puffs commissioned by "Secret Infirmity and Venereal gentlemen": proprietors justified larger fees because the subject matter presented unique challenges for journalists tasked with presenting it as "news."[98] In other cases, consulting surgeons struck deals to make advertising less costly. Drawing on intercepted correspondence, one journalist reported that a surgeon paid a weekly Glasgow newspaper a flat rate of ten pounds for a twenty-one-week run of classified advertising and a weekly puff in the same paper.[99] The proprietors of provincial newspapers seem to have been especially willing to work out bespoke arrangements. In some deals described by this journalist, consulting surgeons gave books and patent medicines to newspaper editors for free in exchange for puffs. The editors sold the goods to customers through their offices and pocketed the proceeds.

Consulting surgeons acknowledged that they spent a lot on advertising, and sometimes offered numbers of their own. In their own publications, however, they framed exorbitant spending on advertising as a sign of their concern for readers' well-being, or of their faith in the efficacy of their remedies, encouraging readers to apply the logic that Rosenberg identifies. According to *The*

94 Reprinted in "Curtis on Manhood," *The Bombay Almanack and Book of Direction for 1858* (Bombay: Bombay Gazette Press, 1858), n.p.

95 For instance, see "Mannheit," *Deutsche Zeitung Frankfurt*, March 4, 1849, 584.

96 Peter Yeandle, "Exotic Bodies and Mundane Medicines: Advertising and Empire in the Late-Victorian and Edwardian Press," in *Paraphernalia! Victorian Objects*, ed. Helen Kingstone and Kate Lister (London: Routledge, 2019), 244–264.

97 Courtenay, *Revelations*, 12. 98 Burn, *Language of the Walls*, 91.

99 Burn, *Language of the Walls*, 91.

Silent Friend, readers should interpret R. and L. Perry & Co's campaign for the Cordial Balm of Syriacum as a sign of the company's confidence in its product. "It requires the strongest conviction of its intrinsic worth and physical excellence, by long and great experience," Perry & Co declared, "to induce the inventor or proprietor of any Medicine to incur the serious expense of making it known by advertisements; an expense of no less than £20,000 annually to Messrs. Perry and Co." Indeed, Perry & Co claimed, "it could be of no avail to enter upon . . . the vast expense of making known such remedies, if their merits would not support their character when they were known."[100]

Efforts at calculating consulting surgeons' advertising costs ultimately foundered because it became clear that they offered limited insight into consulting surgeons' operations. As one group of medical practitioners noted in 1850, even if it was possible to calculate consulting surgeons' total domestic advertising costs, those costs must only scratch the surface of their outlay. Their gross annual incomes needed to be sufficient to cover the costs of printing and distributing their manuals, "binding, storing, the rent of several large houses in expensive parts of London, [and] the employment of numerous agents . . . as far off as Bombay and Calcutta."[101] In the end, medical practitioners generally agreed that the gross annual incomes of the most successful consulting surgeons must exceed £30,000.[102] During a period in which £500 was a typical annual income for a successful general practitioner living in London, and annual incomes of £10,000 could be realized only by elite medical specialists, this was a staggering number.[103]

It was also a number that suggested an alarming disjuncture. Consulting surgeons' position in the regular medical world was at its fringes. Yet, their position in the marketplace could hardly be characterized as "fringe." They were a dominating presence in the Victorian market for advice on sexual and reproductive health issues. Consulting surgeons attracted patients who might otherwise have visited a practitioner who did not engage in "quackish" self-promotion, and they were not necessarily seen as meaningfully different from such practitioners. Branwell Brontë's family consulted physicians and surgeons who would have blanched at being compared to J. L. Curtis, and noted down the names of nostrums supplied by irregulars in a medical encyclopedia that those physicians and surgeons would have considered the epitome of propriety.[104]

In the first decades of the Victorian period, the market for cheap medical print expanded rapidly. The publishing and advertising practices explored in

[100] *Silent Friend* (1841), 75–76.
[101] *A Few Words to News-Readers* (London: W. Eglington, 1850), 3. 7306.df.22, BL. See review of *Brodie's Secret*, *Lancet*, 564 for a similar analysis.
[102] Courtenay, *Revelations*, 2–3. [103] Digby, *Making a Medical Living*, 137.
[104] Shuttleworth, "Female Circulation," 49.

this and the previous chapter challenged regular medical authority in different ways, though the fact that consulting surgeons identified as medical practitioners and competed with regular practitioners for patients meant that regular practitioners perceived them as much more of a problem. As the next chapter emphasizes, they were particularly threatening to regular practitioners because the identity of regular medical practice was unstable, and the differences between its print culture and those that this book has examined thus far were even more ambiguous than I have suggested. Even as the text of regular practitioners' books and articles overlapped with pornographers' and irregulars' publications, so, too, did their publishing and advertising practices. As a new kind of publisher, the specialist medical publisher, entered the book business and looked to the medical profession to cultivate authors and readers, he found himself having to navigate an environment thick with suspicion of medical books, authors, and publishers, and ever-fearful of misidentification.

3 Publishing for Professional Advantage

The Philosophy of Marriage in Its Social, Moral, and Physical Relations (1837) bore all the trappings of respectability. As its title page declares, its author, Michael Ryan, was a member of the Royal Colleges of Physicians and Surgeons in London and an attendant at the Metropolitan Free Hospital. Unlike the other *Marriages* that we have seen in this book, Ryan's *Marriage* was issued by a medical and scientific publisher, John Churchill. At six shillings, it was more expensive than the other *Marriages*, and its smart blue cover would not have looked out of place on a middle-class bookshelf. Yet, the genesis of Ryan's *Marriage* was not unlike the others. Addressing practically everything to do with reproduction, from the processes of botanical fertilization to the benefits of polygamy, much of its text was taken from articles Ryan had written for the *London Medical and Surgical Journal*. Ryan derived most of the text of those articles from lectures that he delivered at various medical schools in the metropolis. The lectures were, as one of his students remembered with a mixture of fondness and exasperation, "totally deficient in originality."[1] Ryan cobbled them together by copying lengthy passages from the works of other authors, which he gradually transported up the publication chain from lecture to article and article to book. Like William Dugdale and Joseph Lambert, Michael Ryan gathered, arranged, and reframed.

Ryan's *Marriage* had another thing in common with the other *Marriages*: many medical men did not consider it a respectable publication. It was certainly a commercial success. At least seven editions of Ryan's *Marriage* were issued in Britain and the United States through the mid-nineteenth century, and the work was renovated, as in Dugdale's *Marriage*, and excerpted, as in Lambert's *Manhood*, countless times. However, it was panned in medical journals for "pander[ing] to the tastes of that portion of the public, to whom the supposed mysteries, which Ryan unveils, are matters of curiosity."[2] "It is melancholy," a writer for the *British and Foreign Medical Review* lamented, "to see

[1] James Fernandez Clarke, *Autobiographical Recollections of the Medical Profession* (London: J & A Churchill, 1874), 133.

[2] "We Promised Our Readers," *Medical Examiner*, May 23, 1838, 174.

a physician and a man of information descend, from whatever reason, to cater such kind of reading for the ill-regulated minds of all who may choose to indulge it; offending the eye of delicacy, like a quack-doctor on the wall."

> The work is divided into three parts: the first treats of Marriage in its moral and social relations, and contains some useful information, intermixing with many topics that look as if they were purely meant to be exciting; the second speaks of the Physical relations of marriage, and may be similarly characterized; the third, which relates to the Morbid relations of marriage, comprehends all the subjects in surgery and midwifery which can offend and disgust, because the information relating to them whilst it is useful, pollutes the minds of those who seek it from curiosity, and without any view to its beneficial application ... there is scarcely an original syllable: the work would be worthless to medical men on this account; for they know all these old stories as well as Dr. Ryan. The novelty is in all this being laid so bare to the general eye; for what object the compiler best knows.[3]

"Dr. Ryan," this writer concluded, "has lamentably forgotten what is due to the public, to the profession, and to himself."[4]

The issue that Ryan's colleagues had with his *Marriage* was not simply that he had written a work that seemed to invite prurient engagement. George Spratt's *Obstetric Tables* (1833), published by Churchill four years earlier, could have been accused of the same thing. *Obstetric Tables* invited readers to explore the female body by manipulating mobile illustrations that would not have been out of place in an album of pornographic images. With the flick of a finger, a reader could reach between a lithographed woman's parted legs and open her labia majora "like doors," revealing a full-colour rendering of her clitoris, labia minora, and vaginal opening.[5] Yet, *Obstetric Tables* was lauded in the medical press as a marvellous pedagogical instrument. Nor was the problem solely that Ryan wrote for readers who were not medical experts. Publishers like Churchill advertised many works on sexual matters in the non-medical press. Such works were often read by, and sometimes written for, audiences beyond the medical, and most aroused no objections of this kind from medical practitioners or the public. Nor was *Marriage*'s derivative nature the main issue. Many medical men scoffed at consulting surgeons' traffic in "stereotyped" knowledge, and some of Ryan's colleagues were offended that he had borrowed their words without attribution.[6] However, compilation – even of the

[3] "Art. VIII. The Philosophy of Marriage," *British and Foreign Medical Review*, April 1838, 442.

[4] "Philosophy of Marriage," *British and Foreign Medical Review*, 446.

[5] Rebecca Whiteley, "Spratt's Flaps: Midwifery, Creativity, and Sexuality in Early Nineteenth-Century Visual Culture," *British Art Studies* 19 (2021): https://doi.org/10.17658/issn.2058-5462/issue-19/rwhiteley. Mobile prints were often advertised in Holywell Street catalogues. For instance, see "Sly Peeps" in Wm. Ward, *Ward's New Catalogue of Parisian Novelties* (Strand: W. Ward, c. 1850), 11. DA 676, box 8, no. 22, MSCE.

[6] Howard Brody, Zahra Meghani, and Kimberly Greenwald, eds., *Michael Ryan's Writings on Medical Ethics* (London: Springer, 2009), 29.

unattributed kind – was still widely practised in medicine, and generally accepted as a lesser mode of authorship.

The problem was that Ryan had done all of these things at once, and that he had done them so obviously, so artlessly. His purpose in "manufacturing" *Marriage* was clear in the eyes of his critics. He was not publishing to advance knowledge or to enlighten the ignorant. He was pandering to prurient curiosity to sell books, and promote his own expertise in the process. Medical journalists constantly alluded to Ryan's allegedly unprofessional motives, as the *British and Foreign Medical Review*'s mock-pondering about his "objects" suggests. In July 1839, when Ryan appeared with the manuscript for a new book on another sexual subject, *Prostitution in London*, Churchill decided to end his partnership with Ryan, fearing for his own reputation as a medical publisher. "I find in reference to the strong feeling existing respecting your publications that I could not have come to any other determination," Churchill wrote to Ryan. "I much regret that I should be compelled in any measure to break my connection with a gentleman from whom I have received kindness and derived profit."[7] Michael Ryan was no Joseph Lambert. He had lectured in medical schools that, while not the best London had to offer, were respected. He had been the editor of the *London Medical and Surgical Journal*, which his colleagues recalled as a "beneficial influence on the Profession."[8] He was a member of the Royal Colleges, and is now remembered as "a seminal figure in the development of medical jurisprudence."[9] But what Ryan's colleagues interpreted as his thirst for profit and publicity caught up with him.

Ryan's predicament illustrates three issues that concern this chapter: overlaps in the ways pornographers, irregular practitioners, and regular practitioners treated medical knowledge in print; concern about those overlaps in medical circles; and the informal and contingent nature of the ways they were policed. To understand the evolving politics of selling sexual knowledge during this period, we need to understand that rapidly growing sectors of the print marketplace situated it into contexts that could be seen as dangerous to morals, to medical authority, and, in some cases, to medical incomes. However, we also need to understand the state of the regular medical profession and its fraught relationship with its own print culture. Medical practitioners had debated how to handle print since the Enlightenment. "Should medical knowledge be free and open? Or were there some occasions for secrecy?" they asked one another. "And assuming knowledge ought to be publicized, what were the proper

7 John Churchill to Dr. Ryan, July 6, 1839. MS 1393 1/M3, Records of the Longman Group, ABPP.

8 Clarke, *Autobiographical Recollections*, 135.

9 Brody, Meghani, and Greenwald, *Michael Ryan's Writings*, 3.

channels? Was all medical knowledge fit for public consumption? . . . Was the publishing doctor a public benefactor? Or a self-serving self-publicist?"[10] These debates had not been resolved at the beginning of the Victorian period, and the chances that they would be resolved looked bleak. Medicine had become an increasingly competitive profession and was essentially at war with itself in the 1830s: left-wing advocates of radical medical reform, "general practitioners" unhappy with low incomes, conservative Oxbridge-educated physicians, and splinter groups within these groups had different visions for medicine and different ideas about what its print culture should look like.

Medical reformers recognized better than most print's power to transform the profession and mediate public perceptions of it. From the 1820s, with the appearance of Thomas Wakley's *Lancet*, they had begun to harness the medical journal as means of calling out corruption, fostering a sense of community among disparately identified medical practitioners, and galvanizing support for legislation to regulate medical practice.[11] Their efforts seemed to be having the desired effect. The divisions that had marked medicine at the beginning of the 1830s began to close in the 1840s and 1850s, as medical men increasingly saw themselves, at least potentially, as part of a "unitary and democratized body of practitioners connected by common ideals, knowledges and practices."[12] Yet, print also threatened to undermine work to unite the medical profession, improve its reputation, and – crucially for medical reformers – "restructure the commercial status of medicine and its relation to the public."[13] Part of the challenge lay in the fact that anyone could copy medical knowledge and use it for their own purposes. As this chapter shows, regular practitioners were especially worried about irregular publications and advertisements, which they thought undermined their credibility. However, neither would not have felt so threatening had the medical profession established a strong corporate identity and clear rules for maintaining it in print.

There were few agreed-upon conventions for publishing and promoting medical books. The overtly commercial style that Joseph Lambert took up and the suggestive ways in which William Dugdale framed medical knowledge were certainly considered beyond the pale. However, the boundaries between

[10] Roy Porter, "The Rise of Medical Journalism in Britain to 1800," in *Medical Journals and Medical Knowledge: Historical Essays*, ed. W. F. Bynum, Stephen Lock, and Roy Porter (London: Routledge, 1992), 6–28.

[11] Geoffrey Russell Searle, *Morality and the Market in Victorian Britain* (Oxford: Clarendon, 1998), 129; Michael Brown, *Performing Medicine: Medical Culture and Identity in Provincial England, c. 1760–1850* (Manchester: Manchester University Press, 2014), 49.

[12] Michael Brown, "Medicine, Quackery, and the Free Market: The 'War' against Morison's Pills and the Construction of the Medical Profession, c. 1830–c. 1850," in *Medicine and the Market in England and Its Colonies, c. 1450–c. 1850*, ed. Mark S. R. Jenner and Patrick Wallis (Basingstoke: Palgrave Macmillan, 2007), 239.

[13] Brown, "Medicine, Quackery," 240.

publishing for the public benefit, publishing to promote one's services, and pandering to prurient readers were uncertain, and how far one could toe the lines between them without damaging one's credibility or that of the profession at large was contested. In this context, medical debates about how publishing should be performed devolved into endless rounds of complaint, and print's function as a means of making authority warped. Medical authority was not guaranteed to survive publication. The medical journal gradually came to offer one solution to these problems, and publishers like Churchill came to offer another.[14] Each offered a means of disciplining professional medical discourse and distinguishing it from other kinds. At this stage, though, what constituted orthodox medical practice was unsettled, the medical journal was young, and publishers like Churchill were still establishing themselves. Such publishers saw themselves as valuable assets to a divided profession that had no idea how to handle print communication. Their critics saw them as mercenaries whose economic interests threatened to compromise medicine's integrity.

The Gentlemanly Monopoly

Victorian retrospectives of medical publishing often recall 1790 as the year of its birth. In that year, John Callow, a watchmaker's apprentice, married a bookseller's widow, whose shop at no. 10, Crown Court, London, stood near a famous anatomical theatre. On their marriage, the shop was a mess. Books overflowed from its shelves and stopped up its narrow corridors. Callow put the shop in order, and soon it became a favourite haunt of the practitioners who passed through the neighbourhood every day. Callow responded by increasing its stock of medical books. "In a few years," the physician Samuel Merriman remembered, "it was recommended to Callow by Dr. John Pearson, the learned and scientific surgeon . . . to establish himself *solely* as a MEDICAL BOOKSELLER AND PUBLISHER." Callow took the doctor's advice. By the 1810s, his shop had become "*the* resort of professional men in search of information." "Not only [were] the best *old* medical works to be found in Crown Court," Merriman reminisced, "but also all the *new* publications connected with medicine," many of which Callow now issued himself.[15]

Publishers used a variety of strategies to establish a foothold in the market for medical books at the dawn of the Victorian period. Callow's story was one of them. Promoted by John Churchill, who had bought Callow's business in 1832, the legend furnished Churchill's business with a legacy, one that connected it with London's medical geography, its history, and some of the most famous medical men of the recent past. It downplayed the reputations for

[14] Porter, "Rise of Medical Journalism," 12.

[15] "John Callow, the Medical Bookseller," *Gentleman's Magazine*, January 1845, 30.

producing excellent medical works that general publishers like John Murray and Thomas Longman had developed in the previous century, and elevated a group of entrepreneurs, including Churchill, H. K. Lewis, J. W. Parker, Samuel Highley, Henry Renshaw, and Hippolyte Baillière, as heirs to a new model of medical publishing founded in a gentlemanly relationship between medics and bookmen.[16] This model was enabled by new commercial opportunities that the expansion of medical practice offered during the first half of the nineteenth century. However, its development was not quite as effortless as the story about Callow's business implied. Publishers had to work hard to integrate themselves into the fabric of medical life.

Although a handful of men, including Callow, Renshaw, and Highley, called themselves medical booksellers and publishers during the first years of the nineteenth century, medical publishing really took off as a specialist niche of the British publishing industry in the 1830s and 1840s. As men like William Dugdale and Joseph Lambert seized the opportunities offered by expanding press and postal infrastructures to build thriving trades in cheap medical print, other publishers started or expanded medical lists aimed at readers with more money and education. These publishers were concentrated largely in London, Edinburgh, and Dublin, all well-known centres for publishing and medical training, where local doctors formed both a ready-made market for medical books and journals and a major source of manuscripts on medical subjects. As in most other areas of publishing, and despite the pre-eminence of Scottish medical training at the beginning of the nineteenth century, London was home to the largest of these publishers, and produced the most medical books and journals. However, London-based publishers frequently partnered with publishers in the other cities, who often created Irish and Scottish editions of London medical publications in addition to issuing their own.[17]

The Strand, the geographic centre of London's publishing and bookselling industry, offered would-be medical publishers an advantageous proximity to medical institutions. Parker's shop at 445 Strand was neatly situated mid-way between the Royal College of Physicians and the Royal College of Surgeons,

16 For discussions of medical publishing in the eighteenth century and further information about its development, see David McKitterick, "Publishing for the Trades and Professions," in *The Cambridge History of the Book in Britain*, vol. 6, ed. David McKitterick (Cambridge: Cambridge University Press, 2010), 500–530; Leslie Chard, "Joseph Johnson: Father of the Book Trade," *Bulletin of the New York Public Library* 79, no. 1 (1975): 51–82.

17 For further information about the geography of British medical publishing, see Elizabeth Lake, "Medicine," in *The Oxford History of the Irish Book*, vol. IV, *The Irish Book in English, 1800–1891*, ed. James H. Murphy (Oxford: Oxford University Press, 2011), 576–584; Robin Myers, "The London Scots," in *The Edinburgh History of the Book in Scotland, Volume 3: Ambition and Industry, 1800–1880*, ed. Bill Bell (Edinburgh: Edinburgh University Press, 2007), 396–408; W. F. Bynum and Janice C. Wilson, "Periodical Knowledge: Medical Journals and Their Editors in Nineteenth-Century Britain," in *Medical Journals and Medical Knowledge: Historical Essays*, ed. W. F. Bynum, Stephen Lock, and Roy Porter (London: Routledge, 1992), 29–48.

and down the street from the *Lancet*'s offices.[18] As Ruth Richardson has pointed out, this was a happy coincidence for Parker when the publisher – a generalist with a large literary list – began to expand his medical offerings in the mid-1840s. H. K. Lewis selected an even more advantageous position from which to publish and sell medical books when he set himself up in Gower Street, steps from University College Hospital, in 1844.[19] From this location, Lewis set out to attract the custom of the medical men who passed through the neighbourhood. His shop offered discounts for cash purchases, and housed a circulating library featuring his own works on hygiene, surgery, physiology, gynaecology, and disease. Although Lewis also issued other kinds of books, these services and the firm's geographic position associated it with the hospital, making it, as Callow's shop was remembered, something of a medical institution itself.

Publishers also integrated themselves into the fabric of medical life by cultivating their social networks. Churchill made many connections by attending medical society meetings and hosting doctors in the back room of his bookshop on Prince's Street, where he gossiped with them by the fire in the evenings, "skimming the cream of general politics and medical scandal."[20] These occasions consolidated his reputation as a man who, while not a doctor himself, had a deep understanding of the profession and its needs. The surgeon James Fernandez Clarke recalled receiving his first medical apprenticeship through Churchill. A friend of Clarke's uncle, the publisher recommended him to a surgeon in St. Giles after conducting a terrifyingly rigorous interview.[21] All the while, Churchill took every opportunity to situate his business within a deeper historical context: at medical society meetings, in the medical press, in his correspondence, in his promotional materials, and eventually in his memoirs, the publisher reminded medical men of the relationships that he had forged with esteemed physicians and surgeons, and of his connection to Callow, the father of medical bookselling who had set him on his path.

Additionally, publishers signalled their belonging in medical communities by linking themselves with the profession's governing structures in print. Just as regular and irregular practitioners alike often highlighted their status (or purported status) as members of the Royal Colleges and other medical

[18] Ruth Richardson, *The Making of Mr. Gray's Anatomy: Bodies, Books, Fortune, Fame* (Oxford: Oxford University Press, 2009), Kindle ed. loc. 1598.

[19] McKitterick, "Publishing for the Trades," 510.

[20] "Westminster Medical Society's Dinner," *Lancet*, June 2, 1849, 600–601. "John Churchill," *British Journal of Dental Science*, October 1875, 573. For details about Hippolyte Baillière's involvement in scientific societies, see Josep Simon, *Communicating Physics: The Production, Circulation and Appropriation of Ganot's Textbooks in France and England, 1851–1887* (London: Routledge, 2016), 142.

[21] Clarke, *Autobiographical Recollections*, 95–97.

institutions on the title pages of their books, publishers who enjoyed the patronage of such institutions frequently noted the fact in promotional material, even in cases when that patronage conferred no particular privilege. Baillière, the London-born son of a French publishing and bookselling family whose firm also had offices in Paris and Madrid, billed himself "Publisher and Foreign Bookseller" to the Royal College of Surgeons, the Royal Society, and the Royal Medico-Chirurgical Society in advertisements.[22] Highley, who had managed John Murray's medical department and took much of its business with him when he and Murray parted ways in 1803, heralded his status as "Bookseller to the Royal College of Surgeons of England."[23]

Situating themselves within these interwoven geographic, social, and institutional spaces, medical publishers portrayed themselves as helpmeets to the profession who worked tirelessly to facilitate medical training and communication between experts. Their activities did greatly assist these enterprises. Churchill's series of medical directories for the United Kingdom, begun in 1846, connected doctors with clients, tradespeople, and each other. The medical journals that he, Highley, and others published, which ranged from specialist periodicals, such as the *Asylum Journal of Mental Science*, to general ones, like the *Medical Times and Gazette*, expedited a more public form of communication between practitioners in different parts of the country. Publishers like Baillière, with his international connections, facilitated exchanges of knowledge between practitioners in different countries by issuing translations and foreign editions. Many books that were adopted as standards for medical training, such as Henry Gray's *Anatomy: Descriptive and Surgical* (1858), issued by Parker, were brought out by specialist medical publishers. And, through circulating libraries like Lewis's, which counted several hospitals among its subscribers, medical men could read these works cheaply and conveniently.

Admittedly, medical publishers' portrayals of themselves as happy servants of the profession sometimes stretched the bounds of credulity. Churchill represented his advertising circular, the *Medical Intelligencer*, as a service devised to keep practitioners informed of the "Progress of Medical Literature," A considerable portion of the second number's cover in 1854 is devoted to illustrating how expensive it was for Churchill to put out, showing through a breakdown of costs that he had spent £156 7*s* 6*d* to print 15,000 copies of the circular, place them in envelopes, stamp them, and send one, unsolicited, to

22 George Gulliver, *Elements of the Minute Anatomy of Man and the Mammalia* (London: Baillière, 1842); Julius Vogel, *The Pathological Anatomy of the Human Body*, trans. George E. Day (London: Baillière, 1847); *Quarterly Review Literary Advertiser* (London: John Murray, 1841), 30.

23 Henry Curwen, *A History of Booksellers, the Old and the New* (London: Chatto and Windus, 1874), 168; *Medical Times*, May 2, 1851, advertising sheet.

"every Medical Man in the United Kingdom whose address can be ascertained."[24] Just as readers of R. and L. Perry & Co's broadcasts about the company's advertising expenditures were meant to conclude that it invested in advertising because it was confident in the efficacy of its patent medicines, readers of the *Medical Intelligencer* were meant to conclude that Churchill was not just in medical publishing for the money. Reading between the lines, it's clear that doctors were not the only beneficiaries of Churchill's medical directories. They were also a useful tool for marketing purposes.

Publishers like Churchill took every opportunity to promote themselves as assets to the profession because doctors regularly questioned their motives and morals. They whinged about the quality of the books that medical publishers put out, and grumbled about prices they charged for them, portraying them as mercenaries who put their own profits over the needs of the profession.[25] Churchill's tireless efforts at self-promotion paid off eventually. On his death in 1875, he was toasted in the medical press for his ability to see "a want, [suggest] the kind of work likely to fulfil that want, and . . . put his finger on the man who has leisure and talent sufficient to write it."[26] However, winning medical men over was not quick or easy. Two decades earlier, a medical journalist had speculated that Churchill commissioned books by "throwing a certain number of subjects into one hat, . . . [and] the names of medical men into another, and draw[ing] forth both at random." Allegedly, "the nominees" – medical men who, this journalist claimed, were asked to write books more for their famous names than for their literary talents – "resort[ed] to mere compilation . . . wholesale appropriation from their neighbours" or ghost-writing to deliver their manuscripts on time.[27]

Medical men wrote more darkly about the existential dangers of giving publishers too much control over medical communication. Some envisioned scenarios in which a small number of publishers came to possess "at one and the same time the copyrights to the chief standard medical works, and also those of the medical periodicals."[28] Such corporate monopolies would not only give outsiders to the profession the power to dictate the prices of medical books and periodicals but also enable them to dictate the terms of publishing them. This state of affairs would surely degrade medical literature and reduce its criticism to puffery. Occasional battles between publishers and medical practitioners, like

[24] See no. II, January 1854, cover page in John Churchill, *The Medical Intelligencer*, nos. I–V (London: John Churchill, 1853–1857), RB.23.b.6723, BL.

[25] For example, see "On the Publication of Works in Parts," *Provincial Medical and Surgical Journal*, November 26, 1842, 78–79.

[26] "John Churchill," *British Journal of Dental Science*, 574.

[27] "European Practitioners," *American Medical Monthly*, December 1855, 448.

[28] "Answers to Correspondents – One of the Disgusted," *Lancet*, February 25, 1854, 234. See also "The Lancet: The Guardian of the Interests of the Profession," *Lancet*, March 18, 1854, 313–315.

one explosive episode between Michael Ryan and the *London Medical and Surgical Journal*'s publisher, Henry Renshaw, lent credence to these concerns. In 1834, Renshaw reportedly pressured Ryan to publish an enthusiastic review of a "quackish, catch-penny, and most absurd work" in order to retain its author's advertising business, and then demanded that Ryan puff nostrums advertised on the journal's wrapper.[29] Ryan may have been accused of dabbling in quackery himself, but he considered this behaviour beyond the pale: he ended the journal's partnership with Renshaw. Furious, he moved to expose the publisher after Renshaw continued to issue a version of the *London Medical and Surgical Journal* under a more malleable editor, and sent threatening letters to booksellers demanding that they stop selling Ryan's version.[30]

Concerns that publishers presented a threat to the profession's integrity were the most frequently raised by, or expressed in the organs of, advocates of radical medical reform like Ryan and Wakley, editor of the *Lancet*. In seeking to "raise up" the profession, medical reformers not only aimed to make over medicine's public image but also aspired to transform it from within by rooting out self-serving behaviour, dismantling hierarchies of governance that fostered inequities among practitioners, and installing a fair system for regulating medical practice.[31] One of the early missions of the *Lancet*, whose initially combative, vernacular style was inspired by radical periodicals like T. J. Wooler's *Black Dwarf* (1817–9), was to expose the corruption of medical elites and fight against the power of the Royal Colleges, institutions that *Lancet* writers argued exerted a "monopoly" over medicine.[32] From 1840, the more subdued *Provincial Medical and Surgical Journal* (later, the *British Medical Journal*), the mouthpiece of the Provincial Medical and Surgical Association (later, the British Medical Association), offered lowly general practitioners living outside London a voice against those same elites.[33] Medical publishers,

29 "Address to Our Readers and the Public," *London Medical and Surgical Journal*, August 30, 1834, 154.

30 "Address to Our Readers," *London Medical and Surgical Journal*, 155.

31 Adrian Desmond, *The Politics of Evolution: Morphology, Medicine, and Reform in Radical London* (Chicago: Chicago University Press, 1989), 169.

32 "The Lancet: The Guardian," 313–315. For further information about the *Lancet* and its early ambitions, see Michael Brown, "'Bats, Rats and Barristers': The Lancet, Libel and the Radical Stylistics of Early Nineteenth-Century English Medicine," *Social History* 39, no. 2 (2014): 185–191; Jean and Irvine Loudon, "Medicine, Politics, and the Medical Periodical, 1800–50," in *Medical Journals and Medical Knowledge: Historical Essays*, 62.

33 The Provincial Medical and Surgical Association was established in 1832 to facilitate the exchange of information among general practitioners outside London. The journal was initially titled *The Provincial Medical and Surgical Journal*. In April 1842 it was retitled *The Provincial Medical Journal and Retrospect of the Medical Sciences*, but reverted to its original title two years later. In 1857 the journal merged with the *Association Medical Journal* (itself a re-branded *London Medical Journal*) and was thereafter called *The British Medical Journal*. For further details, see Peter W. J. Bartrip, *Mirror of Medicine: A History of the British Medical Journal* (Oxford: Oxford University Press, 1990).

who emphasized their connections with elite medical institutions *and* sought to profit from medical expertise, were seen by some writers for these organs as the worst of both the irregular and the elite medical worlds, either in thrall to or aspiring to replace the monopoly of the Royal Colleges with a publishing monopoly.[34]

Just as publishers like Churchill were working to consolidate a foothold in the industry, medical reformers began to argue that only an independent medical press, divorced from the commercial publishing establishment and the oversight of the Royal Colleges, could ensure that communication on medical matters in print was equitable and ethical.[35] In the 1840s, many advocated the formation of private subscription societies to publish many, and even all, of the books required for medical training and reference.[36] As well as ensuring independence, medical reformers claimed, subscription publishing societies could make medical works vastly cheaper and equalize practitioners' access to them. The publishing model they proposed had some promising precedents.[37] Even at the proposal stage, though, reformers quarrelled about exactly what kinds of works medical publishing societies should issue, and worried that they would not attract enough subscribers to sustain them.[38] An appeal to general practitioners for donations to keep the *Provincial Medical and Surgical Journal* running in 1842 was so unsuccessful that the Association was forced to bail it out.[39] The outlook for a subscription publishing society charging a guinea per annum – the subscription rate proposed by most advocates of these societies – did not look good.

34 "The Lancet: The Guardian," 313–315.

35 "Corrupt State of Medical Law," *Lancet*, May 10, 1834, 237–244, 237.

36 See "Republication of Medical Works by a Medical Association," *Lancet*, May 21, 1842, 285–286; "Proposed Society for Publishing Medical Books," *Lancet*, July 23, 1842, 579–580; "Medical Publications Society," *Lancet*, August 13, 1842, 701. For more on this history, see G. G. Meynell, *The Two Sydenham Societies: A History and Bibliography of the Medical Classics Published by the Sydenham Society and the New Sydenham Society (1844–1911)* (Folkestone: Winterdown, 1985).

37 During the eighteenth century, small groups of medical practitioners had formed societies, such as the Pylorus Club and the Society for Propagating Human Nature and Knowledge, to publish medical books, periodicals, and collections of essays. See D. A. Kronick, "Medical 'Publishing Societies' in Eighteenth-Century Britain," *Bulletin of the Medical Library Association* 82, no. 3 (1994): 277–282. During the 1830s and 1840s, other groups organized to issue special-interest publications on a subscription basis. The Parker Society, for instance, published the works of early Protestant writers, while the Camden Society issued historical and literary documents.

38 *Provincial Medical Journal and Retrospect of the Medical Sciences*, September 17, 1842, 483; Meynell, *Two Sydenham Societies*, 2; *Provincial Medical Journal and Retrospect of the Medical Sciences*, August 20, 1842, 383–401.

39 Peter Bartrip, "The *British Medical Journal*: A Retrospect," in *Medical Journals, Medical Knowledge: Historical Essays*, ed. W. F. Bynum, Stephen Lock, and Roy Porter (London: Routledge, 1992), 130–131.

The *Lancet*'s claim, in 1854, that "two or three leviathan booksellers" supplied the country with all of its medical books and journals – "publishing what they please, rejecting what they please, and then puffing their own wares in their own journals" – was not quite true.[40] Medical publishing continued to be performed by a variety of players through the mid-nineteenth century. And although they never achieved the kind of influence that some medical reformers wanted, a few medical publishing societies were established, and one, the New Sydenham Society, was quite successful.[41] The *Lancet* was correct, though, in that two firms, Churchill and Baillière, dominated the market for professional medical books and journals by the middle of the nineteenth century. With its robust international network, including new branches in New York and Melbourne, Baillière was the country's largest supplier of foreign medical books and translations, while Churchill was the largest domestic producer. As the *Lancet* commented in 1857, "the publishing of medical books is now conducted under monarchical government, and … Mr. Churchill holds the sceptre with a firm hand."[42]

The services that career publishers offered proved impossible for medical men to resist. Working without the burden of medical duties, they were able to manage the complicated, time-consuming work of ushering manuscripts into print and organizing their advertisement and distribution – kinds of labour that the organizers of medical publishing societies found very difficult to perform efficiently. However, publishers were not necessarily trusted to put the medical profession's interests above their own. As the next section shows, the same was true for medical authors. In theory, the way regular medical authors typically published books – with the assistance of a publisher – distinguished them from men like Joseph Lambert and William Dugdale. In theory, the publisher's imprint conferred a kind of institutional approval that marked a medical work, and its author, as legitimate and respectable. And in theory, the publisher stood between the author and the market, insulating him from direct contact with it. However, alongside persistent distrust in publishers' abilities to work in medicine's best interests, the economic contexts of medical publishing and medical practice undermined these functions of the publisher, and supported a continuous undercurrent of suspicion, particularly in the reforming medical press, that a great deal of regular medical authorship was only superficially distinct from quackery. This suspicion mediated debate about propriety in publishing works on sexual and reproductive issues within the regular medical community, and intensified concern about how works on these issues were being advertised and sold by those outside it.

[40] "The Lancet: The Guardian of the Interests of the Profession," 313–315.
[41] Meynell, *Two Sydenham Societies*. [42] "Medical Catalogues," *Lancet*, March 21, 1857, 305.

The Publisher as Agent

Publishers like Churchill and Baillière were hardly the ruthless mercenaries that their critics made them out to be. They aspired to establish reputations for issuing books and journals of real quality, and cultivated their lists carefully. They developed relationships with respected doctors, kept their eyes peeled for promising young authors, and tried to steer clear of works that they thought would smack of quackery to the professional readers they courted.[43] But while they prized quality, a book's potential to make a profit, or at least break even, was important. As Churchill declared on several occasions, "a publisher swims or sinks by the exercise of his judgement."[44] Economic considerations weighed heavily in negotiations between authors and publishers, influencing the length of the final product, the quality and number of its illustrations, its material design, and the way it was framed. Observing in 1843 that "small monographs" like one proposed by the surgeon Langston Parker, a specialist in venereal disease, "seldom pay to the publisher," for instance, Churchill suggested printing Parker's work in the same format as his previous book, *Modern Treatment of Syphilitic Diseases* (1839).[45] One hundred and fifty copies of *Modern Treatment* remained unsold. Churchill thought that marketing the new book as a companion to the old one could speed sales of both, and imagined binding them together to create a new work if that strategy failed to raise demand for *Modern Treatment*.[46]

Unfortunately, such adjustments could not always make a worthy book from a professional point of view a sound financial investment. Churchill declined more than one manuscript because he judged it "more calculated to advance [the author's] scientific reputation, and consequently to promote [his] professional status, than repay commercially."[47] Such a book might look too similar to a bestseller to achieve good sales, or its topic might be too specialized to attract much interest. For the authors of such books, however, there was another resort: they could cover the cost of publishing it themselves. Churchill frequently apprised authors of this option during the 1840s and 1850s, when he was establishing himself as Britain's largest medical publisher.[48] After politely expressing doubt that a book would be sufficiently lucrative to justify risking his investment, he would suggest that the author cover the costs of publishing

[43] For instance, see Baillière to A. H. Blackley, April 4, 1873, Baillière MS 1570/1/211, Records of the Longman Group, ABPP.
[44] John Churchill to Dr. Williams, February 20, 1857, Longman 1/381/170, Records of the Longman Group, ABPP.
[45] John Churchill to Langston Parker, August 31, 1843, Longman 1/381/133, Records of the Longman Group, ABPP.
[46] John Churchill to Langston Parker, August 31, 1843.
[47] John Churchill to Dr. Williams, February 20, 1857.
[48] Nos. I (January 1853) and V (January 1857) of Churchill's *Medical Intelligencer* boast of the size of his medical list in relation to that of other publishers.

and advertising it himself. Churchill would take a fee for arranging the publication, and the author would have rights to the profits. If Churchill's instincts were wrong, and the author's "expectations of a successful sale [were] justified, [he] would not be kept long without a return for [his] capital."[49]

Paying the costs of publishing one's own book did not carry the same stigma that it does today. The arrangement, often termed commission publishing, was extremely common for most of the nineteenth century.[50] Even so, it attracted opposition: critics argued that commission publishing exploited authors and fostered the overproduction of books with narrow, and sometimes non-existent, readerships. Commission arrangements did benefit publishers by guaranteeing that they would make a modest profit in exchange for the labour of bringing a book out. They also allowed – and to some extent encouraged – publishers to issue more books than they would have under other circumstances. This effect of publishing on commission could damage a publisher's reputation, if it led to an indiscriminate list, but, in the right hands, it could be beneficial. By increasing his stock of medical books, commission publishing made it possible for Churchill to promote himself as the publisher of "a larger number of Medical Works than are issued by all the other publishing houses" by the early 1850s and situate himself as the most powerful medical publisher in the industry.[51]

The benefits of commission publishing were less straightforward for authors. Although some very successful writers chose to publish on commission to maximize their profits, most risked heavy financial losses.[52] Including the costs of paper, typesetting, and printing; binding and advertising fees; free presentation copies for friends, colleagues, and reviewers; and the publisher's ten percent fee for arranging the book's publication, marketing, and distribution, issuing 500 copies of a typical medical book cost between seventy and ninety pounds. This was a serious investment, given that an income of between £300 and £500 signalled a "fair degree of success" for general practitioners working in London.[53] Authors publishing on commission would have to spend considerably more to bring out a book if it contained charts or illustrations, if it

49 John Churchill to Dr. Williams, February 20, 1857.

50 Royal A. Gettmann, *A Victorian Publisher: A Study of the Bentley Papers* (1960; repr., Cambridge University Press, 2010), 116; Jim Cheshire, *Tennyson and Mid-Victorian Publishing: Moxon, Poetry, Commerce* (Basingstoke: Palgrave Macmillan, 2016), 153; Leslie Howsam, *Kegan Paul: A Victorian Imprint* (Toronto: University of Toronto Press, 1998), 131.

51 See *Medical Intelligencer* no. I (January 1853), cover page.

52 Gettmann, *Victorian Publisher*, 110–111; Cheshire, *Tennyson*, 153.

53 These figures are derived from correspondence in Longman 1/381, Records of the Longman Group, ABPP. The quotation and figures for medical practitioners' incomes are from Anne Digby, *Making a Medical Living: Doctors and Patients in the English Market for Medicine, 1720–1911* (Cambridge: Cambridge University Press, 1994), 137. As Digby notes, country doctors earned less on average, usually between £150 and £250 per annum.

was lengthy, or if it was published in a large format. Commission publishing was also open to abuse. Authors were aware, for example, that publishers could charge posted fees for advertising a book in venues where they were, in fact, able to advertise it at a discount or for free.[54]

Why, then, did so many medical authors publish on commission? It is doubtful that they thought they would make a profit. Publishers readily acknowledged that even the most successful medical writers rarely made enough to live on, and that losses were virtually guaranteed for authors who entered commission arrangements.[55] Many doctors published anyway because they wanted to make a lasting contribution to medical knowledge. Some aspired to shape medical training, and some to influence public policy. But the prospect of "professional advantage" was another incentive.[56] Furnishing a doctor with publicity and cultural capital, authorship could attract new clients to his practice. A book could make him sufficiently known that he might be invited to lecture to medical students, offered a hospital position, and come to the attention of the country's wealthiest patients. Experiences like John Elliotson's, whose annual income soared from £500 to £5,000 in the space of just one year following the publication of a series of influential clinical reports in the *Lancet*, acted as grist for the ambitions of many medical men.[57] (Elliotson's fall from grace after he started to champion mesmerism acted as another, less inspiring, lesson in career strategy.)[58]

The economic context of medical practice further explains the appeal of publishing for professional advantage.[59] From 1815, an over-supply of doctors

54 Gettmann, *Victorian Publisher*, 109. That authors were aware of the potential for this kind of abuse is clear from correspondence. For instance, Baillière felt the need to assure one medical writer that "on no account do we charge [authors], [*sic*] what we do not have to pay the proprietors" of the journals in which the firm advertised its books. See Baillière to [illegible] Browne, February 28, 1878. Baillière MS 1570/5/256, Records of the Longman Group, ABPP.

55 For instance, see John Churchill to Dr. Roberts, January 19, 1858, Longman 1/381/174–175 and Baillière to Dr. Drysdale, October 31, c. 1872, MS 1570/5/268, Records of the Longman Group, ABPP; Curwen, *A History of Booksellers*, 343; Digby, *Making a Medical Living*, 136–148. Baillière's comment to Drysdale is typical: "As a rule, Professional Scientific works do not pay their Authors directly, with some few exceptions . . . generally speaking, Scientific writers must be content with fame, & the diffusion of their views." As Bynum and Wilson, "Periodical Knowledge," 43, show, editors of medical journals did make money doing so, but rarely enough to make a living.

56 Digby, *Making a Medical Living*, 172.

57 "Biographical Recollections of the Medical Profession," *Medical Press and Circular*, August 12, 1874, 141–143.

58 Alison Winter, *Mesmerized: Powers of Mind in Victorian Britain* (Chicago: University of Chicago Press, 2000), 95–100.

59 For further information about the economic issues discussed in this paragraph, see M. Anne Crowther and Marguerite W. Dupree, *Medical Lives in the Age of Surgical Revolution* (Cambridge: Cambridge University Press, 2007), 1–5; Digby, *Making a Medical Living*, 136–169; Irvine Loudon, *Medical Care and the General Practitioner, 1750–1850* (Oxford: Oxford University Press, 1986), 7; Alison Moulds, "'Making your Mark' in Medicine: The Struggling

made it very difficult to become established in private practice. The incomes of established medical practitioners were also woefully unpredictable, partly because they faced robust competition for patients and partly because patients often delayed or neglected to pay their bills. While irregulars demanded that patients pay for consultations in advance, regular practitioners deemphasized the transactional nature of the doctor–patient relationship by billing patients afterward.[60] Authorship was seen as a way for young medical practitioners, and especially young physicians, to distinguish themselves from the fray, and for established practitioners to stabilize their income. Secured on the basis of their status as published experts, hospital appointments could furnish senior medical men with greater economic security as well as higher social status in a status-conscious profession.

Publishing for professional advantage was so widely recognized as a career strategy that it was the subject of innumerable satires. "Having familiarized people with your name," one collection of "Private Hints to a Young Physician" instructs, "it behoves you then to give it notoriety; therefore, lose no time in getting into print . . . A Treatise on Indigestion has gained many a physician a sumptuous dinner . . . the physician of the Irish Viceroy is indebted for his livelihood to a little book on gout."[61] But while such pieces emphasize that publicity was a desired effect of publishing a medical book, they also emphasize that publishing a book for this purpose was not looked on as entirely respectable. It looked dangerously close to advertising. Some medical men considered it little more than a veiled form of quackery.[62] This situation helps explain the virulence of medical opposition to practitioners like Joseph Lambert, particularly in organs for medical reform like the *Lancet*. Consulting surgeons represented serious economic competition and associated a profession trying to portray itself as learned and disinterested with naked commercialism. At the same time, consulting surgeons' publishing practices drew attention to an ambiguity between publishing and advertising in regular medicine that was a source of significant professional discomfort.

In this context, commission publishing was often portrayed as a dangerous practice – under such arrangements, was the medical publisher really anything more than an advertising agent? – and medical authorship was subject to constant, informal policing. Medical journals were run through with gossip that this or that

Young Practitioner and the Search for Success in Britain, 1830s–1900s," *History* 104, no. 359 (2019): 83–104.

60 Digby, *Making a Medical Living*, 174, 193–196.

61 "Private Hints to a Young Physician," *Morning Chronicle*, October 1, 1832, 4.

62 W. F. Bynum, "Treating the Wages of Sin: Venereal Disease and Specialism in Eighteenth Century Britain," in *Medical Fringe and Medical Orthodoxy, 1750–1850*, ed. W. F. Bynum and Roy Porter (London: Croom Helm, 1987), 22; Searle, *Morality and the Market*, 107–133.

practitioner wrote books purely for the purposes of self-promotion. This mode of policing did little more than exacerbate authors' anxieties about being misunderstood, however, because it did not resolve a fundamental problem: the rules for publishing in the right ways were unwritten, contingent, and contested. Authors could not circumnavigate the risk of an accusation by declining to write on certain topics. Works on venereal disease, fertility problems, and male sexual dysfunction often aroused suspicion, since these topics were now tightly associated with quackery, as did medical autobiographies, which highlighted the author's accomplishments.[63] However, even a book on aural disease could be seen as an advertisement in disguise.[64] Nor were there clear rules for *how* to write a medical book. Writing a derivative book could be risky. Compiling was faster than writing from scratch, and some practitioners viewed compilation as the trademark of the self-serving author. Yet, compilations were also praised in the medical press as useful syntheses of established knowledge. Moreover, a book could be too original. If he wrote a book that recommended "some new invention . . . in the shape of an instrument, or a medicine, or a peculiar line of treatment," an author risked being seen as over-eager to promote his ingenuity.[65]

Promoting a medical book was even more fraught. In the eyes of many medical reformers, medical books were less often advertisements themselves than they were excuses for advertising. A respectable practitioner could not advertise his address or fees for consultations or publish testimonials without offending his colleagues. All had been considered quackery in medical circles since the eighteenth century. Publishing a book, however, enabled him to get his name into the press without technically advertising his practice. The *Medico-chirurgical Times* called using a book as a proxy for promoting a medical practice "auto-advertising."[66] In practical terms, however, it was far from clear what distinguished this form of advertising from normal book promotion. Some medical men considered having one's book too widely or too regularly advertised in the non-medical press unseemly, but their opinions about what constituted excessive advertising varied. Some medical men took umbrage at those who paid to have their books listed in certain venues, such as the *Medical Circular*'s "Guide to Living Authors," a directory of medical authors that printed their addresses alongside the titles of their books. Since contact information for medical authors was available through professional

63 "Autobiographical Advertising: Both Sides of the Question," *Association Medical Journal*, December 30, 1853, 1150.
64 Review of *Diagnostics of Aural Disease*, *Dublin Quarterly Journal of Medical Science*, August 1, 1861, 96.
65 Review of *Diagnostics*, *Dublin Quarterly Journal of Medical Science*, 96.
66 "Auto-Advertising and Medical Degrees," *Medico-chirurgical Review*, January 1825, 260.

societies, the guide's critics argued, it had no purpose beyond providing non-medical readers with the addresses of medical men with expertise in particular areas.[67] Yet, the fact that the Guide existed at all suggests that many practitioners did not see it this way.

Balancing regular practitioners' collective disapproval of advertising with medical authors' desire to sell their books and make their names proved to be as difficult for publishers as it was for authors. Anxious to attract authors, medical publishers often broadcast their skills at getting a book noticed. On taking over John W. Davies's medical publishing business in 1864, Robert Harwicke took out an advertisement in the *Lancet* which announced that he had "at his command the requisite means for giving extensive publicity for Works published by him."[68] The largest medical publishers often emphasized the advantages that their status as publishers of journals afforded for publicity. As Baillière put it to one author, "our connection with so many medical journals does give us special advantages [in advertising] . . . + where it is in our power, as is frequently the case, we put adverts of works in which we have a pecuniary interest, in gratuitously."[69] Churchill alluded to this power in print, announcing in one of his catalogues that his journals offered authors "a wide extent of literary announcement, and a medium of advertisement, addressed to all classes of the profession."[70] However, such efforts to highlight a publisher's strengths could be perceived as evidence of underhanded practices. Churchill's boast was interpreted by one writer to the *Lancet* as a scandalous admission of puffery:

> . . . what does this phrase, "a wide extent of literary announcement," really mean? Can anybody doubt but that it is really intended to insinuate and convey the impression that Mr. John Churchill can secure, by his influence as a proprietor and publisher of medical reviews and periodicals, favourable notices of the works of those authors who employ him for their publisher? Can anything be more improper than this?[71]

Medical works on sexual and reproductive matters could be especially tricky to promote in this environment. The topics they addressed were often associated with irregular medical practice and thus with self-promotion, and some were also considered particularly attractive to prurient readers, and thus subject to abuse by publishers and authors alike. The unruly space of the print marketplace, where titles issued by many different kinds of players mixed and mingled, exacerbated these problems.

[67] "The New Advertising Scheme," *Medical Times and Gazette*, June 2, 1855, 544–545.
[68] "Medical Publishing," *Lancet*, May 21, 1864, back cover.
[69] Baillière to [illegible] Browne, February 28, 1878.
[70] "Fair Play," *Lancet*, June 22, 1850, 767. [71] "Fair Play," *Lancet*, 767.

The Medical Publisher's List

Medical publishers issued a wide variety of works that addressed reproduction and sexual health. Because compilation was such a common way of making new books during this period, the content of many of these works overlapped with that of works examined in previous chapters. However, they were distinct from the productions hawked by men like William Dugdale and Joseph Lambert in many respects. They were larger, heavier, and better produced, with thicker paper and more precise illustrations. While they became increasingly affordable over the first decades of the Victorian period, they were often more expensive, too – sometimes dramatically so. The implied audience of these works was also different: they usually addressed medical, or at least professional, readers. Moreover, they had a very different relationship with the state. As well as establishing, extending, and amplifying discourses that regulated sex and the body by setting standards for bodily form and function, sexual behaviour, and sexual desire, some of these works overtly supported state interest in managing sexual and reproductive practices.[72] For all of these reasons, it is not especially intuitive to examine trade in such works alongside the pornography and consulting surgeon trades. As elements of the previous sections suggest, however, distinctions that appear strong from a historical distance looked a lot shakier during the first decades of the Victorian period, and understanding this is key to understanding the politics of selling sexual knowledge at the time. Overlaps in how and why these works and works examined in previous chapters were sold, or were thought to be sold, aroused concern in medical circles, and this concern inspired action.

A general overview of the kinds of works medical publishers issued is helpful for establishing a more expansive understanding of trade in sexual knowledge during this period as well as its politics. Although they did not focus solely on sex or reproduction, medical publishers issued countless lectures, treatises, manuals, textbooks, and atlases on anatomy and physiology that included a great deal of information about the reproductive system and the transformations of adolescence. Such works often served as sources for the cheaper pamphlets and manuals examined in previous chapters. While some were plain, workaday titles intended for students cramming for examinations, others were lavishly illustrated

[72] The scholarship on these issues is vast. For examples, see Peter Cryle and Elisabeth Stephens, *Normality: A Critical Genealogy* (Chicago: Chicago University Press, 2017); Sean Brady, *Masculinity and Male Homosexuality in Britain, 1861–1913*, 2nd ed. (London: Springer, 2016); Anna Clark, *Desire: A History of European Sexuality* (London: Routledge, 2019); Deborah Lupton, *The Imperative of Health: Public Health and the Regulated Body* (London: Sage, 1995); Frank Mort, *Dangerous Sexualities: Medico-Moral Politics in England since 1830*, 2nd ed. (London: Routledge, 2000); Ann Laura Stoler, *Race and the Education of Desire: Foucault's History of Sexuality and the Colonial Order of Things* (Durham, NC: Duke University Press, 1995); Judith R. Walkowitz, *Prostitution and Victorian Society: Women, Class, and the State* (Cambridge: Cambridge University Press, 1982).

works of art. Henry Gray's landmark textbook *Anatomy: Descriptive and Surgical* (1858), which initially sold for twenty-eight shillings and was furnished with stunning wood engravings by the surgeon and artist Henry Vandyke Carter, stood in sharp contrast to cheap pocket editions of *Aristotle's Masterpiece* and even manuals like *Manhood*, whose illustrations of the body were smaller, softer, and often older.

Alongside these works, medical publishers issued many works that focused specifically on sexual and reproductive health issues. Manuals, textbooks, and treatises on reproduction, gynaecology, obstetrics, and midwifery appeared in their catalogues year after year. As with the works on general anatomy and physiology, some of these productions were workaday compilations aimed at synthesizing existing knowledge or spare treatises oriented around describing new methods of treatment. Others were expensive and elaborate showpieces. Readers thumbing through Augustus Bozzi Granville's stunning *Graphic Illustrations of Abortion* (1834), which was published by Churchill and initially cost more than two pounds, could gaze at forty-five lithographs and engravings illustrating embryos floating free against a velvety black background, as if suspended in a starless sky, or peep at the creature nestled in the cradle of the uterus, the organ's layers peeled back to enable viewing like the skins of a shaggy onion.[73] Robert Lee's *Anatomy of the Nerves of the Uterus*, issued by Baillière in 1842, depicts the uterus with such full-colour realism that its illustrations look almost photographic.

Medical publishers also issued many books on the functions, disorders, and diseases of the reproductive organs which had a variety of purposes too. Some instructed practitioners in the aetiology and symptoms of specific health problems and promoted particular methods of treating them. John L Milton's *On a New Way of Treating Gonorrhoea* (1852) is a good representative of this genre. Illustrated solely with tables of notes, it marches readers briskly through a series of case studies, provides instructions for applying Milton's method of treating gonorrhoea, which involved injecting patients with silver nitrate, and argues against courses of treatment suggested by other practitioners.[74] Other works organized and synthesized medical knowledge of reproductive health and disease more generally, or examined it from social, moral, behavioural, economic, or legal angles. William John Anderson's *Hysterical and Nervous Affections of Women* (1853), a collection of lectures initially presented to members of the Harveian Society, examines the relationship between diseases of the uterus and psychological conditions in women, while William Acton's *Functions and Disorders of the Reproductive*

[73] A. B. [Augustus Bozzi] Granville, *Graphic Illustrations of Abortion and the Diseases of Menstruation* (London: John Churchill, 1834).

[74] John L. Milton, *On a New Way of Treating Gonorrhoea* (London: John Churchill, 1852).

Organs (1857) examines male reproductive function and dysfunction over the entire life cycle within a matrix of "Social and Moral Relations."[75]

Additionally, publishers like Churchill and Baillière issued works addressing issues related to sexual and reproductive behaviour that overtly aimed to support or influence the law and public policy. Some provided doctors with information that enabled them to aid the state in managing sexual behaviour. Alfred Swaine Taylor's classic *Manual of Medical Jurisprudence* (1844), published by Churchill, shows doctors how to look for physical evidence of sexual crimes, including rape, sodomy, and bestiality.[76] It also instructs readers how to determine whether a woman had been pregnant or delivered a baby, and how to distinguish cases of miscarriage from deliberate abortions, should medical expertise be called on during inquiries surrounding divorce, inheritance, infanticide, or criminal abortion. Other works were written to galvanize support for new laws, or bring about their abolition. William Acton's *Prostitution, Considered in Its Social, Moral, and Sanitary Aspects* (1857), published in the same year as *Functions and Disorders*, urges state intervention to stem the tide of venereal disease, while Michael Ryan's earlier *Prostitution in London* (1839), published by Baillière after Churchill dropped Ryan and modelled on Alexandre-Jean-Baptiste Parent-Duchâtelet's influential *De la prostitution dans la ville de Paris* (1836), rails against the 1834 Poor Law Amendment Act. The Act, Ryan argues, exacerbated the spread of venereal diseases by forcing unwed mothers into prostitution.[77]

Finally, especially early in the Victorian period, medical publishers issued works that addressed sex and reproduction and their relations to marriage, heredity, and racial difference. These works were often written by radical medical practitioners interested in the political and philosophical applications of knowledge about anatomy, physiology, and reproduction, and sometimes inspired by bestsellers on related topics that had gained a wide general readership.[78] Ryan's *Marriage* was one of these works. *Marriage* was modelled on a proto-anthropological genre that emerged in the seventeenth century and remained popular throughout the nineteenth, which Lisa O'Connell calls the "marriage-rites genre."[79] Including works such as Louis de Gaya's *Cérémonies nuptiales de toutes les nations* (1680) and Lady Augusta

[75] William Acton, *The Functions and Disorders of the Reproductive Organs* [. . .]. (London: John Churchill, 1857) and *Prostitution, Considered in Its Social, Moral, and Sanitary Aspects* [. . .]. (London: John Churchill, 1857).

[76] Alfred Swaine Taylor, *A Manual of Medical Jurisprudence* (London: John Churchill, 1844).

[77] Michael Ryan, *Prostitution in London: With a Comparative View of that of Paris and New York* (London: H. Baillière, 1839).

[78] For more on radical medical reformers and their interest in the politics of sex and reproduction, see Desmond, *The Politics of Evolution*.

[79] Lisa O'Connell, "'Matrimonial Ceremonies Displayed': Popular Ethnography and Enlightened Imperialism," *Eighteenth-Century Life* 26, no. 3 (2002): 99–116.

Hamilton's *Marriage Rites, Customs, and Ceremonies of All Nations of the Universe* (1822), marriage-rites books presented readers with a cornucopia of information about marriage customs around the globe, from "bland descriptions of the minutae of wedding ceremonies and courtship procedures to commentary that reproduced received ideas about other worldly forms of sexuality," such as "the amorousness of the French, the hot-blooded passions of the Italians and the Spanish, and the despotism of the polygamous Turks."[80] Compiled from a plethora of published sources, including previous works in the genre, marriage-rites books framed this knowledge as a cornerstone for understanding the universal nature of humanity, drawing connections between marriage in various traditions even as they exoticized "foreign" practices.[81]

Ryan borrowed from marriage-rites books when he made his own *Marriage*, including passages that match verbatim with passages in Hamilton's *Marriage Rites*.[82] The obstetrician's innovation was to combine the descriptions of foreign bodies, climates, and customs that fill most marriage-rites books with lengthy discussions of anatomy and physiology, obstetric procedures, fertility problems, and medical curiosities, also mostly sourced from previously published works. In *Marriage*, Ryan argues that gaining a complete understanding of marriage as a universal did not just require acquiring cultural knowledge of foreign marriage ceremonies and practices like polygamy and eunuchism. Such a project also demanded gaining an understanding of the biological processes associated with reproductive life, and the medical knowledge and procedures that helped manage them. Physiology and obstetrics, Ryan claims, "materially influence population, morals, public health, disease, mortality; as well as personal reputation, property, legitimacy, and even life."[83] Considered holistically, marriage was cultural *and* biological. This was a perceptive argument – but it meant that Ryan's *Marriage*

80 O'Connell, "Matrimonial Ceremonies," 104–105.

81 O'Connell, "Matrimonial Ceremonies," 101, 110.

82 Most of these borrowings were attributed. To see Ryan's unattributed borrowings, compare Ryan, *Philosophy*, 27, 80–85, and 91 with Hallifield Cosgayne O'Donnoghue, *Marriage: The Source, Stability, and Perfection of Social Happiness and Duty* (London: V. Elkins, 1828), 11, 69, 4, 8, 15, 14, and 45; *Philosophy*, 58, 94, 87, and 105 with Theophilus Moore, *Marriage Customs and Modes of Courtship of the Various Nations of the Universe* (London: John Bumpus, 1830), 171, 73, 183, and 222–223; *Philosophy*, 58, 87, 105 with Lady Augusta Hamilton, *Marriage Rites, Customs, and Ceremonies of the Nations of the Universe* (London: J. Smith, 1822), 198–199, 216, and 238; *Philosophy*, 58 with John Armstrong, *The Young Woman's Guide to Virtue, Economy, and Happiness* (Newcastle: Mackenzie and Dent, 1826), 557; *Philosophy*, 68 with *Poor Inquiry (Ireland). Appendix (H.) – Part II* (London: W. Clowes and Sons, 1836), 15; *Philosophy*, 80–85 with "Prize Essay: Marriage," *The Ladies' Monthly Museum* (London: Dean and Mundy), 1827, 13, 248, and 251; *Philosophy*, 83 with John Morison, *Counsels to a Newly Wedded Pair* (London: F. Westley and A. H. Davis, 1830), 74; *Philosophy*, 83 with Timothy Dwight, *Theology: Explained and Defended, in a Series of Sermons*, vol. 3 (New Haven, CT: S. Converse, 1825), 396–397; *Philosophy*, 105 with Jean Baptiste Léonard Durand, *A Voyage to Senegal: or, Historical, Philosophical, and Political Memoirs* [...]. (London: Richard Phillips, 1806), 104; and *Philosophy*, 105 with M. U. Sears, *The Female's Encyclopaedia of Useful and Entertaining Knowledge* (London: J. Sears, 1830), 296–297.

83 Ryan, *Philosophy*, iv.

contained more explicit discussions of the body than other marriage-rites books. Given this, and Ryan's identification with (medical) radicalism, it is little wonder that William Dugdale sold it and renovated it.

Another example – also connected with disreputable bookselling – is Alexander Walker's *Intermarriage; or, The Mode in Which, and the Causes Why, Beauty, Health and Intellect, Result from Certain Unions, and Deformity, Disease, and Insanity, From Others*, also published by Churchill, in 1838. *Intermarriage* is a sequel to Walker's commercially successful *Beauty: Illustrated Chiefly by an Analysis and Classification of Beauty in Women*, an upmarket reworking of John Joseph Stockdale's publication *Kalogynomia, or The Laws of Female Beauty* (1821) – which itself lifted parts of an 1815 essay of Walker's, raising the possibility that Walker was *Kalogynomia*'s author.[84] Walker, a radical lecturer on anatomy and physiology, imported *Kalogynomia*'s argument and much of its text verbatim when he created *Beauty*. He stitched this material together with a list of "mental defects" in women, lengthy passages evaluating the beauty of foreign and ancient women, and exegeses on biology, art history, and aesthetics. *Kalogynomia* and *Beauty* are very much alike. Where *Kalogynomia* presents readers with a mishmash of illustrations running the gamut of sexual explicitness, however, *Beauty* features an orderly series of engravings of nude women posed like classical statues. And while one is never too far away from a titillating passage in *Kalogynomia*, in *Beauty* these passages are enveloped in a dense cocoon of copied prose.[85]

Intermarriage is, in turn, similar to *Beauty* despite its announced focus on interracial and interclass reproduction. As in *Beauty*, as Rachel Walker notes, a clear "undercurrent of erotic desire" runs through *Intermarriage*.[86] The work lingers on the "insanity" of sexual desire, the physical beauty of women of various "races" (and its defects), and "foreign" practices such as clitoridectomy. In offering this material, *Intermarriage* again recycles a great deal of text from *Kalogynomia* and *Beauty* – essentially offering a reprisal of the former in the middle of the book – as well as passages plucked from marriage-rites books, treatises on phrenology, and works on animal breeding.[87] The book, as Damon Ieremia Salesa observes, represented "the fullest radical account of racial

[84] Lucy Hartley, "Walker, Alexander (1779–1852)," in *Oxford Dictionary of National Biography* (Oxford: Oxford University Press, 2004; online ed. 2011), https://doi.org/10.1093/ref:odnb/56049; M. L. Bush, *What Is Love? Richard Carlile's Philosophy of Sex* (London: Verso, 1998), 35–36; Ch. 1, n. 33.

[85] For a closer analysis of Walker's *Beauty* and its sources, see Alexander Maxwell, Carol Harrington, and Sarah Bracey. "Scientific Eroticism, Beauty Theorists, and the Borders of the Erotic: John Roberton's *Kalogynomia* and Alexander Walker's *Beauty*," *Porn Studies* 8, no. 2 (2021): 138–153.

[86] Rachel E. Walker, *Beauty and the Brain: The Science of Human Nature in Early America* (Chicago: University of Chicago Press, 2022), 71.

[87] Walker, *Beauty and the Brain*, 228.

crossing" at the time, an account that approached intermarriage as a "'reforming science' aimed at . . . maximizing individual ability and preventing disease."[88] Yet, while it communicates original ideas about how to use medical knowledge to improve humanity, *Intermarriage* is also a bursting compendium of information about reproductive bodies and sexual practices, one that bears striking similarities to Ryan's *Marriage*, *Beauty*, and the popular works that inspired them.

Pandering, Auto-Advertising, and Paratextual Contamination

Medical debate about publishing and advertising works in the extremely diverse body of literature that I have sketched surrounded three overlapping issues: "pandering" to prurient members of the reading public, "auto-advertising," and something that I'll call "paratextual contamination." Each was thought to undermine medical authority and the upstanding, "scientific" identity for medicine that medical reformers desperately wanted to consolidate.

Given medical authors' historically anxious attitudes towards publishing on sexual matters and overlaps between some of these works and works connected with the pornography trade, we might expect most of the debate to focus on the problem of pandering. As Ryan's case suggests, medical journalists did level charges that a regular medical author sought to entertain the public with descriptions of sex and the body, or had come dangerously close to looking like they wanted to. Such charges usually surrounded works on topics thought to attract prurient readers, such as prostitution, masturbation, and obstetrics and gynaecology. However, these allegations were so rare by the Victorian period that I have only been able to identify a handful of examples, and they were unpredictable, often seeming to rely more on opinions of the author than assessments of the work. Ryan and Walker were both involved in the radical medical reform movement. *Marriage* and *Intermarriage* were issued by the same publisher only a year apart. Both were commercial successes: they attracted readerships far beyond the medical and were reprinted in several new editions at home and abroad. Ryan was harshly criticized for publishing *Marriage* on the grounds that it pandered to prurient readers. *Kalogynomia*, a work that substantially informs *Intermarriage*, was known for its connection with a scandalous publisher, and, as Chapter 7 shows, eventually seized as an obscene book. However, both *Intermarriage* and its predecessor, *Beauty*, escaped medical criticism: they were not seen as attempts to pander to prurient readers despite their similarities to works that were.

A related but also infrequent charge was that medical publishers pandered to prurient readers by commissioning rapidly knocked-up works on issues like prostitution with sales to the general public in mind. A review in the *Edinburgh*

[88] Damon Ieremia Salesa, *Racial Crossings: Race, Intermarriage, and the Victorian British Empire* (Oxford: Oxford University Press, 2019), 158.

Medical and Surgical Journal that railed against Baillière for publishing an anonymous work called *The Greatest of Our Social Evils, Prostitution* (1857) offers a good example of these kinds of charges.[89] Having published works on "mesmerism, hydropathy, homeopathy, and every other kind of suspicious subject," this writer claimed, Baillière was now commissioning works on sexual matters "for the purposes of the book market."[90] The evidence that the *Edinburgh* reviewer provided was a four-page list of titles. It was not the works themselves, he maintained, but the number of them and the fact that they were clustered on the same page of Baillière's advertising sheet that revealed his unsavoury motives for publishing works on these subjects. It "may be, that all of the books here quoted are . . . innocent of pruriency," the reviewer admitted. "But the reader . . . will agree with us in thinking that the conjunction is ominous."[91]

The exponentially larger number of charges of auto-advertising levelled against authors of works on sexual matters emphasises that the idea that medical knowledge was being exploited to promote medical practice was seen as more of a threat to the profession's credibility during this period than the idea that it was being prostituted to prurient readers, though as Ryan's case suggests, these charges could overlap. Churchill, Baillière, Renshaw, Highley, and other medical publishers all advertised works that addressed sexual issues in non-medical periodicals. During the early 1840s, these advertisements appeared in just a handful of newspapers and magazines. However, they began to appear more regularly, and in a much wider range of venues, from the middle of the decade. By the 1850s, readers saw advertisements for works like Langston Parker's *Treatment of Secondary and Constitutional Confirmed Syphilis* (Churchill, 1850), Samuel Bayfield's *Practical Observations on the Local and Constitutional Effects of Syphilis* (Renshaw, 1858), and Francis Burdett Courtenay's *On Spermatorrhoea* (Baillière, 1858) in the classified pages of conservative newspapers, such as the *Standard*; sporting papers, such as *Bell's Life in London*; and Sunday periodicals, such as *John Bull*. Churchill advertised works on women's reproductive health such as Anderson's *Hysterical and Nervous Affections of Women* (1853) in the *Lady's Newspaper*, an illustrated broadsheet for upper-class women.

Why did medical publishers advertise in these spaces? One reason may be that medical practitioners read non-medical newspapers and magazines, often more frequently than they read medical journals. Another reason may be that the lines between the categories of professional and popular reading material were blurrier than they are today. Just as middle and working-class readers bought manuals that excerpted works aimed at medical practitioners, middle- and

[89] Review of *The Greatest of Our Social Evils*, *Edinburgh Medical and Surgical Journal*, vol. III (Edinburgh: Sutherland and Knox. London: Simpkin, Marshall, and Co, 1858), 79.

[90] Review of *Greatest*, *Edinburgh Medical and Surgical Journal*, 79–80.

[91] Review of *Greatest*, *Edinburgh Medical and Surgical Journal*, 80.

upper-class readers often bought such works themselves. Although the implied audience of George Spratt's *Obstetric Tables* is medical students, for instance, a review in the *Athenaeum* anticipated that monied readers would find it attractive as a collector's item.[92] Readers of all classes also turned to medical textbooks to learn about the body and sexuality. Undigested by editors, textbooks could be difficult to navigate, however. Allen Clarke, the son of provincial textile workers, skimmed through physiology textbooks in the public library in hopes of learning more about sex and reproduction but found them "incomprehensible."[93] Middle-class readers like the novelist George Eliot, who read anatomy and physiology textbooks aloud with her partner, George Lewes, in the evenings, found them easier to work through. However, even Eliot switched to lighter books after dinner.[94]

Interest in capturing crossover readerships may be one of the reasons that prices for medical works dropped precipitously in the first decades of the Victorian period, a pattern that tracks the general trend toward cheap print explored in previous chapters. However, medical practitioners' perennial complaints that books were too expensive are more likely the main reason that medical publishers decided, as Churchill put it, that it was "better to realise a profit from a large number [of books] at low prices, than from the sale of a limited number at high prices."[95] In 1842, the cheapest work on sexual or reproductive issues advertised by a medical publisher in the non-medical press was Francis Burdett Courtenay's five-shilling *Nature and Cure of Strictures of the Urethra*.[96] Twelve shillings was a more typical price, and some works were much more expensive.[97] Between the late 1840s and 1860, however, prices for these works plummeted to a median two shillings and sixpence, matching the prices of many Holywell Street productions.

Although it is possible to interpret medical publishers' newspaper advertisements as attempts to reach practitioners who rarely read medical journals or to capture cross-over readerships, writers in the medical press often interpreted them differently: in their eyes, these advertisements were "auto-advertising" at work. As Milton observed in *A New Way of Treating Gonorrhoea*, the number of works on gonorrhoea and syphilis listed in the catalogue of the library of the Royal College of Surgeons of England had increased exponentially between the seventeenth century and 1844, the year Milton's book was published, despite the fact that knowledge of these diseases and methods of treating them had barely advanced. The sheer number of works on venereal disease

92 Whiteley, "Spratt's Flaps."

93 Jonathan Rose, *The Intellectual Life of the British Working Classes*, 2nd ed. (New Haven, CT: Yale University Press, 2010), 210.

94 George Eliot, *The Journals of George Eliot*, ed. Margaret Harris (Cambridge: Cambridge University Press, 1998), 57.

95 "Obituary: John Churchill," *Medical Times and Gazette*, August 14, 1875, 199.

96 *Satirist; or, the Censor of the Times*, October 12, 1845, 322.

97 For instance, see notices in *Morning Post*, January 1, 1842, 1.

being published each year offered evidence, Milton suggested (apparently unaware of the irony of doing so in a book called *On A New Way of Treating Gonorrhoea*), that most practitioners were publishing simply to promote themselves. "Patients," he lamented, "have been half scalded in hot baths; the penis has been almost frozen with cold lotions; nay, the patient has been enjoined not to make water in the streets lest the penis might take cold," not on the basis of new knowledge but because doctors wanted to make names for themselves.[98]

Even when medical journalists thought that a work made an important contribution to knowledge, they increasingly interpreted its advertisement in the non-medical press as self-promotion: under the proxy of advertising a book, medical men were announcing to readers that they had the expertise to treat their health problems. Medical publishers' book advertisements were notably more restrained than consulting surgeons' notices. They were shorter, and eschewed flowery descriptions of the book's contents and its author's expertise. They provided no information about the location of the author's medical practice or his fees; mentioned no associated medicines or devices; and offered less information, and sometimes none at all, about where one might obtain a copy of the book. Yet, as medical journalists often pointed out, the prevalence of commission publishing arrangements meant that publishers' advertisements for medical books were frequently paid for by authors themselves. In 1851–2, for instance, part of the commission that William Acton paid John Churchill covered fees for advertising his *Practical Treatise on the Diseases of the Urinary and Generative Organs in Both Sexes* (1851) in a variety of periodicals, including *The Times*, the *Athenaeum*, and *Bell's Life in London*.[99] According to their critics, the only thing that separated such authors from irregulars like Joseph Lambert was the fact that the publisher put his name on the advertisement: a prophylactic against the appearance of quackery.

In regular medical circles, then, concerns about selling sexual knowledge had shifted from the turn of the century, when William Burke anxiously informed readers of his *Popular Compendium of Anatomy* (1804) that they would find nothing in his book that would "be in the least offensive to the delicacy of a chastened and correct mind."[100] Regular practitioners' anxieties about presenting sexual information to the public had become more and more interwoven with, and in some contexts almost swallowed by, anxieties about the fact that those who published and advertised books on these issues could be seen as quacks, or were, in

98 Milton, *On a New Way*, 2.

99 Longman 1/386/247–8, Records of the Longman Group, ABPP. To offer another example: Charles Drysdale, the physician and future president of the Malthusian League, whose work is outlined in Chapter 6, paid Baillière to advertise three of his books, *Syphilis*, *Alpine Heights*, and *Medicine for Women*, in *The Times* as well as four medical journals. See Baillière MS 1570/1/184–5, Records of the Longman Group, ABPP.

100 William Burke, *The Popular Compendium of Anatomy: or, A Concise and Clear Description of the Human Body* [. . .]. (London: S. Highley, 1804), 242.

fact, falling into quackery: degenerating from learned and disinterested men of science into low-class exploiters of knowledge for economic gain. This shift in the focus of medical anxieties about presenting sexual knowledge maps on to the increasing number and visibility of irregular publications on sexual health problems and advertisements for them, and medical reformers' increasing determination to distance medicine from market interests. As debates about what I call "paratextual contamination" show, the convoluted geography of the print marketplace compounded and extended concerns about the meanings and effects of advertising medical books in non-medical spaces. Medical men worried that the close proximity of regular and irregular publications in the space of the marketplace fostered confusions of professional identity that seriously undermined the medicine's reputation and legitimate practitioners' incomes.

Medical publishers occasionally issued books for doctors who were associated with irregular practice or who became associated with it over time: Churchill published an anatomical atlas for Joseph Kahn in 1852, for instance, and the Madrid branch of Baillière's firm issued J. L. Curtis's *Manhood* in Spanish in 1853.[101] More frequently, retailers sold regular and irregular medical works alongside each other. In the early 1840s, readers could find *Manhood* and R. and L. Perry & Co's *The Silent Friend* in Baillière's bookshop in Regent Street.[102] During a period in which periodicals multiplied and newspaper advertising skyrocketed, it was the fact that regular and irregular medical works were advertised in many of the same spaces, however, that became a subject of ongoing complaint in the medical press. In the eyes of many regular practitioners, there were very important differences in the content of regular and irregular medical book advertisements. However, these differences were not necessarily obvious to non-medical readers. Medical publishers promoted titles on the same or similar subjects as irregulars, and their advertisements necessarily employed some of the same language: for instance, medical publishers also advised readers that they could purchase books through the mail in exchange for postage stamps (though they did not offer the option to receive purchases in sealed envelopes).

In this context, the spatial proximity of medical publishers' and consulting surgeons' advertisements on the newspaper page became a focus of particular concern in the reforming medical press. Newspaper editors usually grouped the latter together at the bottom of their advertising pages, but they did not, as the *Lancet* complained, draw a "quarantine" around them. As a result, notices for regular and irregular publications often appeared "next door" to each other, bringing them into association on the space of the page (Figure 3.1). Medical

[101] Joseph Kahn, *Atlas of the Formation of the Human Body: In the Earliest Stages of Its Development* [...]. (London: John Churchill, 1852); J. L. Curtis, *De la virilidad: de las causas de su decadencia prematura é instrucciones para obtener su completo restablecimiento* [...]. (Madrid: C. Bailly- Baillière, 1853).

[102] See advertisements in *Morning Post*, January 1, 1842, 1; *Era*, January 16, 1842, 1.

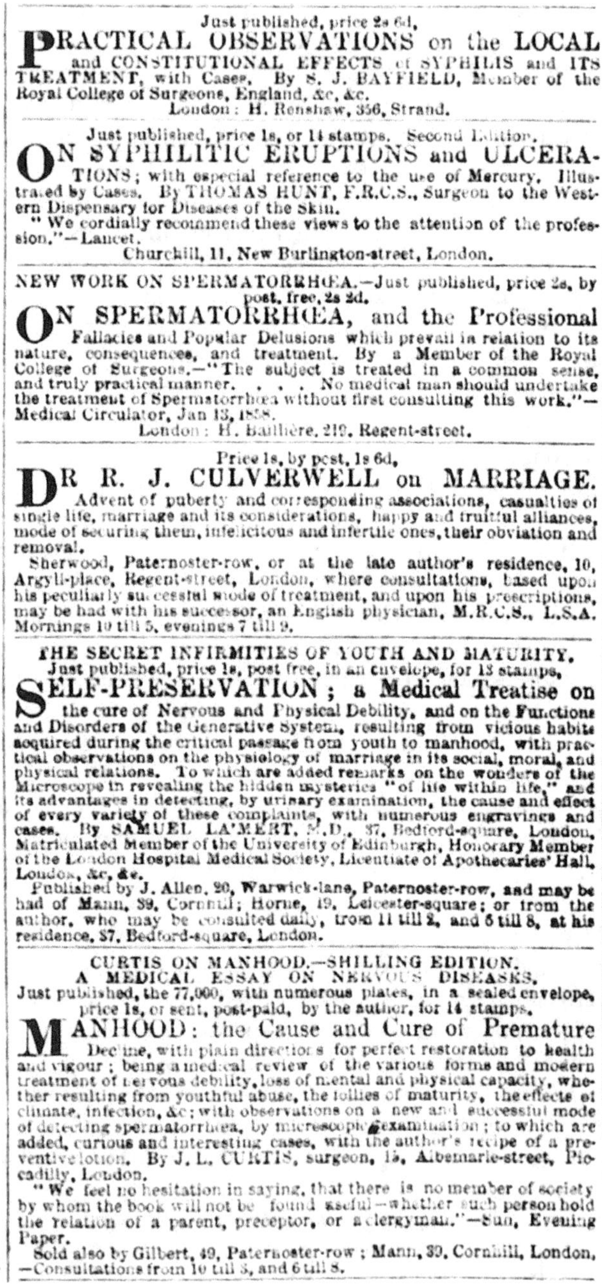

Just published, price 2s 6d,

PRACTICAL OBSERVATIONS on the LOCAL and CONSTITUTIONAL EFFECTS of SYPHILIS and ITS TREATMENT, with Cases. By S. J. BAYFIELD, Member of the Royal College of Surgeons, England, &c, &c.

London: H. Renshaw, 356, Strand.

Just published, price 1s, or 14 stamps. Second Edition.

ON SYPHILITIC ERUPTIONS and ULCERATIONS; with especial reference to the use of Mercury. Illustrated by Cases. By THOMAS HUNT, F.R.C.S., Surgeon to the Western Dispensary for Diseases of the Skin.

"We cordially recommend these views to the attention of the profession."—Lancet.

Churchill, 11, New Burlington-street, London.

NEW WORK ON SPERMATORRHŒA.—Just published, price 2s, by post, free, 2s 2d.

ON SPERMATORRHŒA, and the Professional Fallacies and Popular Delusions which prevail in relation to its nature, consequences, and treatment. By a Member of the Royal College of Surgeons.—"The subject is treated in a common sense, and truly practical manner. . . . No medical man should undertake the treatment of Spermatorrhœa without first consulting this work."—Medical Circulator, Jan 13, 1858.

London: H. Baillière, 219, Regent-street.

Price 1s, by post, 1s 6d,

DR R. J. CULVERWELL on MARRIAGE. Advent of puberty and corresponding associations, casualties of single life, marriage and its considerations, happy and fruitful alliances, mode of securing them, infelicitous and infertile ones, their obviation and removal.

Sherwood, Paternoster-row, or at the late author's residence, 10, Argyll-place, Regent-street, London, where consultations, based upon his peculiarly successful mode of treatment, and upon his prescriptions, may be had with his successor, an English physician, M.R.C.S., L.S.A. Mornings 10 till 5, evenings 7 till 9.

THE SECRET INFIRMITIES OF YOUTH AND MATURITY.

Just published, price 1s, post free, in an envelope, for 13 stamps,

SELF-PRESERVATION; a Medical Treatise on the cure of Nervous and Physical Debility, and on the Functions and Disorders of the Generative System, resulting from vicious habits acquired during the critical passage from youth to manhood, with practical observations on the physiology of marriage in its social, moral, and physical relations. To which are added remarks on the wonders of the Microscope in revealing the hidden mysteries "of life within life," and its advantages in detecting, by urinary examination, the cause and effect of every variety of these complaints, with numerous engravings and cases. By SAMUEL LA'MERT, M.D., 37, Bedford-square, London, Matriculated Member of the University of Edinburgh, Honorary Member of the London Hospital Medical Society, Licentiate of Apothecaries' Hall, London, &c, &c.

Published by J. Allen, 20, Warwick-lane, Paternoster-row, and may be had of Mann, 39, Cornhill; Horne, 19, Leicester-square; or from the author, who may be consulted daily, from 11 till 2, and 6 till 8, at his residence, 37, Bedford-square, London.

CURTIS ON MANHOOD.—SHILLING EDITION.

A MEDICAL ESSAY ON NERVOUS DISEASES.

Just published, the 77,000, with numerous plates, in a sealed envelope, price 1s, or sent, post-paid, by the author, for 14 stamps.

MANHOOD: the Cause and Cure of Premature Decline, with plain directions for perfect restoration to health and vigour; being a medical review of the various forms and modern treatment of nervous debility, loss of mental and physical capacity, whether resulting from youthful abuse, the follies of maturity, the effects of climate, infection, &c; with observations on a new and successful mode of detecting spermatorrhœa, by microscopic examination; to which are added, curious and interesting cases, with the author's recipe of a preventive lotion. By J. L. CURTIS, surgeon, 15, Albemarle-street, Piccadilly, London.

"We feel no hesitation in saying, that there is no member of society by whom the book will not be found useful—whether such person hold the relation of a parent, preceptor, or a clergyman."—Sun, Evening Paper.

Sold also by Gilbert, 49, Paternoster-row; Mann, 39, Cornhill, London, —Consultations from 10 till 3, and 6 till 8.

Figure 3.1 "Next door" advertisements for regular and irregular medical works in *Bell's Life in London and Sporting Chronicle*, February 14, 1858, 2. Content provided by The British Library Board, with thanks to The British Newspaper Archive.

writers worried that this practice made works like *Manhood* and *The Silent Friend* look legitimate, and thus enabled men like Joseph Lambert to make "enormous" incomes, "all filched from the profession . . . or extorted from the public." They also worried that bringing regular medical works "into contact with these abominations" on the page made regular medical works look illegitimate.[103] Medical writers often called on newspaper editors to stop publishing consulting surgeons' advertisements, claiming that it would benefit them by attracting more advertising business. Many authors "have been deterred from advertising books in such papers, in consequence of observing those under the head of 'new publications' placed in juxta-position" with consulting surgeons' notices, one medical journalist argued.[104] Some dreamed up creative solutions that would enable newspaper editors to publish advertisements of both kinds while clearly separating them on the page. The *Lancet* proposed that editors "place blocks of non-conducting puffs between [consulting surgeons' notices] and the better sort of advertisement – Grimstone's snuff, Solomon's spectacles, or any other rubbish, might be used for such a purpose."[105]

Envisioning newspaper editors protecting medical publishers' advertisements from contamination by quarantining consulting surgeons' advertisements on the page, the *Lancet*'s proposal neatly illustrates regular practitioners' anxiety about being associated with quackery even as it reveals how this anxiety competed with their desire to reap the benefits of publicity through print. The image of the "non-conducting puff" also echoes the role that publishers played in mediating these anxieties: they insulated medical authors from direct contact with the market. Yet, this was a precarious arrangement, one threatened by suspicion of publishers' motives, suspicion of authors' motives, and concern about the confusions of professional identity that consulting surgeons actively encouraged and that the crowded geography of the print marketplace helped facilitate. Overlaps in the publishing and advertising practices examined in this and the previous chapters really do seem to have fostered confusions of identity even in the medical community, as a student's letter to the *Medical Times* about a book he had seen Baillière advertising in the press in 1851 illustrates. "Is the author of the 'Philosophy of Marriage' (published by Baillière, Regent-street.) *the* Dr. Ryan," the letter reads, "or does it emanate from some parties assuming his name, in the 'Silent Friend' style?"[106]

The first decades of the Victorian period marked great changes in medical publishing and book advertising. By the middle of the nineteenth century, the print marketplace was awash with medical writing on sexual matters and

103 Review of *Brodie's Secret*, *Lancet*, 564.
104 "The Obscene Medical Sharpers," *Dublin Medical Press*, December 23, 1846, 411.
105 Review of *Brodie's Secret*, *Lancet*, 564.
106 "To Correspondents," *Medical Times*, September 13, 1851, 295.

teeming with different players whose products and practices blurred together in multiple ways. This chapter aimed to demonstrate anxiety about this situation in regular medical circles, where it came from, and where it was directed. There was an increasing sense, particularly among medical reformers, that something had to change if medicine was to develop itself into a coherent, "scientific" profession that was perceived as trustworthy and worthy of public trust in the first place. Initially, this did not involve serious attempts to discipline regular medical publishing or book advertising, however. Instead, as the next chapter shows, amid mounting assaults on the Holywell Street trade by anti-vice crusaders, organs of reform like the *Lancet* attacked consulting surgeons on the grounds that they peddled "obscene quackery." This progression affirms Michael Brown's argument that defining a collective identity for medicine first entailed firmly situating "those deemed 'unorthodox' in knowledge, practice, or education" outside the profession.[107]

[107] Brown, "Medicine, Quackery," 240.

4 Obscene . . . in a Certain Sense

Edward Duncombe was minding his bookshop in Upper St. Martin's Lane when a strange man came through the door. He wore a travelling cloak, as if he had just returned from a journey, and asked Duncombe for "some Songs and a catalogue of obscene Books for a friend in the Country."[1] Money was no object. He was willing to pay two or three guineas apiece for the books his friend was looking for. The stranger had come to the right place. Duncombe, 63, ran a brisk trade in smutty song books, and sold pornographic novels and prints under the name John Wilson. He had recently returned to his business after a two-year stint in Cold Bath Fields Prison, having made the mistake of selling one of those novels to a man who had visited his shop repeatedly, promising to pay an enormous sum.[2] That man had been an agent for the Society for the Suppression of Vice, Britain's longest-running anti-vice society. Duncombe had no appetite for another prison sentence. He told the stranger that he did not sell obscene books, or know anyone who did. The stranger was not discouraged. He returned to Duncombe's shop again and again, asking for specific titles: *The Confessions of Madame Vestris* (c. 1830), an epistolary account of youthful seduction and wedding-night bliss, and *Seraglio Scenes* (1830s), a harem fantasy "by the author of 'The Lusty Turk'."[3] Each time, Duncombe refused.

Duncombe's instincts had not failed him. One day, at the conclusion of yet another disappointing visit, the stranger did not slink away from the bookshop. Instead, he turned to the door and called out to a group of police officers waiting in the street. They crowded in. One of the officers instructed the old bookseller not to move, lest he handcuff him and "strap him down." Then a plain-clothes officer entered with an agent for the Society for the Suppression of Vice. Together, they ransacked Duncombe's shop, rifling through the drawers behind

[1] "Edward Duncombe, of 28 Little Andrew Street, Saint Martins Lane, Charged with Selling Obscene Prints: Defendant's Statements," April 16, 1856, MJ/SP/1856/006, LMA.

[2] "Court of the Queen's Bench, Dec. 7," *Globe*, Thursday, December 8, 1853, 4.

[3] "Edward Duncombe, of 28 Little Andrew Street." It may be significant that this agent's words – at least, as they were recorded by Duncombe – echoed phrases in Duncombe's sales catalogues. The police and anti-vice crusaders seem to have relied on sales catalogues to conduct stings. See Chapter 6 for another example.

the counter and scattering books and papers everywhere. Try as they might, however, they "could not find any obscene or improper Books or Prints."[4] After the search was over, the plain-clothes officer turned to the Society agent and told him to take what he wanted. The agent took one last look around the shop. Eventually, he pocketed a handful of plates from behind the counter, and five or six books that struck Duncombe as unremarkable. "Commonly sold and exposed in Shop Windows," they included three medical titles: "Aristotle's Works, Physiology of Man, and Physiology of Woman." A few weeks later, in April 1856, Duncombe found himself in court, charged with distributing obscene material.

Duncombe had been selling cheap medical works for about twenty years. Among other things, he marketed them as titillating reading material. But would any judge or jury consider them obscene? Duncombe did not believe it. And if there is any truth to this story, which he submitted to support his defence at trial, the leaders of the Society for the Suppression of Vice shared his doubt. The Society did not present *Aristotle's Works*, *Physiology of Woman*, or, indeed, any of the books that Duncombe claimed its agent had seized from his shop as evidence of his crime. Instead, it presented the judge with a lavishly illustrated pornographic volume. The stranger, a paid witness for the Society named Blower Halden, claimed that Duncombe had sold it to him for thirty shillings after a friendly round of haggling. The book wasn't a plant, Halden added hastily: before he entered Duncombe's bookshop, "his pockets were searched by Sargent Thomas of the F. Division to see that he had no book about him, and when he came out he immediately handed the book in question to the officer, who was waiting in the street, and both marked it with their signatures."[5]

Who was telling the truth in this episode is less important than what it emphasizes about the status of cheap medical works on sexual matters at the time. They were assumed to attract prurient readers. Their authors and publishers could be harangued for pandering to those readers. They were sometimes marketed as titillating reading material. However, as the diverse, open trade explored in the previous chapters suggests, selling them was not considered a legal risk. The expansion of the print marketplace had certainly aroused anxieties that extended far beyond regular practitioners' concerns about its effects on the medical profession. Readers now despaired at how to navigate the sheer amount of published material available for sale.[6] The limits of publicly acceptable display also became a more frequent topic of debate. Together with manuals on venereal disease, reprints of old midwifery books, and works on female beauty, the publishing industry boom had made salacious

4 "Edward Duncombe, of 28 Little Andrew Street."
5 "Middlesex Sessions," *Times*, April 17, 1856, 11.
6 Maurice S. Lee, *Overwhelmed: Literature, Aesthetics, and the Nineteenth-Century Information Revolution* (Princeton, NJ: Princeton University Press, 2019).

penny papers, thrilling sensation novels, and gossipy news reports on divorce, inheritance, and sexual assault cases ubiquitous.[7] Stereoscopic slides of Parisian ballet dancers were being displayed in shop windows across London, and advertisements for nude photographs were beginning to trickle into the press.[8]

If the past few chapters have emphasized anything, it is that such materials were subject to a range of interpretations. The same medical work could be considered a shameless piece of self-promotion, a source of scientific knowledge, a means of moral instruction, a guide to a pleasurable sex life, convenient masturbation material, or some combination of these things. Victorian views about what was and was not beyond the limits of public display consequently diverged, sometimes in the extreme. For some Londoners, nude statues on display at the Crystal Palace, the site of Britain's 1851 Great Exhibition of the Works of Industry of All Nations, were grossly offensive. For others, a campaign to have the statues' genitals covered up was a cartoonish display of cultural ignorance.[9] There was only one cultural form that almost everyone, including publishers like Duncombe, agreed was obscene: unrelentingly explicit fiction like *The Confessions of Madame Vestris*, and the kinds of prints it was often packaged with. In a context in which laws against the display and distribution of obscene material existed, but a legal definition of obscenity did not, this meant that throughout the 1830s and 1840s prosecutions for obscenity overwhelmingly focused on pornography, the emergent, as-yet unnamed genre whose production and distribution Duncombe and his competitors were turning into an industry.

That pattern changed in the 1850s. Duncombe's 1856 trial did not surround medical works. However, it was bookended by a series of legal actions that ended in the destruction of cheap medical books and pamphlets and the shuttering of public anatomical museums on the grounds that they were obscene. This chapter examines these developments, and how they were driven by medical reformers' mounting concerns about consulting surgeons and public anatomical museums, and the Society for the Suppression of Vice's determination to shut the Holywell Street trade down. The mid-nineteenth century is often characterized as a watershed moment in which anxieties about print and sex set off a moral panic that established new standards for public display. The events examined in this chapter paint a different picture,

[7] Barbara Leckie, *Culture and Adultery: The Novel, the Newspaper, and the Law, 1857–1914* (Philadelphia: University of Pennsylvania Press, 1999); Thomas Boyle, *Black Swine in the Sewers of Hampstead: Beneath the Surface of Victorian Sensationalism* (New York: Viking, 1989).

[8] Lynda Nead, *Victorian Babylon: People, Streets, and Images in Nineteenth-Century London* (New Haven, CT: Yale University Press, 2000) .

[9] Jan Piggott, *Palace of the People: The Crystal Palace at Sydenham, 1854–1936* (London: Hurst, 2004), 52.

one that affirms Katherine Mullin's recent argument that "the 'Victorian morality' supposedly encapsulated in the 1857 [Obscene Publications] Act and underscored in its 1868 refinement was something of a [modernist] fantasy."[10] They emphasize how tirelessly, and often ineffectually, small groups worked to whip up opposition to publications and displays that were widely tolerated, less out of concern for their specific effects on British citizens than out of opposition to particular kinds of businesses that had grown large and lucrative in the new age of mass print.

In examining how and why these groups argued that medical works were obscene in the hands of certain players, this chapter offers a picture of crystallizing strategies that would impact medical bookselling for decades to come, and influence how regular practitioners and, later, sex radicals contested and produced authority. Medical reformers made allegations of obscenity to undermine a kind of entrepreneur that they considered a threat to the medical profession and its members, while the Society for the Suppression of Vice embraced such allegations amid a flagging crusade against commercial vice culture. While gaps in the historical record make the Society's arguments difficult to access, medical reformers and some members of the judiciary supported these allegations by promoting contextual models of obscenity justified by paternalistic ideas about the reading capacities of women, children, and especially young men, the largest target audience of consulting surgeons and Holywell Street publishers alike. Medical works distributed in certain ways to certain audiences, they suggested, presented a danger to public morals in ways that they would not in other contexts.

By positioning the question of how a publication was being sold as crucial in obscenity cases, contextual models of obscenity addressed two obstacles that the groups I examine ran into. The first was the culture of reprinting and excerption that the Victorian print marketplace was built on, which meant that medical representations that these groups framed as obscene did not simply fall into roughly the same genre as works that they framed as legitimate. They were often very similar textually. The second obstacle was rapid crystallization of pornography's identity in the hands of a new, specialized body of producers. It did not yet have a name. Nevertheless, it was a media form that many people considered instantly recognizable by the 1850s, and it offered a standard against which works like *Aristotle's Masterpiece* would always be compared. The formulation of a legal "test of obscenity" in 1868, examined towards the end of the chapter, established commercial context as vital to determining obscenity in legal cases, affirming arguments examined in this chapter. As we shall see, the test's introduction did not necessarily sway public, governmental,

[10] Katherine Mullin, "Unmasking *The Confessional Unmasked*: The 1868 *Hicklin* Test and the Toleration of Obscenity," *ELH* 85, no. 2 (2018): 495–496.

or judicial opinions as to whether medical works could fairly be called obscene. Many people were not convinced. However, its introduction would prove to be a significant turning point in the history of selling, and authorizing, sexual knowledge.

The Trials of Prosecution

The origins of British obscenity law lie more than a century prior to Duncombe's trial, in an attempt to put the bookseller Edmund Curll in prison. Curll was known for publishing piracies, state secrets, and bawdy books, and tried to barter favour by acting as a political informant. His antics made him powerful enemies in the government, and by the middle of the 1720s they were determined to punish him. In 1725, the Crown had Curll arrested for selling "Lewd and Infamous Books." However, it found it difficult to establish that Curll had committed a crime. The works it presented to the court as evidence were *Venus in the Cloister, or, The Nun in her Smock* (1724), an English version of an anti-Catholic piece of French erotica, and *A Treatise on the Use of Flogging in Venereal Affairs* (1718), a translation of a Latin production framed as a medical treatise. Both works could be considered immoral, but, in England, neither counted as blasphemous, libellous, or seditious. Moral matters were dealt with in ecclesiastical courts under canon law, and Curll's counsel argued that common law had no jurisdiction in the case. Ultimately, a novel counter-argument prevailed and, in 1727, the common-law misdemeanour of obscene libel joined those of blasphemous and seditious libel. What made Curll's actions criminal, judges in the case decided, was that he dealt in *printed* works, which could be distributed "all over the kingdom." Curll's actions constituted a threat to public morality because his publications could spread around and "affect all of the King's subjects."[11]

Recognizing obscenity law's origins in an attempt to punish a single troublesome bookseller is helpful to understanding how it operated in England more than a century on. It did not ban books or censure authors, but targeted isolated acts of publication, display, or distribution. Its highly individualized applications meant that it was enforced very inconsistently and, as we shall see, enabled a certain amount of legal creativity: as in Curll's case, charges of obscenity were often driven by concerns that stretched beyond, and in some cases had little to do with, the works at issue. This origin story also helps explain the state's relatively hands-off stance on enforcement. Obscene libel's status as a misdemeanour rested on the argument that obscene material

[11] *Rex v. Curl* 1727, *English Reports* 93: 850–851. For a thorough account of Curll's career, arrest, and trial, see Paul Baines and Pat Rogers, *Edmund Curll, Bookseller* (Oxford: Oxford University Press, 2007).

endangered all of the monarch's subjects. Yet, the government was never strongly invested in protecting them from it. While the police played an increasingly important role in obscenity cases during the nineteenth century, no public prosecutor was ever charged with bringing them to court. That task was mostly left up to private parties, who were welcomed to prosecute those who dealt in obscene material – and to shoulder the costs of doing so.

For most of the nineteenth century, the Society for the Suppression of Vice primarily enforced obscenity laws in England. On its establishment in 1802, the middle-class Anglican organization outlined some extraordinarily broad goals: it aimed to combat "profanation of the Lord's day and profane swearing; publication of blasphemous, licentious and obscene books and prints; selling by false weights and measures; keeping disorderly public houses, brothels and gaming houses; procuring; illegal lotteries; [and] cruelty to animals."[12] Suppressing so many forms of immorality proved impossible for the Society, whose use of *agent provocateurs* to catch vice in action made it so unpopular with the public that it perennially struggled to attract members. It drifted from campaign to campaign. At various times, it waged war on Sunday trading, blasphemy, racecourses, betting shops, West End prostitution, and sensational journalism, only to give up after a few years. There was one exception to this pattern: the Society's opposition to the Holywell Street trade. The Society had been a stalwart enemy of radical politics in the 1810s and 1820s, bringing fourteen actions for blasphemous libel against Richard Carlile and his family members, and it was a consistent opponent of the raucous trade in sexual material that grew out of radical circles.[13]

The Society's decades-long crusade against Holywell Street publishers was plagued by problems largely caused by the nature of obscenity law itself. One of the most significant was that prosecutions for obscene libel were expensive, time-consuming affairs. The Society relied on regular donations from a small number of wealthy patrons, including Eton College and the Dean of Westminster, and occasional bequests from deceased members to fund its activities.[14] It never had enough money to bring all the prosecutions it wanted to. Aiming to maximize their impact, it tended to target the most successful

[12] M. J. D. Roberts, "The Society for the Suppression of Vice and Its Early Critics, 1802–1812," *History Journal* 26, no. 1 (1983): 159. For further information about the Society and its history, see Roberts, "Making Victorian Morals? The Society for the Suppression of Vice and Its Critics, 1802–1886," *Australian Historical Studies* 21, no. 83 (1984): 157–173 and Colin Manchester, "Obscenity Law and Its Enforcement in the Nineteenth Century," *Journal of Legal History* 2, no. 1 (1981): 45–61.

[13] "Society for the Suppression of Vice (U.K.)," in *Encyclopedia of Censorship*, eds. Jonathon Green and Nicholas J. Karolides (London: Infobase, 2014), 521. See William St. Clair, *The Reading Nation in the Romantic Period* (Cambridge: Cambridge University Press, 2004), 313 for further details about the Society's pursuit of Carlile and his family.

[14] See Society for the Suppression of Vice account records (1802–91), HBM; Manchester, "Lord Campbell's Act," 225.

Holywell Street publishers. All told, it prosecuted William Dugdale nine times. As the fact that the Society repeatedly prosecuted Dugdale suggests, however, its actions had little practical impact. According to the Society, the number of shops known for selling sexual material in London did fall from nearly sixty in the 1830s to about twenty by 1850.[15] However, the massive expansion of Holywell Street newspaper advertising over this period suggests that if this is true, it probably had less to do with the Society's prosecutions than it did with the increasing popularity of postal retailing, and the dominance that Dugdale, Duncombe, and a few other figures came to exert over the trade.

Why were the Society's prosecutions so ineffectual? People often speculated that Holywell Street publishers got charges against them dropped or dismissed by calling on friends made in high places through their trade in luxury pornography. A former compositor of Dugdale's claimed to have bumped into him at his shop just a few months after he had been sentenced to two years in prison.[16] However, it appears that the main problem was, again, the law itself, which did not have the capacity to ban books, nor destroy businesses. A bookseller could be fined or sent to prison for up to two years for distributing obscene publications, and the state could destroy his copies of the works at issue. However, new editions of the same works could and did freely enter the market, as competitors capitalized on the free publicity that obscenity trials generated. In many cases, as the Society's secretary, Henry Pritchard, complained in 1857, Holywell Street publishers' families continued to run their businesses while they were in prison, sometimes issuing copies of the same works they had been prosecuted for selling. These offences would have to be dealt with separately to get the works off the street.[17]

The Society had enduring faith that more legal action would resolve these problems, and repeatedly lobbied Parliament to pass legislation to make it less expensive and more expedient. Thanks to these efforts, a clause in the 1824 Vagrancy Act banned the exposure of "any obscene print, picture, or exhibition" "in any street, road, highway, or public place," and enabled offenders to be summarily tried before a magistrate.[18] Unfortunately for the Society, the clause did not cover material displayed in shop windows (a shop window was not legally a public place), nor material sold inside a bookshop. Prosecution for obscene libel remained the Society's only recourse in these cases. More lobbying eventually secured clauses in the 1838 Vagrancy Act, which made displaying obscene articles in windows an offence, and the 1839 Metropolitan Police Act, which enabled the police to take sellers of obscene articles into

[15] HC Deb August 12, 1857, vol. 147, col. 1480.

[16] Thomas Frost, *Reminiscences of a Country Journalist* (London: Ward and Downey, 1886), 54.

[17] HL Deb June 25, 1857, vol. 146, col. 328.

[18] Quoted in Colette Colligan, *The Traffic in Obscenity from Byron to Beardsley: Sexuality and Exoticism in Nineteenth-Century Print Culture* (Basingstoke: Palgrave Macmillan, 2006), 11.

custody without a warrant. These developments fostered cooperation between the Society and the Metropolitan Police force, and, at first, they enabled more prosecutions.

However, Holywell Street publishers were nothing if not adaptive. Dugdale baited the Society on at least one occasion by displaying racy prints affixed with strategically placed labels in his shop windows, but most cleaned up their window displays.[19] The Society did not consider this much of a victory. Its goal was to kill the trade itself. To keep prosecutions going, it fell back on an old trick: paying young men to visit Holywell Street publishers' shops and purchase items that could be used as evidence for prosecutions. Holywell Street publishers soon caught on. Suspected agents were sent away with bawdy songsters and other merely suggestive material. Recognized agents were packed off with religious pamphlets. By the middle of the 1840s, the Society and its allies in the police force had taken to using the bawdy material to apply for warrants to search their shops for explicit publications. Once again, Holywell Street publishers adapted. They concealed their explicit productions and kept their eyes peeled for police officers. In 1851, one of Dugdale's shop-boys recognized officers approaching his shop at no. 37 Holywell Street, locked them out, and dashed to Dugdale's second shop at no. 16 Holywell Street. By the time the police arrived at no. 16, a mass of books and prints was burning in the fireplace.[20]

The difficulty of procuring evidence to prosecute Holywell Street publishers was deeply frustrating to the Society and its allies in the police force. In their zeal to crack down on the Holywell Street trade in the face of its seemingly unstoppable expansion, they began to ignore the letter of the law. In March 1856, shortly after the alleged ransacking of Duncombe's shop, John Stanton, an agent for the Society, and seven police officers stormed into Dugdale's house while he was out on business. They did not have a warrant to search it. Nevertheless, as a "great crowd" looked on from the street, they did so and seized thousands of books, prints, and stereotype plates on the grounds that they were obscene. Dugdale was incandescent with fury. He was also prepared. William F. Howe, a legal clerk he had hired to get him out of Cold Bath Fields Prison a few years earlier, had been at the house in his absence. With Howe's assistance, Dugdale sued Stanton for entering his residence and seizing his property. The police raid had been illegal, Dugdale argued, and Stanton's actions had been burglary. This time, Dugdale had the law on his side.[21]

[19] "The Queen v. William Dugdale the Elder," MJ/SP/1850/05/010, 2, LMA.

[20] "The Abomination of Holywell-Street," *Morning Advertiser*, September 25, 1851, 6.

[21] "Court of the Exchequer," *Reynolds's Newspaper*, July 13, 1856, 16. For information about Howe, whose later career in New York rivalled Dugdale's for notoriety, see Richard H. Rovere, *Howe and Hummel: Their True and Scandalous History* (New York: Farrar, Strauss, 1947).

The lawsuit embarrassed the Society, the police, and the judiciary. Dugdale and his supporters dredged up mishandling of previous obscenity cases, boldly defended his trade in explicit literature, and ridiculed the Society's claim that all of the items seized in the raid were obscene. Acting as a witness, one of Dugdale's daughters, Frances Thornhill, testified that she – a married woman with three children – did sell "what you [the judge] call obscene books" at her father's shop. However, she declared, "I do not call 'Fanny Hill' obscene. Coloured figures of naked men and women are in that book, but you can also see them at the Crystal Palace." Watchers in the court gallery laughed. Seeing that the judge was unconvinced by Thornhill's views on Dugdale's edition of John Cleland's *Memoirs of a Woman of Pleasure*, Howe took the argument in a more conciliatory direction. He hastened to agree that the work was indecent. But, he pointed out, Stanton and the police had illegally seized "some thousands [of works] . . . which are not so. There are the 'Sam Hall' song books, for instance, with Mr. Robson in *Villikins* (laughter); the 'Fifteen Comforts of Matrimony,' by Sheridan; Dr. Culverwell's works; Lord Byron's 'Cain'; 'Animated Legs'." The gallery roared with laughter.[22]

Howe found support on the witness stand as well as in the gallery. An arbitrator called by the court, a Soho stereotype founder, agreed with Howe's assessment of Dugdale's publications. Having sifted through the mass of books, prints, and stereotype plates seized from Dugdale's house, the founder declared that the "only obscene works amongst it are 'Fanny Hill,' 'Scenes in a Harem,' 'The Trial of Roger for a Game at Romps' and the 'Adventures of a Bedpost'," all well-known erotic titles. "The remainder," he opined, "are mostly medical works and facetious, humourous tales, but are not obscene or indecent."[23] Dugdale won his suit. But the Society refused to back down. It pushed on with its actions, and with lobbying of government. The following year, seizing property suspected of being obscene became legal, and the raid on Dugdale's shop became a model for action against the Holywell Street trade. This shift in strategy brought works like *Aristotle's Masterpiece* and R. and L. Perry & Co's *The Silent Friend* to the centre of courtroom debates about the boundaries of obscenity law.

Medical Works in Court

The Society for the Suppression of Vice found a saviour in the Lord Chief Justice, John Campbell: a man who was both an active politician in the House of Lords and a judge who had ruled for the Society in many obscenity cases over the years.[24] In May 1857, Campbell presided over two obscenity trials.

[22] "Court of the Exchequer," *Reynolds's Newspaper*, 16.
[23] "Court of the Exchequer," *Reynolds's Newspaper*, 16.
[24] For instance, see "Court of the Queen's Bench, Dec. 7," *Globe*, 4.

One was yet another trial for William Dugdale, who was charged with selling "prints of an indecent nature" and an "obscene and disgusting book."[25] The proceedings were memorable. After recounting Stanton's actions the previous year and suggesting that lines in Campbell's staid chronicle *Lives of the Chancellors and Keepers of the Great Seal in England* (1848–50) were grossly indecent, Dugdale cried that he had not had a fair trial, brandished a knife, and threatened to commit suicide on the spot. But the trial that lingered in Campbell's mind was that of William Strange, another printer, publisher, and bookseller connected with radical politics, for selling *Paul Pry*, a flash penny paper that spun its stories about sexual scandal as a campaign to expose metropolitan vice.

Like other flash papers, *Paul Pry* was suggestive, but not sexually explicit. The Society's decision to target a periodical of such "low-level smuttiness" has been interpreted as a sign of its determination to draw a firm "distinction between acceptability and unacceptability" in print culture.[26] The Society certainly found the paper's adoption of its anti-vice rhetoric as a fig leaf for publishing courtesan biographies offensive. However, it is doubtful that it targeted *Paul Pry* solely for its content. Flash papers frequently promoted and were sometimes backed by Holywell Street publishers. *Paul Pry* was printed at Strange's address for a pseudonymous proprietor, and the only person who advertised in it was William Dugdale, who used the paper to spread word about his "extensive Catalogue of Rare and Curious Works."[27] The Society convinced Campbell that comparatively innocent works like *Paul Pry* could be moral poison, and opened his eyes to how interwoven trade in such works was with trade in pornography.[28] Watchers in the court gallery had laughed at the

25 "Law Intelligence," *Morning Chronicle*, May 11, 1857, 8.

26 Nead, *Victorian Babylon*, 221.

27 "Advertisement: Now Publishing," *Paul Pry*, October 11, 1856, 8. It is impossible to know what was really going on in this case. It is unclear whether the William Strange involved was William Strange the elder, a contemporary of Dugdale's, or his son, William Strange the younger. Dugdale may or may not have been involved in *Paul Pry* beyond advertising in it. The only other periodicals I have seen in which Dugdale was the sole advertiser were those he published, but the pseudonym under which *Paul Pry* was issued, Richard Martin, was not identified with Dugdale. Given that the Society never attempted to prosecute figures like William West, a radical publisher-bookseller known for his trade in bawdy material, my guess is that the Society believed that *Paul Pry* and Strange were connected with the pornography trade, a charge that Strange denied in court. For a record in which Strange addressed the idea that he was connected with the "Holywell-street gang," see "The Queen v. Strange," *Saint James's Chronicle*, May 12, 1857, 1. On the question of which Strange was involved, see John Adcock, "A Strange Story – William Strange of Paternoster Row," *Yesterday's Papers*, accessed February 19, 2024, https://john-adcock.blogspot.com/2014/05/a-strange-story-william-strange-of.html. On West's free trade in bawdy material, see Ed Cray, "Introduction," in *Bawdy Songbooks of the Romantic Period: Items Published by William West* (1836–42), ed. Ed Cray (London: Routledge, 2022), xxix–xxxvi.

28 See "The Queen v. Strange," *Saint James's Chronicle*, 1; Campbell's words in HL Deb May 11, 1857, vol. 145, col. 103; and his discussion of Dugdale's business in HC Deb July 9, 1857, vol. 146, col. 1152.

idea that Dr. Culverwell's works were obscene. However, such works were a means through which young men were encouraged to seek out immoral pleasures – and purchase reading material that few Victorians would hesitate to call obscene.

Speaking of the matter in the House of Commons, Campbell cited Dugdale's translation of Alexandre Dumas the younger's romantic novel *La Dame aux camélias* (1848), which the bookselling firm W. H. Smith was then selling across the country in its popular railway bookstalls. Although he personally considered Dumas's novel "of a polluting character," Campbell admitted that few people would consider the novel obscene. However, he pointed out, Dugdale's translation was bound with a catalogue that advertised nearly a hundred publications, "most of which" were cheap and, he opined, "of a very abominable description indeed."[29] A copy at the British Library lists a mixture of pornographic novels, prints and albums, bawdy song books, night guides, medical works, and French letters for sale.[30] The catalogue transformed Dumas's novel into a gateway to iniquity. Advertisements for inexpensive editions of *Fanny Hill* and *The Adventures of a Bedpost* – works which, Campbell pointed out, had been found obscene in court – appeared at the top of its very first page. "What [is] the remedy for all this," he asked, "and how [is] the evidence to be procured?" The Society had told him of the difficulty it had in getting its hands on works like *The Adventures of a Bedpost*.[31]

Campbell's answer was a bill, drafted with the Society's help, that was designed to create exactly what it wanted in the wake of Dugdale's embarrassing lawsuit: a law that would enable the police to seize and destroy obscene material on sworn testimony that it was being sold to the public. Like the clauses in the Vagrancy Acts and the Metropolitan Police Act, Campbell's Obscene Publications Bill did not specify what obscene material was. Unlike those pieces of legislation, sellers whose property was searched and publications were destroyed would have no recourse to a hearing.[32]

The bill horrified many members of Parliament. Some members of the House of Lords argued that in failing to spell out what constituted obscenity, Campbell was making way for the destruction of great art and literature. Before long, an over-zealous police officer would surely mistake a classical nude for an indecent print.[33] In the House of Commons, debate centred on a different

29 HC Deb July 9, 1857, vol. 146, col. 1152.

30 See "Works Sold by H. Smith," in Alexander [*sic*] Dumas, *The Lady of the Camelias* [*sic*] (London: Henry Smith [William Dugdale], c. 1855), C.194.a.447(1), BL.

31 HC Deb July 9, 1857, vol. 146, col. 1152.

32 See Colin Manchester, "Lord Campbell's Act: England's First Obscenity Statute," *Journal of Legal History* 9, no. 2 (1988): 223–241 for a more thorough discussion of the Obscene Publications Bill's design and its passage through Parliament.

33 HL Deb June 25, 1857, vol. 146, col. 328. Nead, *Victorian Babylon*, 193 offers an extended analysis of this argument.

problem: Campbell's bill invited deliberate abuses of the law. Leaving the term "obscene" undefined, some MPs argued, would incite a flood of frivolous lawsuits. Recalling Dugdale's recent performance in court, one predicted that the "literary works of Lord Campbell himself – his *Lives of the Lord Chancellors* . . . would be made the subject of prosecutions."[34] Others worried that frustrated authorities would exploit the bill's provisions to search the property of people suspected of committing other crimes. And others were certain that competitors would use them to attack each other. The MP Richard Monckton Milnes reported that booksellers "entertained a well-grounded fear that, in a trade in which so much competition existed, the Bill, if passed, would enable any man, hostilely disposed towards them, to . . . declare upon an oath, that he knew they had some obscene books in their possession," a claim that could lead to a raid on their businesses and, potentially, the unwarranted destruction of their stock.[35] Campbell aimed to kill a cancer on the book trade, but his cure would poison the industry.

None of these objections was unfounded.[36] But Campbell was stubborn. Although he eventually altered the bill so that a magistrate, judge, or justice of the peace would decide whether works seized by the police were destroyed, and although he insisted that the bill was intended to apply "exclusively to works written for the single purpose of corrupting the morals of youth" – which ensured that it passed in August 1857 – he refused to define the term "obscene."[37] Why? Some scholars have suggested that Campbell, the Lord Chief Justice, was naïve and thought that obscenity was self-evident; others, that he thought defining obscenity too difficult to accomplish without endangering his bill. However, Campbell's zeal to rid England of Holywell Street publishers, and his knowledge of how they operated, suggests a third possibility: Campbell knew that leaving the term open to interpretation was the only way to have a chance at destroying the Holywell Street trade. In isolation, few people considered many of the works that Dugdale sold obscene. He took care to conceal works that were widely seen as offensive from the authorities – and

[34] HC Deb August 12, 1857, vol. 147, col. 1479

[35] HC Deb August 12, 1857, vol. 147, col. 1480. Scholars often do not take Milnes's remarks seriously because he was a collector and author of expensive pornography and thus had a personal interest in blocking Campbell's bill. However, as the next chapters suggest, these remarks were perceptive.

[36] Radicals charged with blasphemous libel had previously sued respected publishers for blasphemous libel in protest. Campbell presided over some of the proceedings. See Jim Cheshire, *Tennyson and Mid-Victorian Publishing: Moxon, Poetry, Commerce* (Basingstoke: Palgrave Macmillan, 2016), 40. Moreover, business owners often weaponized allegations of immorality to attack competitors. For instance, see Lee Jackson's account of skirmishes between brewers and owners of gin palaces in *Palaces of Pleasure: From Music Halls to the Seaside to Football, How the Victorians Invented Mass Entertainment* (New Haven, CT: Yale University Press, 2019), 21, 70–84.

[37] HL Deb June 25, 1857, vol. 146, col. 329.

should they be destroyed, he could sell other material until he could reprint them and use it to advertise them. If the Society found magistrates who could be swayed by the argument that material other than pornography was dangerous in the wrong hands, however, it could strike a much larger blow at his and his competitors' businesses.

That is, at least, what that Society seems to have attempted immediately after the passing of the Obscene Publications Act. Historians often claim that no judgments on works "other than pornographic material" were passed under the Act until 1868, over a decade after it came into effect.[38] However, court records of obscenity trials rarely indicate which titles came under scrutiny, a policy meant to avoid giving them publicity. Since journalists were not bound to conceal titles or refrain from describing the works at issue, newspaper reports often fill in these details.[39] Reports on the raft of obscenity trials that followed the Act's passage in the autumn of 1857 and the spring of 1858 suggest that at the direction of the Society the police systematically raided publishers' and booksellers' shops and warehouses in and near Holywell Street, indiscriminately seizing the stock of players whose main business was sexual material and players who probably sold just a few explicit works alike. The Society then asked magistrates presiding over the cases to order the destruction of many works that would not previously have been considered likely to justify obscenity charges, including medical works.

Reports of the proceedings illustrate serious disagreement over whether these works could fairly be called obscene, not least between the Society and the people whose businesses had been raided. Book trade workers did not bother to defend pornography in these cases. Typical defences for selling an explicit novel or print were that the seller had acquired it in a bulk purchase from another bookseller and not known what it was, or that a Society agent had pressured the seller to procure it. The only possible exception to this pattern was Sydney Powell, a bookseller who challenged the court to prove that stereoscopic slides that he insisted were "intended for medical men . . . and in no respect more indecent than the exposure of living models in our schools of art" were obscene. If the court could assure him "of the point at which the line could be drawn" between science and obscenity, he swore, "he would pledge

[38] Manchester, "Lord Campbell's Act," 234. See also Katherine Mullin, "Poison More Deadly than Prussic Acid: Defining Obscenity after the 1857 Obscene Publications Act (1850–1885)," in *Prudes on the Prowl: Fiction and Obscenity in England, 1857 to the Present Day*, ed. David Bradshaw and Rachel Potter (Oxford: Oxford University Press, 2013), 15.

[39] To reconstruct obscenity trials, I compared all identifiable reports on the trials cited here and in subsequent chapters in *British Library Newspapers 1800–1900*, *19th Century UK Periodicals*, Part I, and *British Newspaper Archive* in addition to examining official court documents. For further information about crime reporting during this period, see Judith Rowbotham and Kim Stevenson, eds., *Criminal Conversations: Victorian Crimes, Social Panic, and Moral Outrage* (Columbus, OH: Ohio State University Press, 2005).

himself to observe the law."[40] Medical books and pamphlets, however, were given a real defence. Sellers protested that such works offered valuable information, had freely circulated for decades, and were being sold in respectable shops all over London. On those grounds, they were clearly not obscene.

At first glance, news reports suggest that these arguments were ineffective. James Thornhill (Dugdale's son-in-law), Edward Morris, Charles Paul, William Winn, and Henry Blacketer each protested when they appeared to summons in the autumn of 1857 that their medical works were "perfectly correct" instructional volumes, only to see them destroyed.[41] Some magistrates seem to have been as eager to destroy their stock as the Society. In one case, in which several booksellers protested the Society's characterization of *Aristotle's Masterpiece* as an obscene publication, the magistrate roared that "the title page alone was enough to condemn the book."[42] Others wrestled with the decision. The magistrate Robert Phillip Tyrwhitt mused that "there were certainly some very indecent things" in an unnamed medical work sold by Blacketer, and that they "were certainly very dangerous to youth," but, being at least "half-medical," the work must have some scientific value. Yet perhaps, Tyrwhitt reasoned, "the medical was only used for the purpose of selling the books." The "book before him was never read by young surgeons." Ultimately, he justified condemning the work to destruction by citing concerns about its circulation. It may have scientific value, he conceded. Yet, Blacketer sold it "into the hands of raw, inexperienced youths." The fact that Blacketer was selling the book to inappropriate readers turned necessary scientific detail into gratuitous representation.[43]

However, some news reports suggest that other magistrates rejected the idea that medical works, or at least some medical works, were obscene. For instance, Winn's expression of bewilderment over what booksellers "may sell and what [they] may not" on one of his court appearances suggests that some magistrates thought medical works put before them unobjectionable, so debates about them never took place in court, or were not reported:

> [A] work called *The Silent Friend*, which was seized last time, and had been returned as unobjectionable, was now seized again. Then *Aristotle* was condemned, but now they had brought out a new edition, which they thought unobjectionable. In fact, *Curtis on Manhood*, which had been returned, had been transmogrified into *Aristotle*, which had

40 "Police Intelligence," *Morning Chronicle*, February 18, 1858, 8.
41 "The Hollywell-Street Nuisance," *Morning Chronicle*, October 14, 1857, 7; "Police Courts: Bow Street," *Daily News*, November 21, 1857, 6; "Police Intelligence: Bow Street," *Morning Post*, November 21, 1857, 7; and "Seizure of Indecent Publications," *Morning Chronicle*, November 27, 1857, 3.
42 "Police Intelligence," *Morning Post*, November 21, 1857, 7.
43 "Seizure of Indecent Publications," *Morning Chronicle*, 3.

been condemned. (Laughter) The magistrate would, therefore, see all they wanted to do was to "keep within the law."[44]

It is also clear that some judges considered even measured decisions like Tyrwhitt's wrongheaded. In November 1857, Justice John Taylor Coleridge spoke out against the "misdirection of the provisions of a statute, doubtless well intentioned, but not therefore the less dangerous."[45] In Coleridge's view, the intended and rightful target of the Obscene Publications Act was trade in pornography, and men of his station knew pornography when they saw it: "common sense," he claimed, enabled them to identify publications whose object was to "excite depraved passions." However, "it was not uncommonly said that this or that picture of some great artist . . . might properly form the subject of a prosecution . . . and it was very easy for ingenious persons to deceive themselves, and perhaps others, by such a tone of argument." Echoing earlier debates in Parliament, Coleridge raised the spectre of a scenario in which Holywell Street publishers turned "the table on the public by prosecuting [such] works and publications under the colour that they are of the objectionable kind." They might claim that an artist's statue of Eve at the fountain in John Milton's *Paradise Lost* was obscene, and prevail on the basis that works of a similar character – works that could be misused by people with "impure mind[s]," but whose purpose was not to excite the passions – had been condemned. This would surely undermine public faith in the law. "Instead of looking at an isolated passage or picture," he argued, magistrates must "look at the book itself, and see whether the general object of it was of the kind represented in the indictment." "Take any medical or surgical book," he went on. Such a book could be misused, of course, but everyone "knew that the author, in dealing with his subject, must tell things for the sake of instruction."[46]

In this uncertain environment, as Winn's comments suggest, some publishers aimed to make it harder for the Society to argue that their medical works were obscene. The title page of one 1857 edition of *Aristotle's Masterpiece* declares that "the whole of these celebrated productions have undergone a complete revision, and every objectionable passage calculated to be offensive to virtue or morality, carefully expunged" (Figure 4.1). Its preliminary Advertisement, dated November 1857, repeats the message, claiming that expurgation has rendered the manual "instructive and entirely free from offence":

44 "Keeping within the Law," *Bell's Life in London*, November 15, 1857, 8.

45 "The objection we made to the *Obscene Publications Act*," *Law Times*, November 14, 1857, 110.

46 "Mr. Justice Coleridge on Obscene Publications," *Beverley and East Riding Recorder*, November 14, 1857, 3.

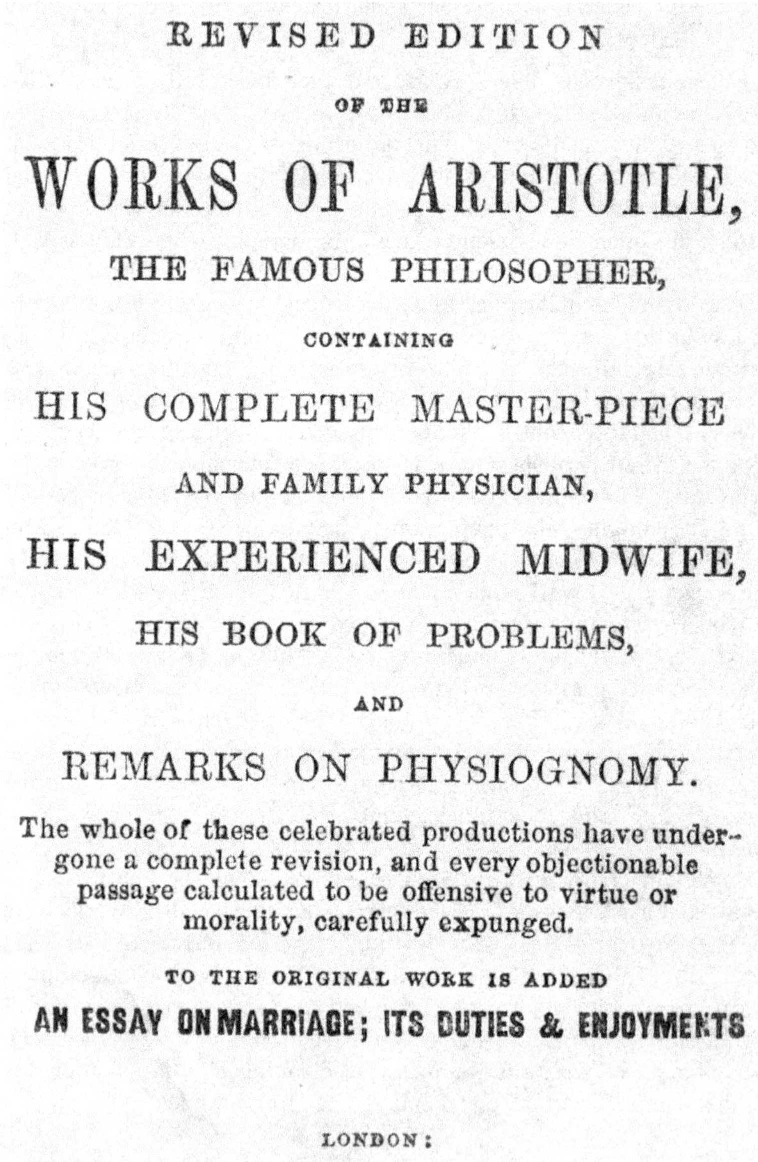

REVISED EDITION

OF THE

WORKS OF ARISTOTLE,

THE FAMOUS PHILOSOPHER,

CONTAINING

HIS COMPLETE MASTER-PIECE

AND FAMILY PHYSICIAN,

HIS EXPERIENCED MIDWIFE,

HIS BOOK OF PROBLEMS,

AND

REMARKS ON PHYSIOGNOMY.

The whole of these celebrated productions have undergone a complete revision, and every objectionable passage calculated to be offensive to virtue or morality, carefully expunged.

TO THE ORIGINAL WORK IS ADDED

AN ESSAY ON MARRIAGE; ITS DUTIES & ENJOYMENTS

LONDON:

PUBLISHED BY J. SMITH, 193, HIGH HOLBORN.

Figure 4.1 Title page with disclaimer. *Revised Edition of the Works of Aristotle, the Famous Philosopher* (London: J. Smith, [1857]). By courtesy of Michael and Anne Bull.

> The odium in which the book has been held by the moral and virtuous, does not apply to the present edition. That which was good and useful has been retained, and that only; the omission being supplied by new matter of an interesting and valuable character.
>
> No one can be more anxious than the Publisher to put an end to the shameful traffic in immoral or obscene books. At the same time, no one can be better aware of the fact, [*sic*] that such books command a large circulation. To supply a good and moral edition of a work hitherto accounted the reverse of either, is, he believes, both good and useful. With this object in view, he issues the present edition of *Aristotle*, as he is able to state with confidence that it contains nothing unchaste or impure.[47]

This edition of *Aristotle's Masterpiece* is, indeed, one of the more buttoned-up versions of the manual, in which the original introductory Masterpiece, which describes puberty and the first stirrings of sexual desire, has been replaced with an essay on "Marriage: Its Duties and Enjoyments," which appears to have been cobbled together out of excerpts from various literary works, conduct books, and Nicholas Venette's *Conjugal Love*.[48] Many of this edition's differences from the 1684 *Aristotle* predate the Obscene Publications Act's passage. It may not really have been censored for the occasion. However, a reference in its chapter on "Monstrous Births" demonstrates that an editor did work on the text after the Obscene Publications Act was passed. Here, a brief description of the hirsute body of Julia Pastrana, an indigenous Mexican woman who was exhibited as "the Bear Woman" and "the Nondescript" in London in August 1857, joins descriptions of other "living curiosities."[49] According to the text, Pastrana's exhibition took place "a few weeks ago." While updating this section, an editor may have deleted material that they considered likely to support obscenity charges.

Luckily for those who issued copies of *Aristotle's Masterpiece*, the manual and other cheap medical works vanished from the courts when the Holywell Street raids ended in 1858. The Society was satisfied with what it had accomplished, and so was Campbell. "Holywell-street, which had long set law and decency at defiance, has capitulated after several assaults," he wrote gleefully in his diary. "Half the shops are shut up, and the remainder deal in nothing but

47 *Revised Edition of the Works of Aristotle* (London: J. Smith, 193, High Holborn, 1857), de.24.07306, BL.

48 For possible sources, compare *Revised Edition*, 26, with Robert Pollack's poem *The Course of Time* (Edinburgh: William Blackwood and T. Cadell, 1827); *Revised Edition*, 31, with Robert Charles Dallas, *Elements of Self-Knowledge; Intended to Lead Youth into an Early Acquaintance with the Nature of Man* [. . .]. (London: B. Crosby, 1805), 255; *Revised Edition*, 39, with *A Manual of the Etiquette of Love, Courtship and Marriage* (London: Thomas Allman, 1853), 53; *Revised Edition*, 40, with "Hood on Matrimony," *Harper's Weekly*, August 8, 1857, 510; and *Revised Edition*, 17–18 with Nicholas Venette, *Conjugal Love; or, The Pleasures of the Marriage Bed* [. . .]. (London: Printed for the Booksellers, 1750), 150–151.

49 *Revised Edition*, 57. For further information about Pastrana and her life, see Nadja Durbach, *Spectacle of Deformity: Freak Shows and Modern British Culture* (Berkeley: University of California Press, 2009), 107.

moral and religious books!"[50] The actions of 1857–8, which Campbell compared elsewhere to the 1857 siege of Delhi, did deal a massive blow to the Holywell Street trade. However, their effects were mostly temporary. Aspects of the trade, and of London's low culture more broadly, were permanently diminished. Although Duncombe and Dugdale carried on selling sexual material well into the 1860s, they advertised in a narrower range of venues, and the raucous commercial culture promoted by flash papers like *Paul Pry* faded along with flash papers themselves.[51] But new players and new forms of entertainment seamlessly filled their place. Businesses oriented around the sale of explicit photographs and stereoscopic slides had begun to emerge in the 1850s. By the early 1860s, they were booming.

Adolphus Henry Judge, alias Adolphus Henry Delplangue, was known as "one of the most extensive and crafty dealers in these publications ... the king of the trade."[52] Judge and his four brothers – one of whom was married to Dugdale's daughter Jessie – created thousands of explicit photographs out of premises in Kentish Town, London.[53] They sold them to customers hearkening from "all classes of society" and "all parts of the country" by post under a variety of trade names, including Delplangue & Co, Megret & Co, Hall & Co, and Rozez, Janin, and Humbert, and probably supplied third-party dealers on a wholesale basis.[54] Like Dugdale a few years earlier, Judge advertised widely in the press. His advertisements often indicated that his images were taken "from life" or "from nature," euphemisms for nudity that served as shorthand for such photographs in advertisements through the rest of the century. In some venues, Judge was more daring: an 1863 notice in *Herapath's Railway Journal* informs readers that Delplangue & Co sold "erotic photographs" alongside the novels of the Marquis de Sade.[55]

As that advertisement suggests, while such pornographers did not deal in the same variety as Holywell Street publishers, they typically offered a handful of explicit novels and medical works alongside visual material, as well as French letters. *Aristotle's Masterpiece*, *Every Woman's Book*, and *Fruits of Philosophy*

50 Quoted in M. J. D. Roberts, "Morals, Art, and the Law: The Passing of the Obscene Publications Act, 1857." *Victorian Studies* 28, no. 4 (1985), 626–627.

51 Dugdale died in prison in 1868. There is no record of Duncombe's death, but his trail vanishes in the mid-1860s.

52 Quoted in Peter Mendes, *Clandestine Erotic Fiction in English, 1800–1930*, 2nd ed. (London: Routledge, 2016), 443.

53 Sheryl Straight, "The Judge Brothers," *The Erotica Bibliophile*; accessed February 19, 2024, www.eroticabibliophile.com/; "Extraordinary Charge of Libel," *Morning Advertiser*, September 26, 1864, 7.

54 "The Trade in Indecent Literature," *Morning Post*, August 30, 1872, 7. By 1872, the Judges had reportedly established six shops devoted to this material in London. See "The Trade in Indecent Literature," *London Evening Standard*, August 31, 1872, 7.

55 "Stereoscopic Slides Taken from Life," *Herapath's Railway Journal*, July 11, 1863, 730.

were the most common medical works advertised.[56] Curiously, Judge also experimented with cultivating another market for his photographs: medical students. In 1861, Delplanque & Co advertised "Photographs showing the Mons Veneris, Labic Pudendi, Perinaeum, Meatus Uranarius, &c." to students in the *Medical Times and Gazette Advertiser* and the *Lancet General Advertiser* for a guinea a set.[57] It is impossible to know whether these images were the same ones that Judge advertised elsewhere as erotic photographs, and hard to say whether medical students, who were known for making bawdy jokes in anatomy theatres, were really meant to use them as instructive material.[58] Either way, Judge's decision to advertise in medical journals suggests new ways in which thin boundaries between the categories of the medical and the erotic could be exploited.

As well as failing to shut down trade in sexual entertainment, the events of 1857–8 failed to establish that cheap, explicit medical works were obscene, even in pornographers' hands. On one raid on Judge's residence in Kentish Town, police officers dismissed what they found as "quasi-medical" productions and speculated that Judge kept his offensive material in another venue.[59] Next to the photographic equivalent of *The Confessions of Madame Vestris*, *Aristotle's Masterpiece* could look awfully tame. And those who did consider such works dangerous to public morals often did not think that they were covered under Campbell's Act. Indeed, a writer for the *Saturday Review* suggested that Campbell's refusal to define the term "obscene" was to blame for an increase in the sale of materials "which are certainly not positively indecent, but which, it is equally clear, are expressly intended for the gratification of that pruriency which Parliament tried to deprive of its coarser stimulants."[60] A writer for the *Solicitor's Journal & Reporter* summed up the situation in 1867: the "definition of the offence [of obscene libel in common law] is very defective," he grumbled, "nor have the statutes, which have supplied a better machinery for suppressing the offence, given

56 For examples, see "Aristotle's Masterpiece," *Reynolds's Newspaper*, February 7, 1864, 8; "Nothing Impossible," *Illustrated Sporting News and Theatrical and Musical Review*, November 20, 1869, 8; "Secret Doings" and "The Forbidden Book," *Illustrated Police News*, December 14, 1872, 4.

57 "To Medical Students," *Medical Times and Gazette Advertiser*, August 11, 1860, [2]; "To Medical Students," *Lancet General Advertiser*, August 11, 1860, [2].

58 Laura Kelly, *Irish Medical Education and Student Culture, c.1850–1950* (Oxford: Oxford University Press, 2017), 189.

59 "Middlesex Sessions," *The Times*, August 31, 1872, 11.

60 "Holywell-Street Revived," *Saturday Review*, August 21, 1858, 180. For further examples, see "Photography and Bad Taste," *London Review*, March 28, 1863, 326–327; "Moral Sewage," *Saturday Review*, December 24, 1864, 776–777; "M. Dupin on the Social Evil," *Saturday Review*, July 8, 1865, 42–43; "Immoral Advertisements," *Pall Mall Gazette*, November 28, 1865, 9–10; "Mr. Swinburne's Defence," *London Review*, November 3, 1866, 482–483; "London Streets," *Saturday Review*, November 16, 1867, 629–630.

any assistance in defining it."[61] For now, the only certain means of securing a victory in obscenity cases was to seize pornography.

Obscene Quackery

The Society for the Suppression of Vice was not the only group eager to persuade the authorities that, in the hands of certain players, medical works were obscene. While the Society was trying to put Holywell Street publishers out of business, a handful of reform-oriented medical journals began to campaign against what they called "obscene quackery." From the early 1840s, following the explosion of consulting surgeons' manuals into the marketplace, the *Lancet*, the *British Medical Journal*, the *Medical Circular*, and, in Ireland, the *Dublin Medical Press* made strident efforts to galvanize opposition to their authors. As we saw in Chapter 2, they ran investigations into the infrastructure of consulting surgeons' businesses, and published bitter exposés of their imitations, exaggerations, and, in some cases, outright frauds. However, these efforts had little effect on consulting surgeons' ability to do business. Indeed, they only became more of a fixture in the market for medical advice. Increasingly, campaigning medical journals rallied around a different charge, one that turned regular practitioners' longstanding anxiety about presenting sexual information to the public into a weapon against irregular medical practice: they claimed that consulting surgeons' manuals and advertisements were obscene.

A typical article on obscene quackery claimed that consulting surgeons represented a grave threat to public morals. Their advertisements exposed vulnerable people to allusions to sexuality without their consent, while their "vile trash" manuals were calculated to incite morbid or prurient engagement. For the good of the nation, newspaper editors *must* ban consulting surgeons' advertisements from their pages. These articles got an enthusiastic reception from medical readers. Doctors often wrote to the *Lancet* and the *British Medical Journal* to praise them for exposing "obscene quacks," to express their anxiety at the prospect of putting "an ordinary newspaper into the hands of a female . . . lest they should be shocked by the disgusting advertisements which are emblazoned on its pages," or to call for the establishment an "Association for the Repression of Quackery" or a "Society for the Suppression of Fraudulent and Obscene Advertisements," which would work to "redeem . . . the periodical press from its present position of hireling servitude to medical swindlers and obscene advertisers."[62] Campaigns against obscene quackery also gained modest support

61 "The Law of Libel – III," *Solicitor's Journal & Reporter*, September 14, 1867, 1019.

62 "The Disgusting Pages of the Newspapers," *Lancet*, July 30, 1842, 622–633; "Proposed Society for the Suppression of Fraudulent and Obscene Advertisements," *Association Medical Journal*, July 22, 1853, 631–633; "The Repression of Quackery," *Medical Press and Circular*, March 3, 1869, 188–189.

in provincial newspapers, whose editors did not stop publishing consulting surgeons' advertisements, but happily attacked their rivals for doing the same.[63]

Regular practitioners may well have found consulting surgeons' manuals and advertisements offensive. However, just as newspaper editors stood to benefit from accusing their rivals of publishing indecent advertisements, charging consulting surgeons with purveying obscene material served their own interests. As Roy Porter emphasized, an accusation of quackery is the very definition of what sociologists of science have called "boundary work": applying to no particular practice, but to any form of behaviour that its wielder deems unorthodox, the term has long served as an instrument to situate certain individuals, groups, acts, or ideas outside the bounds of medicine.[64] Accusations of *obscene* quackery were a twofold strike: at once, they rhetorically situated consulting surgeons outside the bounds of legitimate medicine and outside the bounds of respectable society. More narrowly, they lent medical reform, a project to which journals like the *Lancet* and the *British Medical Journal* were devoted, new currency as an issue of public morals. Writers for these journals had long claimed that legislation to regulate medical practice was the only permanent solution to the scourge of quackery.[65] Now, they framed that legislation as essential to protecting citizens' morals as it was to protecting their bodies.

To support their claims, anti-quackery campaigners promoted a contextual view of obscenity oriented around the issue of circulation. Long-standing concerns about medicine's relationship with commerce had had a powerful effect on the ways quackery was represented in regular medicine. Transparent commercialism was positioned as a form of quackery itself, but it was also portrayed as a calling card of incompetent or dishonest practice since it went against regular medical conventions. If a medical work was advertised through placards, handbills, or cards; if it included testimonials for its author's services or directions to access them; or if its title used vernacular medical terms, the logic went, its author must be a charlatan. Arising during a period in which an encounter with a consulting surgeon's advertisement was utterly unavoidable, campaigns against obscene quackery took this argument in a slightly different direction. Instead of,

63 See "Shameful Impurity of the Hull Advertiser's Columns," *Hull Packet and East Riding Times*, October 27, 1843, 18; "Remarks on the Present State of the Medical Profession in this Country," *Leeds Mercury*, November 2, 1844, 7; "Publications," *Daily News*, May 27, 1846, 7; "Advertisements & Notices: Medical Announcement," *Freeman's Journal and Daily Commercial Advertiser*, September 2, 1854, 1; "Immorality and Quackery," *Derby Mercury*, June 3, 1857, 8.

64 Roy Porter, *Health for Sale: Medicine and Quackery in England, 1660–1850* (Manchester: Manchester University Press, 1989), vi.

65 See Michael Brown, "Medicine, Quackery, and the Free Market: The 'War' against Morison's Pills and the Construction of the Medical Profession, c. 1830–c. 1850," in *Medicine and the Market in England and Its Colonies, c. 1450–c. 1850*, ed. Mark S. R. Jenner and Patrick Wallis (Basingstoke: Palgrave Macmillan, 2007), 238–261.

or in addition to, collapsing charlatanism with commercialism, they collapsed obscenity with commercialism. The "popular" form of consulting surgeons' manuals, their easy accessibility, and the ubiquity of advertisements for them were framed as clues that should apprise readers of offensive content within the manual, and framed as dangerous in their own right.

An 1850 pamphlet issued by the Union for the Discouragement of Vicious Advertisements, an anti-quackery group associated with the *Lancet*, offers a good illustration of this argument in action. The pamphlet begins by decrying the lurid content of works like *Manhood* and *The Silent Friend*. However, it rapidly shifts away from discussing the manuals' main text and images to focus on their bibliographical makeup and the ways they were distributed:

> These are publications which, with a light veil of pretended science, are designed to excite and gratify a morbid curiosity. They propose fallacious modes of illicit indulgence without the risk of the consequences that attach themselves to it. They are filled with pictures, which leave the most pernicious impression on the mind; the very tables of contents are studiously calculated to arouse dangerous ideas. The titles are skilfully worded in insinuating language, and some volumes, which contain no direct obscenity themselves, seem written principally to introduce others more fully immoral by the same author. These books are printed in such a form as to be accessible to the purses of all, and to be capable of being transmitted secretly by post to those who send the required value in postage-stamps. They are obviously addressed not to the sick alone, but to the young and unwary.[66]

According to the Union, it was not the content of these works alone that threatened the "young and unwary." Even seemingly mundane elements of the manuals, such as their tables of contents, were "calculated to arouse dangerous ideas." What made these works especially endangering in the Union's rendering, though, was their material accessibility: obscene quackery is portrayed as a kind of disease in the Union's pamphlet, inexorably creeping into domestic space. "No home is safe," the pamphlet warns its readers, "these publications may be carried, by the facility of modern transport, into each of our nurseries and kitchens, and be perused, perhaps at this moment, by some member of our households in unwary ignorance."[67]

Collapsing commercialism with obscenity was an expedient approach to attacking the consulting surgeon trade. Decrying consulting surgeons' representations of the body and sexuality in specific terms was untenable. Their manuals promoted the same ideas as works by regular medical practitioners, and used similar, and sometimes exactly the same, language to do so. Linking medical works' decency as reading material and legitimacy as science with certain methods of presentation and distribution, on the other hand, enabled

[66] "A Few Words to News-Readers" (London: W. Eglington, 1850), 1–4, 1–2. 7306.df.22, BL.
[67] "Words to News-Readers," 3.

anti-quackery campaigners to draw a line between medical orthodoxy and medical heterodoxy rooted in commercial practice at a time when consulting surgeons' exploitation of print for commercial gain was exactly what alarmed them.

Although tales of doctors' sexual misconduct circulated in the press (and, inevitably, in the pornography trade), anti-quackery campaigners do not seem to have worried that charges of obscene quackery would arouse concern that regular practitioners were being corrupted by their own reading material.[68] They diffused this possibility by appealing to the same paternalistic model of reading that Tyrwhitt had cited to condemn Blacketer's book: a model of reading that framed women, children, and young men as vulnerable to the influences of print in ways that established professional men like themselves were not. What campaigns against obscene quackery did risk arousing was concern that regular medical authors endangered public morals. The commercial dividing line that they drew between medicine and quackery was precarious. As we have seen, the differences between regular and irregular medical book advertisements could be subtle to the uninitiated, and the regular and irregular medical works' prices and modes of distribution were often the same or similar. Arguably, if no home was safe from contamination from *Manhood*, no home was safe from the influence of works on sexual matters issued by John Churchill and Hippolyte Baillière.

Initially, anti-quackery campaigners simply aimed to convince newspaper editors to stop publishing consulting surgeons' advertisements.[69] Their efforts were spectacularly unsuccessful: irregular medical advertisements represented a significant and reliable stream of income that newspaper editors did not want, and in many cases could not afford, to lose. The law became an increasing focus of campaigns against obscene quackery in this context, following events in 1853 and 1854 which saw local authorities charge three figures connected with travelling anatomical museums with displaying obscene models under the Vagrancy Acts: Joseph Woodhead, the owner of Woodhead's Museum, in Sheffield; J. W. Reimer, the owner of Reimer's Anatomical Museum, in Hull; and James Lang, a demonstrator at Henry's Anatomical Museum, in Barnsley.[70] Lang pled guilty to exhibiting "indecent representations of the human body," and was released on the condition that he close the museum.[71]

[68] On the doctor figure as an increasing fixture of pornographic literature, see Coral Lansbury, "Gynaecology, Pornography, and the Antivivisection Movement," *Victorian Studies* 28, no. 3 (1985): 413–437.

[69] "Is It Possible to Redeem the Newspaper Press from its Servitude to Fraud and Obscenity?" *Association Medical Journal*, August 12, 1853, 697.

[70] "Magisterial Proceedings: Indecent Exhibition," *Sheffield Independent*, December 31, 1853, 8; "Henry's Anatomical Museum," *Association Medical Journal*, March 17, 1854, 255; "Local and Other News," *Leeds Intelligencer*, February 25, 1854, 5.

[71] "Henry's Anatomical Museum," *Association Medical Journal*, March 17, 1854, 255.

Reimer was found guilty, but only fined a nominal 2*s* 6*d* – less than the cost of three tickets to his museum – because the magistrate was convinced that the museum had "educational potential."[72] Woodhead was fined ten shillings and moved his museum to London, where his models had been displayed without complaint in the 1851 Great Exhibition at the Crystal Palace, only to be fined again for displaying "filthy, obscene, and indecent figures."[73]

The sources of the complaints against these museums were never made public. Reports only indicate that "some individuals" were offended by what they saw and decided to report it to the authorities.[74] However, Woodhead claimed that medical men conspired to bring charges against him in London, and it is not unlikely that medical men were the complainants in some, and even all, of these cases. As Alan Bates has demonstrated, public anatomical museums were enormously popular in the early 1850s, selling up to a million tickets a year. Bates argues that their sheer popularity galvanized opposition to them among medical practitioners even before they started advertising medical services: what had once looked like a welcome means of promoting medical expertise was beginning to look like an unwelcome challenge to it.[75] Even if they were not the source of the complaints against the museums, it is significant that medical practitioners contributed to efforts to shut them down. In all of these cases, local doctors testified against the defendants, claiming, as one practitioner did in the Lang case, that their displays "were calculated to excite the errotic [*sic*] desires of the people, and ... make a profit by pandering to those desires."[76]

Apprised of the Vagrancy Acts' efficacy as a mechanism for shutting down public anatomical museums, anti-quackery campaigners began to consider obscenity law as a means of combating the consulting surgeon trade. Campbell's introduction of the Obscene Publications Bill during the summer of 1857 attracted close attention from writers for the *Lancet* and the *British Medical Journal*. While some of these writers viewed the bill's introduction ahead of legislation for medical reform as evidence of misplaced government priorities, others urged their colleagues to embrace it as an instrument to suppress quackery.[77] Like the Vagrancy Acts, the Obscene Publications Bill did not cover advertisements in newspapers. However, if it was passed, a complaint could enable the police to seize consulting surgeons' manuals. If a magistrate deemed them obscene, they would be destroyed, and their authors could be prosecuted for obscene libel. The popular weekly *Punch*, which

[72] A. W. Bates, "Anatomy on Trial: Itinerant Anatomy Museums in Mid Nineteenth-Century England," *Medical History* 9, no. 2 (2016): 192.
[73] Bates, "Anatomy on Trial," 193.
[74] "Obscene Exhibitions," *Dublin Medical Press*, April 26, 1854, 14.
[75] Bates, "Anatomy on Trial," 199. [76] "Magisterial Proceedings," *Sheffield Independent*, 8.
[77] "It Would Be Difficult," *Lancet*, August 8, 1857, 146.

counted several ex-medical men among its staff and often reported on medical debates, promoted these views to the public, going so far as to deem a crackdown on consulting surgeons the "chief case for Campbell's Act."[78]

On the eve of the Act's passage, anti-quackery campaigners pressed the Society for the Suppression of Vice to prosecute consulting surgeons. The *Lancet* argued that there was "abundant ground to warrant the interference of the Society." "Worrying the Holywell-street vendors is good sport enough," the journal coaxed, "but scarcely more successful than lopping off the heads of a Hydra . . . Surely [obscene quackery is] more deserving of [the Society's] attention, as being calculated to engender that miserable depravity of mind which induces men to purchase the poison vended by traders in obscene publications."[79] The Society did not acknowledge the *Lancet*'s words. Months passed, and a parade of cheap medical works passed through the courts. The *Lancet* and its allies stepped up their appeals. By the winter of 1857–8, *Punch* was equating consulting surgeons with Holywell Street publishers, dubbing them "Holywell Doctors" and "Holywell quacks," and arguing that they were as, or more, dangerous to public morality as men like William Dugdale:

> A clean sweep has been made of Holywell Street. The obscene pigeons have been turned out of the dirty dove-cotes. But while the pigeons have been vexed, censure spares the crows. The rookery of the quacks is undisturbed, and their vile and lying advertisements still pollute the country newspapers and some of the London journals, and lie upon the tables of fathers of families to afford Sunday reading to their sons and daughters. To go through Holywell Street or not was optional; but it is impossible to avoid seeing that which is thrust under one's nose. The Society for the Suppression of Vice is evidently afflicted with partial blindness.[80]

The Society ignored these appeals.

[78] "The Chief Case for Lord Campbell's Act," *Punch*, August 22, 1857, 73. According to *The Curran Index to Nineteenth-Century Periodicals* (Research Society for Victorian Periodicals, 2002-), www.curranindex.org/, Percival Leigh, who studied medicine at St. Bartholomew's Hospital, wrote most of *Punch*'s stories on obscene quackery, including this article; "Quacks of Advertising Columns," *Punch*, October 3, 1857, 144; "Downing-Street and Holywell-Street," *Punch*, November 7, 1857, 188; and "Quack! Quack! Quack!" *Punch*, December 5, 1857, 227. For more on *Punch*'s relationship with medicine, see Richard Noakes, "Punch and Comic Journalism in Mid-Victorian Britain," *Science in the Nineteenth-Century Periodical: Reading the Magazine of Nature*, ed. Geoffrey Cantor, Gowan Dowson, Graeme Gooday, Richard Noakes, Sally Shuttleworth, and Jonathan R. Topham (Cambridge: Cambridge University Press, 2004), 91–122.

[79] "The Action against Kahn, of Coventry Street, for Extortion: Suppression of Obscene Quackery," *Lancet*, August 15, 1857, 175.

[80] "Quack! Quack! Quack!" *Punch*, 227. See also "Quacks of Advertising Columns"; "Downing-Street and Holywell-Street"; "Medical Annotations," *Lancet*, November 7, 1857, 478; [Henry Silver], "A Good Opening for Quacks," *Punch*, January 2, 1858, 7; [Henry Silver], "A Queerer for the Quacks," *Punch*, May 5, 1860, 187.

The campaign against obscene quackery temporarily died down around the passage of the 1858 Medical Act, which finally gave "legally qualified Medical Practitioners" statutory recognition.[81] The Act established a General Medical Council to form and maintain a public register of qualified medical practitioners, monitor standards for medical training, and de-register practitioners found guilty of committing criminal acts or engaging in unprofessional conduct. For years, medical reformers had claimed that such legislation would eradicate quackery. However, the Medical Act was not designed for this purpose, and it quickly proved to be an ineffectual instrument for it. Many general practitioners could not afford to pay fees to be included in the Medical Register, which meant that it did not list many medical men who would have been considered "regular." And practitioners who practised medicine in ways that offended their colleagues often declined to register themselves, which left them free to practice as they wished. It was possible to prosecute such practitioners for falsely claiming medical qualifications or using titles such as "surgeon" or "physician" in advertising material. However, they could easily dodge a guilty verdict by purchasing a foreign diploma. Some irregulars didn't bother to purchase one, resigning themselves to paying the maximum five-pound fine for committing the offence in the event they were prosecuted.

As medical reformers began to recognize that the Medical Act could not suppress the consulting surgeon trade, screeds against obscene quackery surged back into the medical press.[82] The surgeon Francis Burdett Courtenay's melodramatic exposé *Revelations of Quacks and Quackery* (1865), first published as a series of reports in the *Medical Circular*, warned parents that if their daughters sent away for a consulting surgeon's manual, "irreparable moral contamination" would ensue.[83] The *Lancet* claimed that "vile quack advertisements" had led to the suicide of a young man in Kent. The "books to which they refer contain every element of pruriency, of vile suggestion, and of cunning terrorism which can work upon the mind," it cried.[84] The general outline of these arguments was not novel. Irregulars had been accused of damaging minds and morals for a long time. However, anti-quackery campaigners made their accusations in ever more brutal terms, framing consulting surgeons and, increasingly, the owners of public anatomical museums as sexual predators and shadowy anarchists. Now, their

[81] See M. J. D. Roberts, "The Politics of Professionalization: MPs, Medical Men, and the 1858 Medical Act," *Medical History* 53 (2009): 37–56 for further details about the passage of the Medical Act and its perceived deficiencies.

[82] "Has the Medical Act Failed as Regards the Suppression of Illegal Practices?" *BMJ*, May 26, 1860, 400–401.

[83] Frances Burdett Courtenay, *Revelations of Quacks and Quackery: A Series of Letters by "Detector" reprinted from "The Medical Circular,"* 3rd ed. (London: Baillière, Tindall & Cox, 1865), 26.

[84] "Purification of the Press," *Lancet*, January 28, 1865, 101.

works did not simply weaken public morals or set off hypochondria. They fostered "loathsome debauchery," violence, and social disorder.[85]

In 1860, local authorities charged William and Louis Lloyd, the owners of a public anatomical museum in Leeds, with displaying models "dangerous to public morality." The Lloyds' defence that their anatomical models were educational was rejected, and they were destroyed on the grounds that they were "utterly useless for any scientific object" and "pandered to the worst passions of human nature."[86] Five years later, Reginald Rudd, described as "a medicine vendor," was charged with distributing obscene books in Bolton. Rudd's solicitor argued that "everything recorded in the publications might be met with in medical books," but agreed that they "had unquestionably a degrading effect."[87] Rudd was only fined twenty shillings, but campaigning medical journals framed this and the Lloyd case as important precedents that portended sweeping action against consulting surgeons under Campbell's Act.[88] They were wrong. Eight years after the Lloyd case, the *Lancet* was still calling on the police and the Society for the Suppression of Vice to do their duty, and lamenting obscenity law's weak enforcement.

Several issues impeded organized action against consulting surgeons under obscenity laws during the 1850s and 1860s. One was that anti-quackery campaigners were unwilling to act themselves. (It is notable that most charges against irregulars on the grounds that they were displaying or distributing obscene material during this period were under the Vagrancy Acts, which cost complainants little time or money.) Instead of taking the law into their own hands, they aimed to persuade others to prosecute consulting surgeons. However, there was not much practical support for such a project. The General Medical Council refused to admit proprietors of "unseemly" exhibitions into the Medical Register, and removed prominent consulting surgeons from it: in 1863, Robert Jacob Jordan was struck off the Medical Register for "conduct unbecoming of a physician," and Samuel La'Mert was struck off for publishing an "indecent and unprofessional treatise."[89] However, neither the Council nor any other major medical institution supported prosecuting such practitioners for distributing of obscene material.

85 "The Museum Nuisance," *Lancet*, August 27, 1864, 243.

86 "The Week," *BMJ*, January 7, 1860, 15.

87 "Suppression of Quackery," *Lancet*, November 4, 1865, 518.

88 I have found reports of only two other cases in which people were charged for selling or displaying indecent medical works during this period. See "The Late Serious Charge against a Doctor of Medicine," *Illustrated Police News*, September 14, 1867, n.p. and "Indecent Quack Publications," *Lancet*, July 18, 1868, 99.

89 Lesley A. Hall, "'The English Have Hot-Water Bottles': The Morganatic Marriage between Sexology and Medicine in Britain since William Acton," in *Sexual Knowledge, Sexual Science: The History of Attitudes to Sexuality*, ed. Roy Porter and Mikulas Teich (Cambridge: Cambridge University Press, 1994), 351–353.

There was also little support for prosecuting consulting surgeons under obscenity laws outside the medical community. "The 'fine line of demarcation' ... between us and them," as one medical writer put it, presented a difficult roadblock.[90] While anti-quackery campaigners framed consulting surgeons' publications and advertisements as fundamentally different from those of legitimate medical practitioners, many people did not perceive meaningful differences between them. Cataloguing medicine's wars with itself, the *Saturday Review* quipped that medical men "avow that their object is to clear the profession of quacks ... before we assist them in their undertaking, we should like to know, in common with a large part of the public, what it is they include in their definition of quackery."[91] Relatedly, many people were skeptical of the claim that consulting surgeons' publications endangered public morals. It is difficult to interpret its silence in the face of endless entreaties from the *Lancet*, but it is plausible that the Society for the Suppression of Vice considered it neither necessary nor desirable to prosecute consulting surgeons since they warned people against sexual vice in such strident terms. And finally, many people did not think that obscenity laws applied to medical works, even though medical works had been seized and condemned under them. In a yet another skirmish involving Woodhead's Museum, Bates notes, authorities in Derby called the museum "disgusting and demoralizing," but did not think they had any legal power to shut it down.[92]

The 1860s drew to a close with the stink of failure, at least for the groups examined in this chapter. Several public anatomical museums shut down around 1857, possibly out of fears that the Obscene Publications Act would be used against them. Yet, others appear to have benefitted from the notoriety of being called obscene, and the consulting surgeon business continued to thrive.[93] And while the Holywell Street trade was seriously diminished by the end of the 1850s, a new kind of trade in sexual material – trafficking in some of the same products, and some that anti-vice crusaders considered even worse – was flourishing. At the same time, to the consternation of legal experts, there remained no consensus about what the term "obscene" meant in a court of law. Campbell's refusal to define the term in his bill may have been meant to facilitate the Society for the Suppression of Vice's fight against the Holywell Street trade, but it fostered a great deal of confusion.

The Circumstances of the Publication

In 1868, the legal meaning of the term "obscene" was resolved, after a fashion, with a ruling in the trial *R.* v. *Hicklin*. The *Hicklin* case surrounded *The Confessional Unmasked*, a pamphlet first published under a pseudonym in 1836

[90] "Medical Parasites," *Lancet*, August 3, 1861, 127.
[91] "Doctors and Quacks," *Saturday Review*, July 10, 1858, 30.
[92] Bates, "Anatomy on Trial," 195. [93] Bates, "Anatomy on Trial," 200.

that purported to expose the "Depravity of the Romish Priesthood." An evangelical group called the Protestant Electoral Union – whose founders included the solicitor Charles Hastings Collette, soon to be the new secretary of the Society for the Suppression of Vice – had issued 25,000 copies in 1865.[94] The *Confessional* was deliberately shocking: adopting a common structure in pornographic literature, its author arranged passages culled from various Roman Catholic theological manuals in order of sexual explicitness, beginning with fairly tame questions that priests might put to the young about courtship and ending with answers to questions about specific sex acts, such as whether a husband might "introduce his —— into the mouth of his wife."[95] Whether the Union aimed to protest state tolerance for Roman Catholicism or, as Mullin has suggested, make a steady stream of income from those who recognized the pamphlet's utility as a sex manual, it promoted the *Confessional* in towns with large Catholic populations and set off a "sectarian, political, and regional uproar."[96] In 1867, authorities in Wolverhampton charged Henry Scott, a metalworker who had been selling the pamphlet for a shilling, with distributing obscene material. A drawn-out legal skirmish ensued, and the case ended up on the Queen's Bench in 1868.

The defence claimed that the *Confessional* could not be obscene because it was a religious work. This argument was widely ridiculed in the press: picking "out every foul passage" from theological manuals and selling "them in a penny pamphlet to boys in the streets," the *Pall Mall Gazette* cried, rendered them unfit for their original purpose.[97] According to Mullin, the outcry forced the new Lord Chief Justice, Alexander Cockburn's, hand. He ruled for the prosecution, declaring, "I think the test of obscenity is this, whether the tendency of the matter charged as obscenity is to deprave and corrupt those whose minds are open to such immoral influences, and into whose hands a publication of this sort may fall."[98] In outlining this "test of obscenity," Cockburn made history: the *Hicklin* test, as it became known, became the standard legal method of determining obscenity in Britain, the United States, and most British colonies for nearly a century, influencing the outcome of obscenity trials all over the world.[99]

As Mullin has emphasized, Cockburn's test of obscenity was formulated to address a difficult and unanticipated local predicament.[100] However, as this chapter is shown, it also addressed a decade of debate in Parliament, among legal experts, in the courts, and in the press about what kinds of material

94 See Mullin, "Unmasking *The Confessional Unmasked*," 477.
95 Quoted in Mullin, "Unmasking *The Confessional Unmasked*," 475.
96 Mullin, "Unmasking *The Confessional Unmasked*," 476–477.
97 "The Legality of the 'Confessional Unmasked,'" *Pall Mall Gazette*, July 13, 1867, 10.
98 Regina v. Hicklin, *Law Reports 3: Queen's Bench Division* (1868), 371.
99 While the *Hicklin* standard was replaced in most of these countries in the 1950s and 1960s, it remained the standard in India until 2014. See Indian Penal Code, "Sale, etc, of obscene books, etc.," section 292:1.
100 Mullin, "Unmasking *The Confessional Unmasked*," 472.

obscenity laws covered. By the mid-nineteenth century, as one writer for the *Solicitor's Journal & Reporter* suggested, it was difficult for many experts to view common-law understandings of obscenity as covering anything other than pornographic material. The photographs that Adolphus Henry Judge advertised as erotic were clearly created with "lewd" or "licentious" intent.[101] Medical and theological works were not. But the print world of the mid-nineteenth century was a complex and convoluted one, a world in which sexual discourse was constantly being broken down, stitched together, reframed, and redistributed in new ways. For different reasons, anti-quackery campaigners and some members of the judiciary had argued that how a publication was sold, and to who, mattered. In defining obscenity not in relation to authorial intent but in relation to audience – "into those whose hands a publication of this sort may fall" – Cockburn's test of obscenity affirmed those arguments.

It is important to recognize that in practice, however, Cockburn's test of obscenity did not rest on a work's audience, not precisely. What those who sought to apply the test, including Cockburn himself, relied on was an idea of readership or potential readership, grounded in analyses of various features of a work's commercial context: who had published it, how much it cost, where and how it had been advertised, how it had been distributed, and so on. Cockburn made his test's reliance on these kinds of contexts more explicit earlier in the case when he addressed the issue of "necessarily" obscene works: like a theological manual or a legal textbook, a "medical treatise, with illustrations necessary for the information of those for whose education or information the work is intended, may, in a certain sense, be obscene, and yet not the subject for indictment," he declared, "but it can never be that these prints may be exhibited for any one, boys and girls, to see as they pass. The immunity must depend upon the circumstances of the publication."[102] Cockburn suggested that certain forms of advertisement and distribution legitimately served medical needs, that others did not, and that a judge could tell the difference.

The formulation of the *Hicklin* test of obscenity marked a crucial turning point in the history this book traces. In practice, it made medical works obscene no more than the Holywell Street raids had. Many authorities continued to be skeptical of the idea that medical works were covered under obscenity laws, even when they were cheap, popular works that could easily fall into the hands of young and female readers. However, alongside the 1858 Medical Act and regular practitioners' increasing efforts to professionalize their own print culture, the test created a more stable framework for arguing that medical works were obscene in court. This had a significant impact on trade in medical works on sexual matters. Sellers were intermittently prosecuted under

101 "The Law of Libel – III," *Solicitor's Journal & Reporter*, 1019.

102 Regina v. Hicklin, *Law Reports 3*, 367.

obscenity laws as part of efforts to combat quackery, pornography trafficking, fraud, and political organizing, and the circumstances of their works' publication and distribution were used to argue that they were obscene. These actions helped fuel myths about censorship that were applied to sell sexual knowledge in its material form and as a programme of scientific enquiry.

5 Dull Instead of Light

The 1870s and 1880s witnessed major shifts in the trade in sexual knowledge. Public anatomical museums dwindled, and advertisements for consulting surgeons' manuals faded from view. Textbooks and treatises on sexual subjects grew dense with technical vocabulary, and advertisements for them vanished from non-medical periodicals. Popular writing on many of the same subjects became briefer and more euphemistic. At the same time, the production and distribution of some cheap, frank genres, such as the contraception manual, skyrocketed. These developments were intertwined with medical and emerging activist groups' efforts to consolidate coherent collective identities and establish their authority in and through contests over print. Regular medical practitioners sought to separate "medicine" from "quackery" once and for all by developing stricter conventions for writing, publishing, and advertising medical works. At the same time, allegations of obscenity offered a means through which both groups contested authority and sanitized sexual knowledge from associations with the irregular medicine and pornography trades.

This chapter focuses on developments in regular medicine. The first section examines how medical groups experimented with using obscenity laws to police medical practice in the first half of the 1870s, viewing them as more viable alternatives to the 1858 Medical Act in the wake of the *Hicklin* test's formulation. In the eyes of some experts, this was a risky use of the law. Although the *Hicklin* definition of obscenity was commonly thought to apply only to cheap, popular medical works, Alexander Cockburn had not clearly specified "under what circumstance the publication of obscene matter is justifiable."[1] Theoretically, government blue books and textbooks and treatises aimed at practising medics could be dragged into obscenity trials. Theory never really became practice, however. Most actions against sellers of medical works under obscenity laws were like those examined in this and the previous chapter: they were aimed at people

[1] Arthur Powell, *The Law Specially Affecting Printers, Publishers, and Newspaper Proprietors* (London: Stevens and Sons, 1887), 183. See also "The Law and the Lawyers," *Law Times*, August 5, 1871, 248; Robert George Glenn, *A Manual of Laws Affecting Medical Men* (London: J & A Churchill, 1871), 240.

and publications situated at what regular practitioners considered the fringes of legitimate medical practice, or outside it altogether. Medical groups ultimately found it impossible to suppress irregular trade in treatments for sexual and reproductive health problems. By the end of the 1880s, however, they had collapsed the boundaries of indecency, fraud, and certain forms of medical practice so effectively that they were joined in new legislation aimed at the drug trade. In a different form than that examined in the previous chapter, obscene quackery became a widely accepted concept.

Amid, and in some cases because of, these actions, regular medicine's own systems of communication came under increased scrutiny. Prominent members of the profession argued that going after irregulars was not enough to root out the scourge of quackery: medicine's own systems of print communication needed to be professionalized to wrest the temptation of falling into quackery out of doctors' hands and shore up public trust in medical expertise. The second and third sections of the chapter examine the haphazard emergence of better-defined conventions for medical writing, publishing, and book advertising during this period, and debates that surrounded them. While regular medical practitioners had been developing more distinctive publishing conventions for some time, concerted attention to the need for them hastened this process and established a more robust, if largely unwritten, framework for legitimating medical knowledge and its producers. In establishing this framework, regular practitioners belatedly met the expectations of readers like Alexander Cockburn.

The efforts to discipline medical communication examined in this chapter were not "about" sex or protecting readers from discussions of it. Like the actions against irregular practitioners under obscenity laws, they were responses to interrelated professional concerns about competition, status, credibility, and ethics. Yet, they are interconnected with the history of sexual knowledge and deserve serious attention here. Concerted efforts to discipline medicine's systems of print communication had their roots in longstanding concerns about how medical knowledge could be exploited, and how its exploitation could undermine trust in medical expertise. The fact that writing on fertility, male sexual dysfunction, and venereal disease had become so associated with quackery made questions about how to write, publish, and advertise works on sexual and reproductive issues a fixture of debates about propriety in medical writing, publishing, and book advertising. The outcomes of these efforts also had important implications for access to sexual knowledge. Resolving blurry boundaries between "popular" and "professional" and "medicine" and "quackery" required changing how medical practitioners wrote and how they advertised their publications. These changes expanded divides in the kinds of sexual knowledge that medical practitioners and non-medical readers enjoyed easy access to.

Obscenity Law as an Alternative Instrument

The anti-quackery campaigns examined in the previous chapter were just one element of mounting attempts to suppress irregular medical practice during the mid-nineteenth century. Medical groups sued irregulars for libel and fraud, and, after the passage of the 1858 Medical Act, for falsely claiming formal titles and qualifications. However, it was difficult to police medical practice under these laws. Libel laws, as the legal historian Anat Rosenberg has pointed out, "did not serve a single interest group": irregular practitioners could, and did, employ them for their own purposes.[2] Fraud was difficult to prove in court, and lawsuits frequently collapsed.[3] Actions under the Medical Act often failed on technicalities. Moreover, the maximum penalty for violating the Medical Act – a five-pound fine – did little to deter practitioners from making false claims. The idea that obscenity laws offered an alternative means of policing medical practice had often met with skepticism in the 1850s and 1860s. After 1868, however, several medical groups and at least a handful of friendly magistrates came to believe that, in some cases, the *Hicklin* test's emphasis on context over content made obscenity laws viable alternatives to other legal instruments. In the 1870s, these groups openly used obscenity laws to try to police medical practice and make the case that irregular medical practice was illegitimate and harmful to the public.

One of the first and most well-documented of these efforts emerged out of attempts to censure Charles Watson, a London-based practitioner who published pamphlets promoting his expertise in treating venereal disease and male sexual debility under a variety of aliases.[4] Watson falsely claimed to be a governor of the Male Lock Hospital, a storied London institution that specialized in the treatment of venereal disease in men.[5] Patients believed him, and those that he disappointed often wrote to the hospital to complain about him.[6] One man reported that he had sent away to a Dr. Hammond – a suspected alias of Watson's – for a "self-adjusting curative" belt, which was supposed to prevent nocturnal ejaculations. Instead, he received several bottles of medicine. When he wrote to Hammond and demanded the belt, Hammond insisted that his payment had only covered the medicines and a consulting fee. The belt would cost two guineas more. The patient paid up, only to receive "a

[2] Anat Rosenberg, *The Rise of Mass Advertising: Law, Enchantment, and the Cultural Boundaries of British Modernity* (Oxford: Oxford University Press, 2022), 2019.

[3] Rosenberg, *Rise of Mass Advertising*, 231–236.

[4] See advertisements in *Caledonian Mercury*, November 3, 1858, 1; *Investor's Chronicle and Money Market Review*, December 17, 1870, 602; *Medical Press and Circular*, March 6, 1872, 219.

[5] James Bettley, "Post Voluptatem Misericordia: The Rise and Fall of the London Lock Hospitals," *The London Journal* 10, no. 2 (1984): 167–175.

[6] "Unqualified Practitioners," *Medical Times and Gazette*, June 8, 1872, 600.

common suspensory bandage, with three or four pieces of metal surrounding the waist" and another string of metal pieces through which he was supposed to pass his penis. The device chafed the patient's penis, and the experience embarrassed the patient, who was incredulous that the hospital would associate itself with a charlatan.[7]

The hospital's directors worried that Watson's claims were undermining its reputation. An action against him for similar claims under the Medical Act had failed on a technicality a decade earlier.[8] Nevertheless, they asked one of the hospital's surgeons, Shirley Deakin, to look into pursuing Watson and other irregulars who claimed to be affiliated with the hospital again. In June 1872, Deakin consulted a sympathetic magistrate, who reportedly told him that the hospital could choose between two courses of action: it could prosecute Watson under the Medical Act again for practising under false pretences, or it could prosecute him for obscene libel.[9] By the autumn, the hospital's directors seem to have decided against pursuing Watson, at least officially. However, Deakin had assembled a group of doctors associated with the hospital and several allied institutions to pursue actions against Watson and several other medical entrepreneurs. Deakin had also found a partner with a wealth of experience to bring the actions: the Society for the Suppression of Vice.

At first glance, the Society's involvement is surprising. It had ignored anti-quackery campaigners' appeals in the 1850s and 1860s. By 1872, however, the Society was mired in debt.[10] Under the leadership of a new secretary, the solicitor Charles Hastings Collette, it operated at least occasionally as a for-hire outfit, exchanging prosecutions for generous donations.[11] When Deakin approached the Society's leaders and asked them to prosecute Watson and the

[7] Frances Burdett Courtenay, *Revelations of Quacks and Quackery: A Series of Letters by "Detector" reprinted from "The Medical Circular,"* 3rd ed. (London: Baillière, Tindall & Cox, 1865), 16.

[8] "Legal Intelligence," *Medical Times and Gazette*, November 12, 1864, 530.

[9] "The Lock Hospital and Advertising Charlatans," *BMJ*, June 8, 1872, 616; "Unqualified Medical Practitioners," *Medical Times and Gazette*, June 8, 1872, 660; "The Medical Act and the Quack Fraternity," *Medical Times and Gazette*, June 22, 1872, 714.

[10] M. J. D. Roberts, "Making Victorian Morals? The Society for the Suppression of Vice and Its Critics, 1802–1886," *Australian Historical Studies* 21, no. 83 (1984): 171. See Society for the Suppression of Vice account records (1802–1891), HBM for original financial records.

[11] In addition to this case, see "Society for the Suppression of Vice," *Morning Post*, July 9, 1875, 3, in which Collette broadcast that the Society would prosecute distributors of "medical works and pamphlets" in exchange for donations, and the publisher Henry Bohn's testimony in *The Queen v. Charles Bradlaugh and Annie Besant* (London: Freethought Publishing Company, 1877), 230, which suggests that Catholic priests backed an action against him. This change in the Society's operations could account for the oddly heterogeneous focus of its prosecutions in the 1870s. These prosecutions are outlined in Katherine Mullin, "Poison More Deadly than Prussic Acid: Defining Obscenity after the 1857 Obscene Publications Act (1850–1885)," in *Prudes on the Prowl: Fiction and Obscenity in England, 1857 to the Present Day*, ed. David Bradshaw and Rachel Potter (Oxford: Oxford University Press, 2013), 11–29.

other individuals that his group had identified, they agreed in exchange for funds to pay for the prosecutions and keep the Society running.[12] The money was funnelled to the Society through a newly formed Quack Prosecution Fund, set up by Deakin and Matthew Berkeley Hill, another specialist in venereal disease, in hopes that other medical men would donate to their cause.

In each case, the Society worked closely with the group that Deakin had assembled (hereafter referred to as the "Lock group") throughout the long march from investigation to arrest to indictment. It gathered evidence that figures identified by the group were distributing obscene material by paying young men to visit their premises, purchase their publications, and record observations.[13] After confirming that this evidence could support obscenity charges, the Society printed summaries of its findings and sent them to its backers. Together, they developed arguments to present in court.[14] After this process was concluded, the Society alerted its allies in the police force, who raided the targets' premises and confiscated allegedly obscene material under the Obscene Publications Act. The Society then went to court to argue that the seized material was obscene.

These cases illustrate an evolution of arguments initially employed against consulting surgeons and owners of anatomical museums in anti-quackery campaigns. Although they continued to use terms like "disgusting" to describe the works at issue, after the *Hicklin* judgement medical groups no longer tried to argue that they were as or nearly as dangerous to public morals as pornography, nor did they labour to evoke images of the impressionable youths, blushing wives, and innocent children who might be damaged by them. "Obscene quackery," in other words, was no longer explicitly collapsed with sexual deviance. Instead, medical groups focused on demonstrating something that the passage of the 1858 Medical Act had made easier: that the sellers of the publications at issue were not legitimate medical practitioners. If they were not genuine medical men, the argument went, then the "circumstances of the publication" that had been so important to Cockburn were clearly illegitimate. The defendants must have some nefarious motive for distributing the works at issue: defrauding readers, inciting immoral behaviour, or both.

Intent was supposed to be meaningless under the terms of the *Hicklin* test: all that mattered was whether a work was being distributed in ways that enabled it to fall into the hands of readers who could be damaged by it. However, this argument enabled medical groups to accomplish several things at once. First, it diffused the defendants' claims that they were simply circulating medical information for professional reasons – their only major defence after the

[12] See "Quack Prosecutions," *Lancet*, February 15, 1873, 250–251. A list of actions backed by the Lock group appears in *Clinic*, February 8, 1873, 69.

[13] *Davidson, Dennison, and Romilly*, 1873. Old Bailey Proceedings Online (t18730203-167); "Obscene Prints," Lancet, November 30, 1872, 797.

[14] "Quack Prosecutions," *Lancet*, February 15, 1873, 250–251.

Hicklin ruling, which stressed the importance of the context in which obscene material was being sold. Second, it enabled medical groups to use the courtroom as a public stage to repudiate the defendants' claims to medical expertise, situate irregular medical practice as dangerous, and assert their own authority. The gist of their arguments was always some version of the following: A medical practitioner who made inaccurate claims about himself had bad intentions. If the intent was not to defraud customers, it was to incite vice; if it was not to incite vice, it was to defraud. Perhaps it was both. Irregular medical practice was illegitimate practice. And in illegitimate hands, sexual knowledge was always harmful to the public.

The Lock group's most high-profile success was the shuttering of Joseph Kahn's Museum in London. In November 1872, a bevy of police officers stormed the museum, now located in Tichbourne Street, at the direction of the Society for the Suppression of Vice. They seized nearly nine thousand copies of Kahn's pamphlet *The Philosophy of Marriage* on the basis of the Society's claim that it was a "lewd and filthy book."[15] Forty cases of anatomical models were later seized from the museum on charges that they, too, were "indecent, disgusting, and demoralising."[16] Kahn had absconded to New York a decade earlier after a patient sued him for extortion, and was therefore absent when the police arrived.[17] However, the museum's proprietors, Henry Romilly, John Davidson, and John Dennison (who reportedly took turns impersonating Kahn for visitors), were charged with unlawfully "selling indecent pictures, for having in their possession 8,700 obscene libels with intent to publish the same, and for a conspiracy to publish."[18]

At first, the trio defended themselves. They argued that the museum was "of a scientific and medical character," and that works that it had displayed and distributed for fifteen years were obviously not obscene.[19] But the Society for the Suppression of Vice refused to quibble over the character of Kahn's works. Citing the absence of Romilly, Davidson, and Dennison's names from the Medical Register, Collette and another solicitor for the Society, a Mr. Besley, argued that they were not medical practitioners. The trio's lack of formal qualifications, they maintained, offered proof that their publications and displays had no legitimate purpose. Indeed, they implied, the fact that these men did not have formal qualifications was evidence that they aimed to "excite the

15 "Marlborough Street," *Morning Advertiser*, December 13, 1872, 7.

16 "Kahn's Museum," *Lancet*, March 8, 1873, 354–355.

17 Ellen Bayuk Rosenman, *Unauthorized Pleasures: Accounts of Victorian Erotic Experience* (Ithaca, NY: Cornell University Press, 2003), 36. For details about Kahn's trial for extortion, see "Appendix: Exposure of the Quack System: Bloomsbury County Court, July 30, 1857" in William Acton, *The Functions and Disorders of the Reproductive System in Youth, in Adult Age, and in Advanced Life*. 2nd ed. (London: John Churchill, 1858), 117–123.

18 *Davidson, Dennison, and Romilly*, 1873.

19 *Davidson, Dennison, and Romilly*, 1873.

imagination and create fears, with the view of trading on both for profit."[20] James Lank, a senior surgeon at the Lock Hospital, testified in support of this argument. Kahn's *Philosophy of Marriage* was not "in any sense a medical treatise for the education or information of medical students," he opined. Its sole purpose was titillating museum visitors and inducing them to pay large sums for dubious cures.[21]

It was only after airing these opinions that Collette and Besley admitted that legally the defendants' intentions were beside the point: what mattered was that they were distributing an explicit work to the public, and that "the case of R. v. Hicklin fully explained the law in such cases." When the magistrate said that he would refer the case to trial, where a jury could decide "whether such publication had a tendency to corrupt minds" likely to come into contact with it, the trio pled guilty.[22] Perhaps they suspected that a jury would not return a favourable verdict, or perhaps they simply did not want to face the agony of a jury trial. The seized copies of Kahn's *Philosophy of Marriage* were burnt along with over a million handbills, catalogues, and other pamphlets in February 1873.[23] The following month, Collette and two police officers took turns with a hammer and smashed the models to smithereens. Dennison and Davidson were ordered to pay fines of 500 pounds each, and Romilly 100 pounds, as the magistrate determined that he was merely a "servant of the establishment."[24] All three were released on the condition that they not display or disseminate such works again.[25]

Romilly, Davidson, and Dennison never claimed to work for the Lock Hospital. However, the attraction that prosecuting them had for a group of medical practitioners who specialized in treating venereal disease is not difficult to understand. It enabled them to publicly repudiate a venue that not only seemed to undermine medics' claims to exclusive authority over anatomical knowledge, as Alan Bates has argued, but was also a popular competing source of information about and treatment for venereal disease.[26] Journalists were eager to report on obscenity cases, and the Kahn case was no exception: Collette and Besley's arguments about the proprietors' falsified qualifications and scurrilous motives were widely reported in the press. That Romilly, Davidson, and Dennison pled guilty before the case was turned over a jury, leading to the destruction of their stock and the

20 "Marlborough Street," *Morning Advertiser*, 7.
21 *Davidson, Dennison, and Romilly*, 1873.
22 "Marlborough Street," *Morning Advertiser*, 7.
23 A. W. Bates, "Dr. Kahn's Museum: Obscene Anatomy in Victorian London," *Journal of the Royal Society of Medicine* 99 (2006): 621. See also "Society for the Suppression of Vice," *Lancet*, June 12, 1873, 56–57.
24 *Davidson, Dennison, and Romilly*, 1873.
25 "Last Week's Latest News," *Reynolds's Newspaper*, February 16, 1873, 5.
26 Bates, "Dr. Kahn," 622–623.

museum's closure, was a marvellous stroke of luck. The action was, the *Lancet* declared, a triumph.[27]

The emphasis on illegitimate practice intensified in the Watson case. Acting on the Society's claims that Watson was selling obscene publications, the Metropolitan Police seized 4,200 books and pamphlets from his residence in Bedford Square around the same time that it raided Kahn's Museum in November 1872.[28] At Bow Street police court later that month, Collette and Besley disabused Watson's claim that he was a governor of the Lock Hospital and argued that his publications "induce[d] weak-minded men to believe that they were suffering from certain illnesses," leaving them vulnerable to fraud and extortion.[29] Indeed, Collette and Besley focused so much on Watson's alleged charlatanism that no report of the case indicates that they argued that his publications presented a moral danger to the public, beyond their broad characterization of the works as obscene according to the terms of the *Hicklin* test. Watson's fraudulence was simply offered as evidence that his publications were dangerous.

Watson's counsel countered that although it was true that he was not a governor of the Lock Hospital, he did have medical credentials in New York. Moreover, if his publications were offensive, so, too, were works by "English medical men of well-known ability."[30] Reportedly, he read extracts aloud to the magistrate, Frederick Flowers, to drive his point home. After Flowers announced that he would leave the verdict to a jury, however, Watson pled guilty. Like Dennison, Davidson, and Romilly, he seems to have thought that a jury trial would not be worth his while.[31] Watson's publications were destroyed, and he was fined 1,000 pounds. Notably, Flowers instructed Watson "not to issue any similar publication, or any advertisements in the papers, or otherwise ... [be involved in] the publication or distribution of such works, or *even [point] to himself as practicing as indicated in these works*."[32] This last directive, which had nothing to do with Watson's publications or their alleged effect on public morals, offers further evidence that some magistrates recognised and approved of obscenity law's use as a means of policing medical practice.

The final case demonstrates that even Flowers's support for this use of obscenity law was limited, however: magistrates were only supportive in cases where they believed that the defendant was defrauding the public. This case, which targeted a man called Isaac Louis Pulvermacher, was different than

27 "A Plague-Spot Obliterated," *Lancet*, December 27, 1873, 913.
28 "Obscene Prints," *Lancet*, November 30, 1872, 797.
29 "Central Criminal Court: Charge against a Medical Practitioner," *Reynolds's Newspaper*, December 22, 1872, 6.
30 "Central Criminal Court," *Reynolds's Newspaper*, 6.
31 *Watson*, 1872. Old Bailey Proceedings Online (t18721216-62).
32 "Summary of this Morning's News," *Pall Mall Gazette*, December 18, 1872, 6. Emphasis added.

the others. Pulvermacher did not practise medicine or claim medical qualifications. Trained in Vienna as an electrical engineer, he identified himself as an electrician or inventor in advertisements, and held patents for a number of devices, including a current regulator, an electric generator, and several galvometers.[33] He was best known for his Volta-Electric Chain-Bands, portable batteries that he claimed could treat a wide variety of ailments.[34] Pulvermacher advertised his Chain-Bands in medical periodicals, offered discounts to hospitals, and hosted private demonstrations in London in 1871–2. Leading medical journals covered the demonstrations, and reported that they impressed famous medical men.[35] Less impressive to these men was Pulvermacher's subsequent use of their names and extracts from their private letters in advertisements.[36] This behaviour embarrassed doctors who had held him in high regard, and seems to have made him a target for prosecution.

Pulvermacher had made himself vulnerable to obscenity charges in 1870 by publishing a pamphlet that addressed the efficacy of electricity as a treatment for "diseases of a private nature."[37] At the direction of the Lock group, the Society for the Suppression of Vice attempted to prosecute Pulvermacher for distributing the pamphlet by post. The case immediately followed Watson's in the same police court, with the same magistrate. Unfortunately, the details of Collette's argument were never reported. However, he clearly failed to convince Flowers that Pulvermacher's pamphlet was dangerous to the public in any capacity. Flowers opined that it was not "within the same category as those of the medical 'quacks'," and adjourned the case for six months.[38] The Society dropped its charges after Pulvermacher withdrew the pamphlet from circulation and threatened to sue Deakin and Collette for slander.[39]

[33] Robert Waits, "Gustave Flaubert, Charles Dickens, and Isaac Pulvermacher's 'Magic Band'," *Progress in Brain Research* 205 (2013): 219–239.

[34] Waits, "Gustave Flaubert," 225–228. See also J. L. Pulvermacher, *Medical Electricity: Its Use and Abuse; or How to Cure Rheumatic, Nervous, Muscular, and Functional Disorders by Self-Application* (London: J.L. Pulvermacher, 1873), 8.

[35] For examples of these advertisements, see "Pulvermacher's Improved Patent Flexible Batteries," *Medical Press and Circular Advertiser*, March 1, 1871, viii and "Electricity Is Life," *Illustrated London News*, March 23, 1871, 302. For details about Pulvermacher's demonstrations, see "Medical Electricity," *BMJ*, February 17, 1872, 191. For more on Pulvermacher, see Takahiro Ueyama, *Health in the Marketplace: Professionalism, Therapeutic Desires, and Medical Commodification in Late-Victorian London* (Palo Alto, CA: Society for the Promotion of Science and Scholarship, 2010), 138–146.

[36] Waits, "Gustave Flaubert," 225–228; Ueyama, *Health in the Marketplace*, 145.

[37] See advertisement in Pulvermacher, *Medical Electricity: Its Use and Abuse*, 8.

[38] "The Medical Prosecutions," *Lloyd's Weekly Newspaper*, December 1, 1872, 7. The pamphlet at issue has not survived, so we cannot know exactly how it differed from Watson's works. However, it is worth noting that Pulvermacher's other publications are less detailed in their descriptions of health issues than Watson's, and that he never claimed to be able to cure them.

[39] "The Medical Prosecutions," *Lloyd's Weekly Newspaper*, 7; "Prosecution of the Quacks," *Medical Press and Circular*, November 27, 1872, 468.

Deakin, Berkeley Hill, and their friends were disappointed with the outcome of the Pulvermacher case, but they were thrilled that Watson and Kahn's associates had capitulated. They wanted to continue their work. Writing on the Watson case, the *Medical Press and Circular* reported that there were at least "eight or ten [individuals] singled out against whom proceedings will be taken, nominally by the Society for the Suppression of Vice, actually by some members of the Profession attached to the Lock Hospitals and kindred institutions."[40] To do so, however, they would need donations. The 1872–3 actions were exceedingly expensive, as the Society demanded large payments for its expertise, detective work, legal services, and overhead. The Watson case alone cost the Lock group 354 pounds.[41]

Deakin and Collette, who had a financial stake in the project as both the Society's secretary and its chief solicitor, appealed for donations to offset the expense of these actions and cover future ones. They sent letters outlining their ambitions to a variety of medical journals, and wrote to several organizations, including the Royal College of Surgeons, asking for funding. "If we are adequately supported by the public," Collette claimed in one letter to the *Lancet*, "we shall clear the country of these pests to society."[42] The *Lancet* supported these appeals, trumpeting the efficacy of obscenity law for combating quackery in the wake of the *Hicklin* ruling.[43] However, the Lock group and its partners were nearly as unsuccessful at attracting practical support as the *Lancet* had been a decade earlier. Few medical men opened their wallets for the Quack Prosecution Fund, and the Royal College of Surgeons refused Collette's request for a donation.[44] Berkeley Hill reported that total donations barely amounted to 100 pounds.[45]

Tepid financial support put an end to the Lock group's ambitions. By the summer of 1873, it had disbanded.[46] Over the next few years, several other medical groups brought similar actions against irregulars, though the time and money it took to bring them meant that they, too, had to temper their goals.[47] Local police forces sometimes assisted these groups by surveilling irregulars and raiding their homes and consulting rooms, and, in a few cases, seem to have

40 "Prosecution of the Quacks," *Medical Press and Circular*, 468.

41 "The Prosecution of Obscene Quacks," *BMJ*, July 12, 1873, 44. The Society's bank records do not record payments from the Lock group. However, they do record several payments of between three and four hundred pounds marked "cash."

42 "Society for the Suppression of Vice," *Lancet*, January 4, 1873, 33–34.

43 For examples, see "Prosecution of Indecent Quacks," *Medical Times and Gazette*, February 22, 1873, 204; "Notices to Correspondents: Quack Prosecution Fund," *Medical Press and Circular*, January 8, 1873, 37; "A Plague-Spot Obliterated," *Lancet*, December 27, 1873, 913.

44 Minute Book, vol. 12, March 13, 1873, 145–146, RCS-GOV/2/1/8, RCS.

45 "Notices to Correspondents: Quack Prosecution Fund," *Medical Press and Circular*, 37.

46 "The Prosecution of Obscene Quacks," *BMJ*, July 12, 1873, 44.

47 "Obscene Quackery and the East London Medical Defence Association," *Lancet*, March 3, 1877, 328–329.

acted of their own accord.[48] The slippage between policing the medical marketplace and policing the print marketplace on stage in the Lock cases was fully in view in these episodes. In one case, in 1876, the Medical Act and the Obscene Publications Act were employed against irregular practitioners simultaneously. Twelve medical practitioners were summoned to a Manchester police court following a series of raids under the Obscene Publications Act. All were fined under the Medical Act for practising under false pretences, and those who had distributed publications advertising treatments for sexual health problems saw them destroyed on the grounds that they were obscene. Professional misconduct and moral endangerment were collapsed into a single, unofficial crime in these cases: obscene quackery.[49]

It is difficult to separate fact from fantasy about the effect that these actions had on trade in sexual health manuals. According to the *Lancet*, the 1872–3 cases panicked prominent irregulars. Many pulled their advertisements from the newspapers, the journal alleged. A few, it claimed, turned their publications over to the Society for the Suppression of Vice, hoping to avoid prosecutions.[50] The *Lancet*'s reports were almost certainly embroidered: the idea that Joseph Lambert or Samuel La'Mert would dump thousands of publications at the threshold of the Society's headquarters like a stockpile of bombs about to denotate is not very plausible. However, advertisements for consulting surgeons' manuals did decline steeply from the mid-1870s.[51] By the beginning of the 1880s, British readers no longer encountered crowds of notices for works like *Manhood*, *Self-Preservation*, or *The Silent Friend* in the quack's corner of the newspaper. Foreign and colonial advertisements for these kinds of manuals also dwindled. Although they continued to circulate into the early twentieth century, most extant examples published after 1880 are foreign translations and reworkings, not British originals.

The decline of the consulting surgeon's manual and the businesses that relied on it to connect with patients was probably influenced by the legal actions I have described. However, other developments are likely as, or more, significant to this history. First, the most prominent consulting surgeons, who had established their businesses in the early 1840s, published manuals under several aliases, and sold them on a global scale, were elderly men by 1870. Lewis Jacob Jordan, the patriarch of the Jordan family firm, died in 1874.[52]

48 For instance, see "A Caution to Quack Doctors," *Manchester Evening News*, October 26, 1877, 4.

49 "The Raid on Quack Doctors," *Manchester Courier*, November 1876, 6.

50 "Quack Prosecutions," *Lancet*, February 15, 1873, 250–251.

51 Virginia Berridge also notes this pattern "Popular Journalism and Working Class Attitudes, 1854–1886: A Study of *Reynolds's Newspaper, Lloyd's Weekly Paper*, and *The Weekly Times*" (PhD thesis, University of London, 1976), 274.

52 "Wills and Bequests," *Illustrated London News*, July 25, 1874, 22.

Joseph Lambert died in 1875, and his brother, Samuel La'Mert, died in 1876.[53] The passing of these powerful figures represented a major disruption to the trade. Second, new technological developments were fostering the massive expansion of drug and rubber manufacturing. Just as the decline of the Holywell Street trade coincided with the rise of a thriving trade in pornographic photographs, the decline of the consulting surgeon business coincided with the proliferation of new medical products that promised to treat impotence, venereal disease, menstrual problems, and, in veiled terms, unwanted pregnancies.[54] Sexual knowledge was not suppressed. However, trades that had facilitated its distribution through print did change, with trade in information about how to treat impotence and venereal disease, in particular, becoming more closely aligned with the drug trade than the book trade.

Anti-quackery campaigners shifted focus accordingly: they gave up campaigning against obscene medical publications and displays almost entirely and concentrated on lobbying the government for legislation to regulate trade in drugs and medical devices.[55] However, arguments that regular medical groups had developed to bend obscenity laws to police medical practice lived on in new legislation. The Indecent Advertisements Bill was introduced in the late 1880s to combat "pernicious pamphlets and circulars issued by quacks ... which make statements (frequently untrue) as to secret and loathsome diseases, and which are mainly intended to frighten readers into consulting the medical quacks in whose interest they are issued."[56] The subsequent Indecent Advertisements Act of 1889 banned "any advertisement relating to syphilis, gonorrhoea, nervous debility, or other complaint or infirmity arising from or relating to sexual intercourse," including pregnancy.[57] Notably, it did not ban advertisements for sexual entertainment. Medics had succeeded in collapsing indecency, fraud, and certain forms of irregular medical practice: the term "indecent advertisement" was now shorthand for "quack advertisement relating to sexual or reproductive issues."

Convincing the state that certain modes of selling advice and treatments for these issues were illegitimate and harmful to the public was a significant victory for anti-quackery campaigners. However, as the proliferation of new

[53] Doreen Berger, *The Jewish Victorian: Genealogical Information from the Jewish Newspapers, 1871–1880* (Whitney, Oxfordshire: Robert Boyd, 1999), 296; "Deaths Registered in January, February, and March 1876: Samuel Lamert, " *England & Wales, Civil Registration Death Index, 1837–1915* (Provo, UT: Ancestry.com Operations, 2006-) www.ancestry.ca/search/collections/8914/.

[54] For instance, see "Hughes's Blood Pills," *South Wales Echo*, December 24, 1885, 2; "Higson's Female Pills," *Nuneaton Chronicle*, January 30, 1885, 8.

[55] Ueyama, *Health in the Marketplace*, 25–58.

[56] Indecent Advertisements Bill [H.L.] Memorandum. HO 45/9086/B6217, TNA.

[57] Nicholas Daly, *The Demographic Imagination and the Nineteenth-Century City: Paris, London, New York* (Cambridge: Cambridge University Press, 2015), 120–121.

kinds of businesses hawking treatments for sexual and reproductive health complaints emphasizes, they failed to suppress public interest in irregular treatments, and the Indecent Advertisements Act failed to suppress the businesses that sold them. Although the penalties for violating the Act were fairly significant – offenders could be fined up to five pounds or imprisoned for up to three months with hard labour – it was difficult to enforce because it was riddled with loopholes. Legislators had worried that making the Act applicable to material in newspapers would give rise to accusations of press censorship.[58] Newspaper advertisements were therefore not covered by the Act, and irregulars continued to advertise widely in newspapers. Some pasted advertisements on sandwich boards and hired young men to carry them around town on their bodies, another method of display not covered in the Act.[59] Others simply adapted copy for posters and handbills to avoid terms specified in the legislation. As the free-love advocate George Bedborough recalled in the 1930s, the Act "stimulated the invention of decent substitutes for phrases made illegal ... 'Social Diseases' 'Secret Diseases' 'Skin Complaints of all Kinds' came to be common expressions."[60]

For a while, anti-quackery campaigners held out hope that the Indecent Advertisements Act would deliver. Some wrote to the Metropolitan Police's Executive Branch demanding that the police do more to enforce it.[61] Others lobbied Parliament to plug loopholes in the Act. In the end, though, the legislation was not altered, police officers' commitment to enforcing it was erratic, and irregular treatments for sexual and reproductive health problems continued to be advertised widely. Laws addressing the print marketplace could be leveraged to police medical practice. They could even be created for this purpose. However, they could not suppress irregular trade in treatments for sexual and reproductive health problems, nor could they destroy those treatments' credibility in the eyes of many Victorians. They also could not raise an impermeable wall across the borders of "medicine" and "quackery." Doctors would need to attend to their own systems of communication to further their ambition of distancing medicine from the market and its moral quagmires.

58 David J. Cox, Kim Stevenson, Candida Harris, and Judith Rowbotham, *Public Indecency in England, 1857–1960: 'A Serious Growing Evil'* (London: Routledge, 2015), 68–70. British legislation aimed at the print marketplace was always influenced by legislators' concerns about being accused of censorship, which they saw as antithetical to democratic liberalism. See Lisa Z. Sigel, "Censorship in Inter-War Britain: Obscenity, Spectacle, and the Workings of the Liberal State," *Journal of Social History* 45, no. 1 (2011): 63.

59 "The Indecent Advertisements Act," *Lancet*, December 13, 1890, 1282–1283; "Indecent Advertisements," *Lancet*, May 3, 1890, 379; "Indecent Advertisements," *BMJ*, January 10, 1891, 79.

60 George Bedborough to Havelock Ellis, February 22, 1930, ADD MS 70556.14, 2, BL.

61 For example, see Leslie Phillips to the Chief Commissioner of Police, Scotland Yard, November 14, 1890, HO 144/238/A52539 Mepol.2/237, No. 104380, TNA.

Elevating Medical Print Culture

Many questions about how to handle print that had preoccupied regular practitioners in the 1840s and 1850s were still not easily answered in 1870. How could the medical profession firmly distinguish its own literature from quack productions? And how could it prevent regular practitioners from exploiting medical knowledge for personal gain and dragging the profession into the mire of quackery? Now that medicine had been granted statutory recognition as a profession – and the Medical Act had proven to be an ineffectual instrument for eradicating quackery as regular practitioners defined it – addressing these issues became a more intensive focus of debate.

Specialized publishing formats, such as the medical journal, and publishers, like the ones we saw in Chapter 3, were now better-established. In practical terms, they increasingly functioned as frameworks through which knowledge and expertise were legitimated, at least in medical circles.[62] However, the journal was still not the dominant format of medical communication, as it is today, and medical practitioners still took it for granted that even specialist publishers did not prevent abuses of publishing or confusions of professional identity. Debates about how medical books should be written, published, and advertised were consequently a significant focus of debates about how to "raise up" regular medical print culture during the 1870s, and no books were the focus of more debate than those that addressed venereal disease, masturbation, sexual dysfunction, and prostitution. These topics had long been associated with quackery or (in the case of prostitution) pandering to prurient readers: misuses of knowledge that advocates of a more professionalized medical print culture wanted to distance medicine from.

That anxieties about ambiguities between "medicine" and "quackery" drove debates about how to treat these topics more than concern for readers' morals is not just indicated by the content of these debates, which incessantly return to the subject of "charlatans" and how their uses of print undermined legitimate medical discourse. It is also indicated by the striking absence of discussions about how to present information about sodomy. British medics were often reticent to discuss sodomy at all. The topic was subject to censorship in the Bourdieuian sense that unspoken cultural pressures discouraged medical authors from engaging with it outside works on venereology and forensic medicine, or reviews of such works.[63] Yet, precisely because of those cultural pressures, writing that addressed sodomy did not present the same problems for

62 Roy Porter, "The Rise of Medical Journalism in Britain to 1800," in *Medical Journals Medical Knowledge*, ed. W. F. Bynum, Stephen Lock, and Roy Porter (London: Routledge, 1992), 12.

63 Ivan Dalley Crozier, "The Medical Construction of Homosexuality and Its Relation to the Law in Nineteenth-Century England," *Medical History* 45, no. 1 (2001): 61–82; Pierre Bourdieu, *Language and Symbolic Power*, trans. Gino Raymond and Matthew Adamson (Cambridge, MA: Harvard University Press, 1991).

the medical profession as writing about mundane phenomena like venereal disease. Few people claimed authority over medical knowledge about sodomy during this period. Propriety in publishing works that addressed same-sex sex and most other forms of non-reproductive sex therefore did not become a matter of open debate in medical circles until the late 1890s, when the proliferation of sexual-scientific works on variant sexualities and their circulation through diverse channels made this necessary.[64]

Recent accounts of the professionalization of publishing in the natural sciences emphasize that it was a gradual, haphazard process.[65] This was also true of medicine even during a period in which practitioners were actively trying to "raise up" medical print culture. Medical men suggested a variety of ways that this could be accomplished in medical journals, public lectures, and medical society meetings. As I show in this section, some argued that authors should adopt certain editorial practices or styles of writing, or that their publishers should issue books with (or without) certain design characteristics, to clearly mark out legitimate medical literature and burnish medicine's emerging identity as a scientific field. None of these arguments seems to have gained a significant following; yet, the content of medical books certainly changed over the course of the late nineteenth century. Other medical men, as the next section shows, advocated establishing rigid conventions for advertising medical books to remove the temptation of exploiting knowledge from medics' hands and clearly differentiate legitimate medical works from quack productions. These arguments garnered more consistent engagement.

Debate about how books themselves might be altered to accomplish these goals was discontinuous partly because the task seemed to many medical men to be impossible: no aspect of a book was immune to misreading, nor to copying and abuse. This was a lesson that medics had learned all too well from the now greatly degraded use-value of paratextual defences of sexual content. Prior to the Victorian period, medical authors routinely inserted such defences into the prefaces to their books, and sometimes into other places as well. Those who wrote works on venereal disease and male sexual dysfunction additionally littered them with complaints about these topics' popularity with quacks, often claiming that few authoritative writers addressed them for fear of associating themselves with charlatans. Such statements were not, or at least not merely, expressions of personal anxiety. They were established rhetorical devices aimed at mitigating the risk of being charged with quackery or

[64] See Chapter 7 for further details.

[65] Alex Csiszar, *The Scientific Journal: Authorship and the Politics of Knowledge in the Nineteenth Century* (Chicago: University of Chicago Press, 2018); Melinda Baldwin, *Making Nature: The History of a Scientific Journal* (Chicago: University of Chicago Press, 2015); Aileen Fyfe, Noah Moxham, Julie McDougall-Waters, and Camilla Mørk Røstvik, *A History of Scientific Journals: Publishing at the Royal Society, 1665–2015* (London: UCL Press, 2022).

pandering to prurient taste by framing the text as serious medical writing and its author as a serious medical man.

Laments about the topics' popularity with quacks remained a common feature of works on venereal disease, male sexual dysfunction, and related topics into the 1870s. However, lengthy justifications for writing about sexual matters had virtually disappeared from regular medical works by this period. When editors recycled material from works published prior to the Victorian period, they often discarded *apologia*s for sexual content, or severely truncated them. A medical encyclopedia that reproduced sections from William Burke's *Popular Compendium of Anatomy* (1804) reduced his three-paragraph *apologia* for writing on the generative organs to three lines, and shoved it into a footnote.[66] Disclaimers published at the beginning of a book, such as "It must be clearly understood that this is a work belonging to the category of 'adult literature'," would not gain traction in Britain until the turn of the century, and were mainly used by sexologists, sex reformers, and their publishers.[67] Although American medical authors continued to employ them, British authors typically dismissed paratextual defences and justifications for writing on sexual matters as worse than useless, partly because irregulars could, and sometimes did, copy them, and partly because they drew attention to sexual content, an effect that disreputable booksellers had long exploited. Counterintuitively, these devices could therefore be interpreted as unprofessional. Reviewing an American work that trumpeted its author's "elaborate delicacy" in dealing with sexual matters in 1869, one English medical journalist complained that the intervention was "almost as suggestive as absolute obscenity."[68]

Medical men occasionally advocated translating explicit passages into Latin as a "scientific" means of elevating works on topics associated with quackery during this period, one that could diffuse authors' anxieties about writing on topics popular with charlatans by demonstrating that they did not wish to parade their knowledge before the public. An 1874 review in the *Medical Press and Circular*, for instance, praised the French physician Guéneau de Mussy's use of Latin to veil "delicate passages" in an article on sterility and impotence in the French journal *L'Union Médicale*. "Mussy," the *Circular* explained, desired to give his work a "scientific character . . . [and] not . . . mere exciting reading to his readers, as if medical periodicals were written for schools of girls or monasteries." Latin covered "as with a veil certain crudenesses of expression which the French language is unable to do," and

[66] Keith Imray, *A Popular Cyclopedia of Modern Domestic Medicine*, American ed. (New York: Gates, Stedman and Company, 1850), 91.

[67] Quoted in Phillip Kuhn, "The Sexual Life of Our Time: Medical Censorship in Early-20th-Century England," *History of Psychology* 23, no. 1 (2020): 52. See Chapter 7 for further details.

[68] "A New Direction for Medical Literature," *Medical Press and Circular*, December 8, 1869, 469.

transformed a work on a topic "shamefully abused by charlatans" into a demonstration of its author's erudition. Mussy's use of Latin affirmed that he was "not merely a physician of the normal school, and has penetrated into the sanctuary of rhetoric in writing an article worthy of Martial and Petronius."[69]

If British medical writers had adopted Mussy's practice, they would have been in good company. Translators of literary texts often veiled risqué passages by leaving them in the original language.[70] Natural scientists – most famously, Charles Darwin – sometimes translated earthier passages into Latin to protect the sensibilities of middle-class readers.[71] However, medical authors rarely used this strategy in Britain, even when addressing taboo topics like sodomy. Some medical men considered selective Latinizing a silly over-performance of respectability. Even medics who railed against obscene quackery sometimes snickered at authors who issued "expurgated editions."[72] Others objected that Latinizing was impractical in an applied field like medicine, where misunderstandings could have mortal consequences. British medical practitioners, as even the *Medical Press and Circular* conceded, were far less fluent in Latin than their Continental counterparts.[73] Other medical writers opined that Latinizing was as prone to abuse as paratextual defences of sexual content: it was just another device that could be copied and misused. Any attempt to invest science with "the veil of secrecy," they worried, was "apt to degenerate into charlatanism."[74]

A more feasible means of elevating medical print culture was making it as dull as possible. Some doctors opined that medical knowledge should always be packaged up in an austere material form that firmly signified its author's professionalism. A review of Baker Brown's *On the Curability of Insanity, Epilepsy, and Hysteria in Females* (1866), which addressed female masturbation, opined that such a book should not be emblazoned with gilt letters (a common feature of irregular manuals in the 1860s) and other "outward *facies* which belong to the class of works which lie upon drawing-room tables": its design should clearly signify its author's restraint in dealing with such topics, not make it an object of desire.[75] Reviewers also recommended leaching medical works' text of colour to

69 "Functional Disorders of the Reproductive System," *Medical Press and Circular*, February 4, 1874, 96.

70 For further details, see Stephen Harrison and Christopher Stray, eds., *Expurgating the Classics: Editing Out in Latin and Greek* (Bristol: Bristol Classical, 2012).

71 Gowan Dawson, *Darwin, Literature, and Victorian Respectability* (Cambridge: Cambridge University Press, 2007), 37–39.

72 "Indecent Advertisements," *Medical Times and Gazette*, December 18, 1852, 624–625.

73 "Functional Disorders," *Medical Press and Circular*, 96.

74 Review of *Atlas of Venereal Diseases, Edinburgh Medical Journal*, vol. XXXI (Edinburgh and London: Oliver and Boyd and Simpkin, Marshall, & Co, 1886), 860.

75 Quoted in Lesley A. Hall, "'The English Have Hot-Water Bottles': The Morganatic Marriage between Sexology and Medicine in Britain since William Acton," in *Sexual Knowledge, Sexual*

achieve these goals. In the same review that praised Mussy's use of Latin, the *Medical Press and Circular* lauded the Scottish surgeon Donald Campbell Black's *On the Functional Diseases of the Renal, Urinary, and Reproductive Organs* (1872), calling it "perhaps, the best work of reference respecting [these diseases] for medical men."[76] However, it was unimpressed with Black's "vivid style," which still makes for entertaining reading:

> Suppress prostitution! Turn the Mississippi! Pluck Jupiter from the studded vault of Heaven! The canker is in society. Prostitution is an appanage of an advanced civilisation. The attempt [to suppress it] is Utopian and unphilosophical, while its causes are permitted to remain; and if possible, could not fail to be productive of greater evils.[77]

The *Circular*'s writer opined that if a second edition of *Functional Diseases* was required, Black should "entirely re-write it and rigidly exclude every phrase that is not necessary to his meaning." This editorial makeover would undoubtedly make the book "dull instead of light," but it "would greatly increase its real value to professional men, for these topics are very delicate ones, and much as we admire fluency and eloquence we would see them reserved for other occasions."[78]

In the eyes of some practitioners, a medical author's reserve needed to extend beyond style alone: he should shear his writing of extraneous or evocative details, lest he appear to be pandering to prurient curiosity. The *Lancet*'s 1870 review of the second edition of the surgeon William Acton's *Prostitution, Considered in Its Moral, Social, and Sanitary Aspects* (1857) praised the book, but scolded Acton for introducing "sensational matter into his history." Among other things, the *Lancet* took issue with his inclusion of "picturesque descriptions of evenings spent in the Cremorne."[79] As Walter Kendrick has noted, Acton's descriptions of the London pleasure-garden were drawn from his visits with the "intention of taking notes on 'the demeanour of London prostitution,' and nothing in his rather disgruntled account would suggest any lapse from sobriety."[80] Even so, his descriptions of the "temples, 'monster platforms,' and 'crystal circle' of Cremorne" are "lush . . . as if [Acton] found it a relief to turn from gray statistics to the evocation of actual sights and sounds."[81] For the *Lancet*, and for a later reviewer for the *British*

Science: The History of Attitudes to Sexuality, ed. Roy Porter and Mikulas Teich (Cambridge: Cambridge University Press, 1994), 352.

76 "Functional Disorders," *Medical Press and Circular*, 96.

77 Donald Campbell Black, *On the Functional Diseases of the Renal, Urinary, and Reproductive Organs, with a General Review of Urinary Pathology* (London: J & A Churchill, 1872), 268.

78 "Functional Disorders," *Medical Press and Circular*, 96.

79 Review of *Prostitution*, *Lancet*, January 29, 1870, 161.

80 Walter Kendrick, *The Secret Museum: Pornography in Modern Culture* (1987; repr.,Berkeley: University of California Press, 1996), 30.

81 Kendrick, *The Secret Museum*, 30.

Medical Journal, however, Acton's inclusion of these details skirted the bounds of professionalism.[82]

In proposing these means of elevating medical print culture, their advocates were suggesting that authors of works aimed at medical practitioners and other professionals adapt methods of self-censorship that authors of medical encyclopedias and other domestic medical reference books, which were usually issued by general publishing firms, had already begun to adopt. At the beginning of the Victorian period, these reference works typically contained lengthy entries on sexual and reproductive matters, usually excerpted and lightly adapted from textbooks aimed at medical students. The information these works offered was not comprehensive. Editors assumed, for example, that like medical students, the married women who were their target audience would already know about heterosexual intercourse (an assumption that perennially disappointed their children, who combed medical encyclopedias for information about where babies came from).[83] Even so, the information they offered was quite extensive. Thomas Andrew's *Cyclopedia of Domestic Medicine and Surgery* (1842) – a work addressed to "mothers and nurses" – frankly defines anatomical terms for the reproductive organs, and includes robust entries on puberty and the onset of menstruation, menstrual problems, the symptoms and progress of pregnancy, miscarriage, and the symptoms and treatment of venereal disease.

From the 1860s, however, entries in medical encyclopedias and other domestic medical reference books were written to order more and more often, and they became less and less informative. Lengthy sections on pregnancy and venereal disease remained a staple of these works. However, their focus shifted from explaining these phenomena to equipping readers with the knowledge required to manage them at home or communicate with a medical practitioner. Descriptions of body parts also became shorter and more euphemistic. The entry for "Vagina" in *Haydn's Dictionary of Popular Medicine and Hygiene* (1874), reproduced in its entirety below, demonstrates the circuitous language and selective detail that its author thought necessary to describe female reproductive organs to an audience of middle-class women, and potentially their servants and children:

> VAGINA. The anatomical name for the female passages, and necessary to be explained because it sometimes occurs that in states of disease applications or injections are ordered to be applied to this part of the body, which is mentioned only by this term. Sometimes, a slight membrane exists at the entrance to this passage, which prevents the proper and natural monthly discharge. When it is discovered it should at once be

[82] "A Grave Social Problem," *BMJ*, December 5, 1881, 904.

[83] See anecdotes in Kate Flint, *The Woman Reader, 1837–1914* (Oxford: Clarendon, 1993), 215.

removed, and it is well if such an accident should be perceived and remedied at infancy, before any evil consequences can result from it.[84]

This brief, apologetic discussion of the vagina, rendered awkwardly in the passive voice, equips readers with the minimum of information necessary for seeking out and interpreting medical advice. Nobody could accuse *Haydn's Dictionary* of pandering.

Conservative doctors approved of works like *Haydn's Dictionary*. In the 1890s, the *British Medical Journal* even lavished praise on *Baby Buds* (1895), a "little manual . . . intended as a guide to mothers and teachers in answering the inconvenient questions of children as to the procreation of the human species."[85] Written under the pseudonym Ellis Ethelmer by either Elizabeth Wolstenholme Elmy, a vocal advocate of women's economic and sexual emancipation, or her husband, the free-love advocate Benjamin J. Elmy, the book was an unlikely recipient of the journal's admiration.[86] However, its editors saw in *Baby Buds* a model for communicating about sex that medical men could learn from. *Baby Buds*' discussion of the reproductive process is filtered through the lens of botanical imagery and narrated by a mother speaking to her child:

You will perhaps ask – "Then, are the male flowers of a vegetable marrow plant needless, or do they lead a useless life; seeing that they bear no fruit?"

No so, my child; neither the male flowers of the vegetable marrow nor of any other plant, are useless; for they produce the peculiar yellowish dust, or grains, called pollen, about which I have already said a few words.

And indeed, if you will notice one of the vegetable marrow flowers attentively, you will see inside it a thickish white stalk, whose top is covered with this yellow dust, of which some must find its way to the female flower and to reach each of the ovules in her ovary; or if any ovule misses being mingled with the contents of the grain of pollen, that particular ovule will not become a really living seed, capable of growing into a plant.[87]

In the *British Medical Journal*'s eyes, Ethelmer was highly successful in writing on a "very difficult and delicate matter" where doctors had failed.[88]

By and large, medical men agreed that works for women and children should be as delicate as possible. However, they were divided on the question of

[84] Edwin Lankester, ed., *Haydn's Dictionary of Popular Medicine and Hygiene* (London: Ward, Lock, 1874), 620.

[85] "Notes on Books: *Baby Buds*," *BMJ*, January 4, 1896, 28.

[86] On *Baby Buds*' uncertain authorship, see Maureen Wright, *Elizabeth Wolstenholme Elmy and the Victorian Feminist Movement: The Biography of an Insurgent Woman* (Oxford: Oxford University Press, 2014), 25.

[87] Ellis Ethelmer [pseud.], *Baby Buds* (Congleton: Buxton House, 1895), 26–27. For more on the familiar and maternal traditions of popular science writing that influenced this book, see Bernard Lightman, *Victorian Popularizers of Science: Designing Nature for New Audiences* (Chicago: University of Chicago Press, 2007), 21.

[88] "Notes on Books: *Baby Buds*," *BMJ*, 28.

self-censorship in works aimed at other practitioners. Donald Campbell Black's foreword to the second edition of *Functional Diseases* (1875) rails at his critics' "confusion ... between the moral and the physical," which, in his opinion, made it "extremely difficult to examine or discuss certain questions relating to sexual matters."[89] For Black, the very idea of self-censorship was antithetical to medical progress:

> It appears to me . . . that one thing should be paramount in the mind of the physician . . . that he should know neither restraint nor impulse but that of truth, and the consciousness that under this guidance neither science nor human well-being will ever be prejudicially assailed. As in the former edition, I assume in the present the responsibility of giving expression to what I believe to be fact. To succeed in elevating the literature of the subjects herein treated, from the mire in which it has been permitted for too long to remain, would have been no unworthy triumph – to hasten the accomplishment of this end, ample reward for the trouble which the present undertaking has entailed.[90]

By the end of the century, though, the text and illustrations in medical books aimed at medical audiences largely adhered to the maxim "dull instead of light."

Text and images from Alfred Cooper's *Syphilis* (1895) are typical of textbooks on venereal disease at the end of the nineteenth century. The book opens with a coloured frontispiece depicting the body of a young adult male with syphilis (Figure 5.1). Although nobody could call it censored (the penis and testes are on full display), the visual codes for moral weakness that made earlier depictions of venereal disease so compelling, particularly in consulting surgeons' manuals, are absent. The head is outside the frame, and remainder of the body has been excised from its social and spatial contexts: it stands against a uniform brown background. Moreover, the body is not wasted or drooling, but fit and otherwise healthy. This image of a diseased body is a performance in "objectivity," firmly leading the eye to visual signs of syphilis and those signs alone.

The text aims for the same brand of "objectivity," making fulsome use of the passive voice. *Syphilis*'s discussion of the transmission of syphilitic infections between sexual partners, for example, reads:

> . . . it is not to be expected that uncreative lesions, the result of sexual intercourse, should invariably preserve and exhibit the pure and simple characters to be found in sores produced by experimental inoculations. The vagina often contains morbid secretions, from its own mucous membrane and from that of the uterus, to conceive that these secretions, inoculated upon the male organ, should be able to give rise to inflammation without any syphilitic virus being present.[91]

89 Donald Campbell Black, *On the Functional Diseases of the Renal, Urinary, and Reproductive Organs*, 2nd revised ed. (London: J & A Churchill, 1875), vi–vii.

90 Black, *On the Functional Diseases*, vi–vii.

91 Alfred Cooper, *Syphilis*, 2nd ed., ed. Edward Cotterell (London: J & A Churchill, 1895), 4.

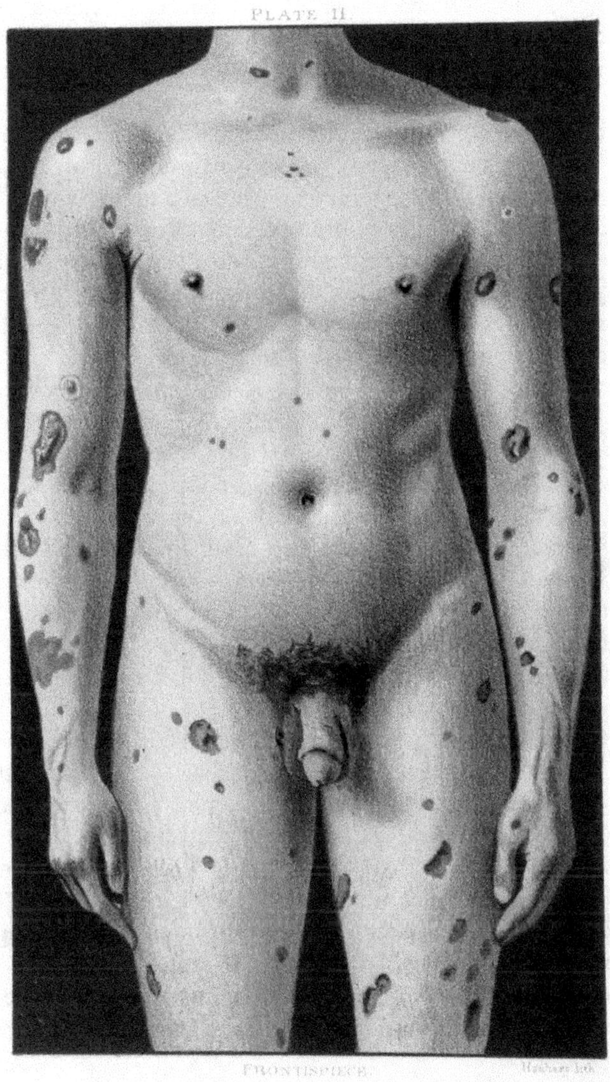

Figure 5.1 Frontispiece depicting a nude male with syphilis, Alfred Cooper, *Syphilis*. 2nd ed, ed. Edward Cotterell (London: J&A Churchill, 1895). Wellcome Collection, CC BY-NC 4.0.

Syphilis displays none of the circuitous avoidance of detail present in family-oriented reference books like *Haydn's Dictionary*. However, it eschews the chattiness and the moralizing characteristic of many early Victorian medical works on venereal disease, and in the reprints and reworkings of consulting surgeons' manuals that continued to circulate in the late nineteenth century. Popular and professional writing on sexual matters was now far more distinct stylistically.

Debates about how to present medical information in the 1870s and 1880s were shaped by persistent concerns about performing professionalism in a context in which medical works on many sexual and reproductive matters had long and deep associations with profiteering. The fact that the stylistic trends I have described evolved gradually and the discontinuity of the debates I have surveyed emphasize, however, that these concerns were among many factors driving changes to medical writing. The increasing specialization of medical practice encouraged authors to embrace ever-more technical language in works intended for their peers.[92] At the same time, writing for the public was becoming a more professionalized enterprise itself, one that involved less and less cutting and pasting from works written for medical practitioners and more and more customized writing for non-medical audiences.[93] In this context, ideas about the capacities of children and women – who were increasingly framed as unable to cope with bodily knowledge during a period in which they were working to gain the right to become doctors themselves – had more of an influence on works for non-medical readers than they had previously.[94]

The stylistic developments that I have sketched had some important implications for access to sexual knowledge. We have seen that medical terms for body parts were not universally understood earlier in the century: some readers needed help to understand that "labia," for instance, meant something like "cunt."[95] However, readers with no medical training were more equipped to understand professional medical textbooks and treatises at the beginning of the Victorian period than they were at its end, and they would have encountered the contents of those works in domestic reference books, manuals, pamphlets, and periodicals aimed at readers like themselves more often. As authorship became a more professionalized activity, "popular" and "professional" medical works became more discrete entities. They used more distinctive language, and the kind and detail of the information that they offered drifted further and further

92 Sally Frampton, "'A Borderland in Ethics': Medical Journals, the Public, and the Medical Profession in Nineteenth-Century Britain," in *Science Periodicals in Nineteenth-Century Britain: Constructing Scientific Communities*, ed. Gowan Dawson, Bernard Lightman, Sally Shuttleworth, and Jonathan R. Topham (Chicago: Chicago University Press, 2020), 312.

93 See Lightman, *Victorian Popularizers*.

94 Lena Wånggren, *Gender, Technology, and the New Woman* (Edinburgh: Edinburgh University Press, 2017), 138.

95 *A Select Catalogue of Books; Facetious and Amorous* ([London]: s.n., n.d.), DA 676, box 6, no. 51, MSCE.

apart. Professional knowledge was being cordoned off. The introduction of new rules for advertising medical publications amplified that effect.

The Frame of Convention

Medical debates about how to present information about sex and reproduction in print were born of concerns about being tainted by quackery and, to a lesser degree, pandering. They were mostly oriented around the desire to clearly mark out medical writing as *professional*: to rid it of unwanted associations with profiteering and firmly associate it with expertise, objectivity, trustworthiness, and social responsibility. If these debates primarily focused on how to avoid confusions of identity or motive, parallel debates about how to publish and advertise medical information were mainly oriented around an overlapping problem: how to force regular medical practitioners to be as restrained and high-minded, as *different* from quacks, as they claimed to be. The old suspicion that many practitioners published mainly to promote themselves was alive and well, and any new kind of publication – especially one aimed at a non-medical audience – attracted concern. As Sally Frampton has recounted, for instance, the rise of popular health periodicals in the 1880s set off a firestorm of medical debate about the propriety of writing for them. Popular articles on medical subjects could be interpreted by the public – or worse, might deliberately function – as "a surreptitious form of advertising" one's practice.[96]

The old suspicion of medical book advertising was also, if anything, more acute than it ever had been. Prominent medical men viewed book advertising in the lay press as a veiled means of self-promotion, and they were now determined to rein it in. In 1869, the *Lancet* proposed the following set of rules for all medical authors and publishers to follow:

> 1st. No work should be advertised with the author's name and titles placed before the title of the book itself.
> 2nd. No review or opinion of the value of the work or the treatment recommended should be appended to the advertisement.
> 3rd. The work should be advertised by the publisher with his other works, and never in the column devoted to quackery.
> 4th. The frequency of the advertisement should be strictly limited to such publicity as a medical publisher would afford a medical work which was his *own* property for the purposes of *bona fide* sale.[97]

The first and second of these recommendations refined longstanding medical opposition to publishing the address of a medical author's practice, his fees, the

[96] Frampton, "'A Borderland in Ethics'," 324.
[97] Quoted in "Salus Populi Suprema Lex," *Medical Press and Circular*, June 23, 1869, 526.

times when he practised, or endorsements of his practice in advertisements for books and pamphlets. The *Lancet* now suggested that the author subordinate his name to that of the book, reducing the advertisement's focus on the author, and collapsed book endorsements with endorsements of the author's talents as a practitioner.

The third recommendation addressed persistent concerns that placing advertisements for medical works "next door" to irregular advertisements in newspapers legitimated irregular medical practice and degraded works issued by legitimate practitioners. Advertising all of a medical publisher's works in a block could ameliorate these effects. The fourth recommendation, that medical book advertising should be limited to that which the *publisher* deemed necessary, derived from opposition to the common practice of authors paying publishers to advertise their books. This was, as Chapter 3 emphasized, by far the most controversial aspect of medical book advertising, because it underscored medical authors' interest in gaining publicity, and was often cited as evidence that publishing was all too frequently used a vehicle for promoting medical expertise.

The *Lancet*'s proposal was hotly criticized in the medical press. The *Medical Circular* charged the journal with hypocrisy – it did not follow some of its rules in its advertising – and suggested that the journal's objection to practitioners advertising books in non-medical venues was a ploy to increase its own advertising revenue.[98] But maintaining the status quo in a context in which medical groups had railed against "obscene quackery" for so long and with such fervour proved impossible. In an 1875 address to the Harveian Society, the surgeon James Lane charged men in the room with indulging in obscene quackery themselves. Observing that medical works on sexual matters were more frequently advertised in non-medical periodicals than works on many other medical subjects, Lane maintained that there was no "*essential* difference" between the practices of their authors and those of consulting surgeons. Their advertisements, too, subjected women to allusions to sex by trumpeting titles "hardly decent to parade upon the daily breakfast-table." Their advertisements, too, promoted their expertise, and they, too, paid for the advertisements. That the content of their books might well be "an honour alike to their authors and to science" was irrelevant. "It cannot be contended that there is any demand for works of this class amongst non-medical readers," Lane claimed. "The only real effect, then, of such advertisements is to bring the names of their authors prominently before ordinary newspaper readers, an aim hardly worthy of those whose acquirements fit them to be our leaders and our teachers, of whose reputation and fair fame we

[98] "Salus Populi Suprema Lex," *Medical Press and Circular*, 526.

are jealous, and whose character and motives we wish to see not only without reproach, but above suspicion."[99]

For Lane, then, advertising medical works in the lay press did not simply risk tainting medicine's reputation by facilitating confusions of professional identity. The practice suggested that regular medicine was tainted by the same self-serving interests as "obscene quackery."[100] What medicine needed, he argued, was a ban on advertising medical books in the lay press. A ban would not only raise medicine's fortunes by increasing public trust in the profession but also make the profession worthy of public trust by wresting the temptation to self-promote out of doctors' hands. "The public is by degrees learning to look to us for the solution to some of the most intricate and important social problems of the day," Lane observed. To retain that confidence, medical practitioners must prove themselves worthy of it. The road to advancing the profession "must be by the abandonment of individual self-seeking, at the expense of the character of the general body; it must be by the cultivation of a thorough loyalty to our order," he thundered, "combined always with the consciousness that the profession is for the public, and not the public for the profession."[101]

By the time Lane made his speech, bans on advertising in the lay press were already coming into effect. The Royal College of Surgeons and Royal College of Physicians had passed resolutions against "advertising medical works in non-medical journals" in 1873.[102] In the case of the Royal College of Surgeons, the resolution followed a debate aroused by the surgeon-electrician Henry Lobb's insertion of advertisements in *The Times* the previous year. Most of the College's fellows considered Lobb's advertisement, which filled an entire column of *The Times*' classified page and listed his address twice, "denigrating to the honour of the College" and "disgraceful to the Profession of Surgery."[103] A complaint against the surgeon Francis Burdett Courtenay, who had paid Baillière to advertise his book *On the Functional Derangements of the Generative System* (1871) in a wide range of weekly newspapers, made up their minds.[104]

These actions, and Lane's speech, motivated further resolutions across the English branches of the British Medical Association, and smaller medical societies throughout the country.[105] By 1877, most English doctors were prohibited from publishing advertisements for medical books or pamphlets in non-medical periodicals, even if the advertisement was placed by the

[99] James R. Lane, "Medical Advertising and Medical Reviewing," *BMJ*, January 16, 1875, 72.
[100] Lane, "Medical Advertising," 72. [101] Lane, "Medical Advertising," 73.
[102] "Medical Advertising," *Lancet*, June 28, 1873, 913.
[103] Minute Book, vol. 12, March 13, 1873, 147, RCS-GOV/2/1/8, RCS. The advertisements referred to are in *The Times*, November 15, 1872, 12.
[104] Minute Book, vol. 12, March 13, 1873, 144.
[105] "Medical Advertising," *BMJ*, July 10, 1875, 56; "Advertisement of Medical Books," *BMJ*, April 8, 1876, 454.

publisher.[106] These prohibitions did not enjoy uniform support. Some medical men argued that zeal to raise up the profession had blinded men like Lane to legitimate reasons for advertising medical books in non-medical venues.[107] Just as non-medical readers sometimes scanned the pages of the *Lancet*, for instance, medical men often read *The Times*.[108] Advertising in the lay press helped authors reach practitioners who seldom read medical periodicals.

Other medical men protested that bans on advertising medical books in the lay press hurt less established practitioners while failing to abolish other covert means of advertising medical practice. Donald Campbell Black, the surgeon whose "vivid" style the *Medical Press and Circular* criticized, pointed out that newspapers were filled with announcements for new hospitals which vaunted their attending practitioners' expertise and appealed to the public for donations.[109] Were those not advertisements? And what of notices like one Black had seen in a number of Glasgow newspapers, which advised readers that "Lord Kelvin, who has been suffering from facia neuralgia, has so far recovered that he hoped to be in Glasgow yesterday evening, but Dr. Ferrier, who has been attending him, prefers that he should remain in London for another week." These notices clearly promoted Dr. Ferrier's practice, spreading the word that he was Lord Kelvin's doctor. "It is perfectly absurd and unfair, in these days of keen competition . . . to lampoon and vilify honest, struggling young men for honourably making known their existence," Black complained, "when this and kindred practices are constantly indulged in, and connived at, in the higher ranks of the profession."[110]

Medical publishers were not pleased with the bans either. An anonymous writer to the *Medical Press and Circular* spoke for one when he lambasted those who dared "propound the duties of medical publishers to the profession . . . medical publishers . . . are supposed to know how to conduct their own business, and certainly do not require or seek to obtain editorial advice gratis on matters of which they are by far the best judges."[111] Ultimately, though, medical authors and medical publishers rapidly accepted limitations on medical book advertising. Medical authors did not want to be cast out of their professional associations, and medical publishers did not want to alienate the field that they relied on to make a living. Indeed, J. & A. Churchill (as the firm was known after John Churchill's sons, John and Augustus, took it over in 1870) took pains to establish its willingness to cooperate with advertising

106 "Cash and Credit – Professional Book Advertisements," *Lancet*, 894.
107 "Medical Advertising," *Medical Examiner*, March 9, 1876, 177–178.
108 Frampton, "'A Borderland in Ethics'," 319.
109 "Medical Advertising," *BMJ*, July 31, 1875, 149.
110 Donald Campbell Black, "Medical Advertising in the Lay Press," *Lancet*, November 21, 1898, 149.
111 "Medical Advertising and Lay Critics," *Medical Press and Circular*, 77.

restrictions. In a letter to the *Medical Times and Gazette*, John and Augustus claimed that their firm had "no idea of profit in . . . advertisements in daily papers, which are issued solely to please the authors. It is the authors who seek this advertisement, and [the firm] will have no difficulty in staying a proceeding which the voice of the profession energetically condemns."[112]

In early 1870s, Churchill, Baillière, and other medical publishers had frequently advertised medical books – including many books on reproduction and sexual health – in the non-medical press. By the early 1880s, as the *Students' Journal and Hospital Gazette* put it, advertisements for medical works had "almost ceased" in such venues, "the exceptions being some few specialists who would . . . have no patients at all except for advertizing [*sic*] their clap-trap publications."[113] Practitioners who violated the new rules were often attacked in the medical press and unceremoniously ejected from medical societies. In a few cases, prosecutions under the Medical Act followed: transgressing restrictions on book advertising was now seen as an indication of improper medical practice, and triggered investigations of the authors and their activities.

Publishers who violated the new advertising standards also faced backlash. In 1882, Smith, Elder & Co placed five columns advertising medical and scientific books in *The Times* without the authors' permission, and was savaged in the medical press for risking their reputations.[114] John and Augustus hastened to assure *Lancet* readers that J. & A. Churchill would not make the same mistake. "Since the Royal College of Physicians passed a resolution to the effect that it was unbecoming on the part of its fellows to permit their works to be advertised in non-professional papers," they wrote, "we have carefully abstained from inserting our announcements in lay papers . . . We entirely agree . . . that advertisements of strictly medical books are out of place in a general newspaper, and we do not insert them ourselves unless specially ordered to do so by our authors."[115]

Like debates about how to present medical knowledge in print, debates about how to publish and advertise medical works extended beyond those that addressed sex and reproduction, and they had more to do with medics' concerns about their own credibility than they did with concern about public access to sexual knowledge. However, restrictions on medical book advertising had some significant implications for access to sexual knowledge. First, they reorganized the system for promoting many works that contained it. While the development of new conventions for writing on medical topics intensified differences between "popular" and "professional" works and the kinds of information they offered, crack-downs on lay advertising narrowed the kinds of venues in which readers

[112] "Advertisement of Medical Books," *BMJ*, April 8, 1876, 454.

[113] "Medical Advertising in the Lay Press," *Students' Journal and Hospital Gazette*, June 10, 1882, 242.

[114] "Medical Advertising," *Students' Journal*, 242.

[115] J. & A. Churchill, "Medical Advertising in the Lay Press," *Lancet*, May 27, 1882, 874.

could encounter works that covered certain medical subjects, or covered them in a lot of detail. This development discouraged a crossover audience for professional works on sexual matters, which was certainly not nonexistent, as Lane claimed, and cut off a means through which people seem to have identified experts to treat sexual and reproductive health issues.

The developments I have sketched in this chapter had other implications for the history of sexual knowledge that will become clear over the course of the next chapters. Most significantly for the purposes of this book, they collectively articulated a negative blueprint for communication through print that medical authors, publishers, and readers were coming to recognize. A legitimate medical work was written by a formally qualified medical practitioner. It had an austere material design. Its text did not draw attention to sexual details by overapologizing for them. It was tightly focused on information understood to be medical in nature, and the amount and kind of information it included was adapted to its audience. Unless it was expressly written for non-medical readers (as with a domestic reference book), a legitimate medical work was not advertised in non-medical venues, and it was not issued by any but a known publisher of medical works. Just as a doctor's education and qualifications, social networks, dress, comportment, and sex had traditionally combined to endorse him as a credible medical practitioner, this array of textual, bibliographical, and commercial features endorsed a work as a legitimate medical publication. To be clear, no single deviation from these conventions necessarily unmade a medical book. Even spelled-out rules could sometimes be broken. However, the link between a medical work's legitimacy and this array of features was becoming ever more sharply defined.

The holistic model of legitimation that I have described relied on roughly the same principle as Alexander Cockburn's test of obscenity in that commercial context – who made a medical work and how it was advertised and how it was sold – strongly influenced determinations of legitimacy. Increasing agreement as to what kinds of features marked out a legitimate medical publication enabled practitioners to begin to leave behind the paranoia about print and its affordances that had plagued the medical profession for many years. However, these conventions were not compatible with the goals of progressive medical authors who sought to bring new kinds of sexual knowledge to the public, and they did not do away with the perceived need to police medical publishing and advertising or protect medical print culture from contamination. The next two chapters illustrate these issues. However, their focus shifts away from the regular medical profession. While examining the publishing activities of activists working at the fringes of regular medical practice in the last decades of the nineteenth century, these chapters consider how the meanings that publication context made influenced efforts to define new collective identities and consolidate their authority.

6 Branding Birth Control

In November 1880, members of the Malthusian League, Britain's first organization dedicated to promoting contraception, gathered in London to honour D. M. Bennett, a vocal free-love advocate and editor of the radical American periodical *The Truth Seeker*. Bennett had just finished serving an eleven-month prison sentence in New York for publishing *Cupid's Yokes: or, The Binding Forces of Conjugal Life* (1876), a tract that called for abolishing marriage. At the event, League members bonded with Bennett over their mutual "struggle for the freedom of the press."[1] In her toast to the hero of the evening, one of the League's founders, Annie Besant, hammered home similarities between conditions in the United States and conditions in Britain, where the *Hicklin* test had made distributors of birth control pamphlets vulnerable to prosecution. Toward the end of her speech, she entreated the crowd to gaze at another League member, Edward Truelove. "He is crowned with the glory of the jail," she declared, referring to a four-month sentence that the elderly bookseller had endured in 1878. To his company, Besant admitted "our friend (Mr. D.M. Bennett) . . . prison had to him no dread."[2]

While doctors were prosecuting irregulars for distributing obscene material as part of ongoing efforts to disambiguate "medicine" from "quackery," Britain was witnessing the rise of sex radicalism. During the second half of the nineteenth century, secularists, spiritualists, socialists, anarchists, and free-thinkers took on a variety of causes associated with sex and reproduction, including contraception advocacy, legal equality for illegitimate children, more liberal divorce laws, and "free unions" outside traditional marriage. As Elizabeth Miller has emphasized, the emergence of this loose, diverse movement marked a major turn in Victorian radical politics, in which the domains of the body and sexuality became central to arguments for freedom of expression.[3] Early nineteenth-century radical agitators had railed against blinkered sexual ideologies. However, their arguments for freedom of speech and freedom of the press had primarily been oriented around their right to criticize the state and the

1 "Reception of Mr. Bennett, of New York, in London," *Malthusian*, December 1880, 179.

2 "Reception of Mr. Bennett," *Malthusian*, 179.

3 Elizabeth Carolyn Miller, *Slow Print: Literary Radicalism and Late Victorian Print Culture* (Stanford: Stanford University Press, 2013), 259.

Church, and this focus continued to dominate free speech discourse into the early 1870s. By the end of the 1870s, however, sex was framed in progressive circles as the primary domain of suppressed speech.

Few progressive causes became as strongly associated with suppressed speech as contraception advocacy. Yet, as the birth control campaigner Marie Stopes would announce in her 1922 history of the contraception movement in Britain, neither the state nor social purity groups mounted significant opposition to trade in contraception literature prior to this turn.[4] And after it, open trade in cheap, practical works on contraception increased exponentially. Some people were arrested for selling these works, and Truelove was imprisoned for it. However, as this chapter shows, arrests were rare, geographically scattered, and often entangled with attempts to crack down on the pornography trade, where birth control pamphlets like Charles Knowlton's *Fruits of Philosophy* continued to circulate. Why, then, did Victorian censorship become so tightly associated with contraception that Stopes was shocked when, while undertaking research for her book, she discovered open discussions of family planning in an 1868 copy of the London *Daily Telegraph*?[5]

This chapter argues that the identification of contraception and censorship was partly the result of an audacious effort to rebrand the cause. At the beginning of the 1870s, many people, including many social protestors, associated contraception with promiscuity – an association that birth control pamphlets' circulation through the pornography trade only encouraged. Framing contraception as a free speech issue offered a way for activists like Besant to distance it from sex itself, and situate it as a respectable cause that a diverse and often quarrelling body of social protestors supported by default. At the same time, this way of framing contraception attracted enormous publicity to the cause and helped brand its representatives as brave freedom-fighters, willing to take on a society that had lost its way. Although they disavowed their shared texts and histories with pornographers, social protestors like Besant were more than willing to exploit their shared understanding that censorship, or perceived censorship, could be useful.[6] From the 1870s, sex radicals took up a strategy that disreputable booksellers used to frame works like *Aristotle's Masterpiece* as rare and desirable reading material to promote causes that they believed in and define a new identity for the contraception movement.

While I emphasize the benefits that framing contraception advocacy as a free speech issue had for birth controllers, it is important to recognize that they were not necessarily being disingenuous when they claimed to worry about arrest. The practical risks of selling literature on birth control methods depended on

[4] Marie Stopes, *The Early Days of Birth Control* (London: G.P. Putnam, 1922), 6–22.
[5] Stopes, *Early Days of Birth Control*, 8.
[6] See Joss Marsh, *Word Crimes: Blasphemy, Culture, and Literature in Nineteenth-Century England* (Chicago: University of Chicago Press, 1998) for details about how freethinkers, whose complicated relationship with the law is only briefly examined in this chapter, invited and exploited blasphemy charges along similar lines.

geographic context. They could also be difficult to gauge in the wake of the prosecutions against irregular practitioners examined in the previous chapter, and the police and anti-vice crusaders' intermittent use of medical material as evidence in crackdowns on trade in pornography, which play a key role in this chapter. Tactical uses of the law, and news from the United States, where birth controllers were zealously prosecuted for distributing obscene material, sowed confusion about the risks of selling works on contraceptive techniques and shaped the Malthusian League's publishing and advertising practices. Simultaneously, these uses of the law supported birth controllers' claims that knowledge about contraception was being suppressed, and reshaped how the movement was understood in retrospect, even – perhaps especially – by its own members.

Reframing Contraception Literature

The Malthusian League was founded in 1877 by a number of figures affiliated with freethought, a worldview that rejected traditional social and religious systems as bases for personal beliefs and embraced skepticism and independent reasoning.[7] Like Holywell Street publishers, freethinkers traced their roots back to early nineteenth-century radical movements that had advocated the abolition of the aristocracy and universal suffrage; embraced deism, agnosticism, and atheism; and agitated for a print sphere freed from government regulation. Miller has argued that freethinkers were more skeptical about print's facility for social change.[8] Even so, they celebrated their lineage to Republican heroes like Thomas Paine and Richard Carlile, and exalted their willingness to be censured for distributing incendiary material. The first number of the *Secular Chronicle*'s 1878 issue presents readers with a large woodcut of Carlile's shop front "as it appeared during the imprisonment of that brave struggler for the liberty of the press."[9] Freethinkers' right to speak out against the influence of the Church was, the *Chronicle* argued in an accompanying article, a direct result of Carlile's sacrifice.

That freethinkers issued works on contraception was another legacy of their roots in these circles. Through the mid-nineteenth century, as Holywell Street publishers printed their own editions of contraception manuals by Carlile, Robert Dale Owen, and Charles Knowlton, so, too, did a number of figures associated with freethought, including James Watson, Austin Holyoake, Edward Truelove, Charles Watts, and George Reddalls. They also dealt in a handful of new works

[7] For further information about the history of freethought, see Michael Rectenwald, *Nineteenth-Century British Secularism: Science, Religion, and Literature* (Basingstoke: Palgrave Macmillan, 2016); Edward Royle, *Radicals, Secularists, and Republicans: Popular Freethought in Britain, 1866–1915* (Manchester: Manchester University Press, 1980) and *Victorian Infidels: The Origins of the British Secularist Movement, 1791–1866* (Manchester: Manchester University Press, 1974); Laura Schwatz, *Secularism, Religion, and Women's Emancipation, England 1830–1914* (Manchester: Manchester University Press, 2015).

[8] Miller, *Slow Print*, 221.

[9] "Carlile's Shop Front," *Secular Chronicle*, January 6, 1878, 1.

on family planning.[10] They sold these works themselves and through a handful of retailers, advertising them in radical books and periodicals and, more sporadically, in mainstream newspapers.[11] Compared to pornographers, however, freethinkers were small-time players in the sale of contraception literature. Michael Mason has estimated that they sold less than a thousand copies of Knowlton's *Fruits of Philosophy*, and even fewer of Owen's *Moral Physiology*, annually.[12]

This strand of the trade was modest partly because freethinkers disagreed about whether they should promote contraception at all, which discouraged those who did sell birth control pamphlets from making their dissemination a central focus of their work. Debate surrounding Truelove's publication of the physician George Drysdale's *Physical, Sexual, and Natural Religion* (1855), which advocated both contraception and sex outside marriage, offers a good sense of arguments on both sides. Some freethinkers, including a number of feminists associated with the narrower Secularist movement established by George Jacob Holyoake in the 1850s, argued that conventional views about sexual morality stemmed from Christian ideologies that they rejected. Criticism of those ideologies was central to the movement's purpose. Therefore, freethinkers should not shrink from debate about sex, marriage, and reproduction. Other freethinkers worried that supporting a book that advocated sexual emancipation was too dangerous. It would encourage outsiders to associate irreligion with immorality, crushing the movement's hopes for meaningful social influence.[13]

The pornography trade's traffic in contraception literature seems to have exacerbated these concerns. By and large, early Victorian freethinkers had distanced themselves from men like William Dugdale, declaring that they were disgusted with the way such publishers "degrade[d] philosophy by allying it with

[10] Other works on contraception issued, reprinted, or sold by freethinkers during this period include M. G. H., *Poverty: Its Cause and Cure* [1854] (London: Edward Truelove, 1860), Cowan Tracts 3, no. 9, Robinson Library, Newcastle University; [George Drysdale], *Physical, Sexual, and Natural Religion* (London: Edward Truelove, 1855); Russell Thatcher Trall's *Sexual Physiology* (New York: Wood & Holbrook, 1866), and John Henry Palmer's *Individual, Family, and National Poverty* (London: E. Truelove, 1875), 7306.aa.15.(6.), BL.

[11] For examples of these advertisements, see "Cheap and Useful Knowledge," *Poor Man's Guardian*, June 6, 1835, 8; "Liberal Books on Politics, Theology, and Social Progress," *Northern Star and Leeds General Advertiser*, November 7, 1846, 4; "Books on Free Enquiry," *Reasoner*, August 13, 1854, 111; "Truelove's Reformer's Library," *People's Paper*, March 10, 1855, 8; "Now Ready," *Glasgow Sentinel*, December 10, 1859, 5; "Poverty: Its Cause and Cure," *Bee-Hive*, January 16, 1869, 8; "Reformers' Library," *Republican*, February 1, 1872, 8; "Works Published by Austin & Co," *Christianity in Relation to Freethought, Skepticism, and Faith* [...]. (London: Austin & Co, 1873), 66–67; "G.H. Reddalls, General Printer and Publisher," *Secular Chronicle*, January 1, 1874, 11; "Books, Pamphlets, Etc., Published by Charles Watts," in *Disestablishment and Disendowment of the English Church* [...], ed. C. Bradlaugh and W. Simpson (London: Charles Watts, 1876), n.p.

[12] See Michael Mason, *The Making of Victorian Sexual Attitudes* (Oxford: Oxford University Press, 1994), 185.

[13] Royle, *Radicals, Secularists*, 263.

obscenity."[14] But outsiders often confused them. As Joss Marsh has noted, smutty and irreligious books often *looked* the same, and were regulated under similar laws: freethinking booksellers were often prosecuted for obscene libel's sibling offence, blasphemous libel.[15] Pornographers and freethinkers also operated bookshops on the same streets, and sold many of the same works. Both dealt in radical and cheap literature, including "Flash Songsters" and "dirty milksop French novels," and at least one freethinking bookseller was caught selling Dugdale's racy periodical *The Exquisite* behind the counter (licentious publications, freethinkers grumbled, sold better than irreligious ones).[16] Moreover, some freethinkers dabbled in provocative publicity stunts, such as advertising the Bible as an obscene book, that were easily misread. People would stop in at freethinkers' shops and ask "not for 'God v. Paterson,' 'Trinity of Trinities,' [or] 'God-ology,'" one bookseller complained in 1844, "... but for *Fanny Hill, The Exquisite, Aristotle*, &c."[17] While some risks of identity confusion faded from the late 1850s, when the pornography trade shed most of the remnants of its roots in radical politics, contraception manuals remained tightly associated with the trade. People referred to Carlile's *Every Woman's Book* as a "Holywell-street publication" in the 1860s and early 1870s.[18] Concerns about being tainted by association lingered on in freethought circles. Holyoake initially refused to advertise Drysdale's book in his periodical *The Reasoner* because he felt that its title was "liable to confound it with Holywell Street productions."[19]

The legality of publishing and distributing contraception manuals did not figure into these debates, nor was it questioned until the 1870s, when a series of events connected with these overlapping publishing histories pushed Knowlton's *Fruits of Philosophy* into a series of obscenity trials.[20] The second of these trials,

14 "The Scotch God," *The Oracle of Reason* 1, no. 86 (1842): 265. See also allusions to Dugdale, publisher of *Voltaire's Philosophical Dictionary*, in *London Investigator*, August 3, 1843, 166 and *Reasoner*, January 9, 1850, 2.

15 Marsh, *Word Crimes*, 208.

16 Quoted in Robert G. Hall, "A Bookshop of Their Own: Reading and Print in Chartism, 1838–1850." *English Historical Review* 136, no. 581 (2021), 910. See also *London Investigator*, July 6, 1843, 130; *Discussion on Secularism: Report of a Public Discussion between the Rev. Brewin Grant, B.A., and George Jacob Holyoake, Esq* [. . .]. (Glasgow: Robert Stark, 1854), 155.

17 "Scotland," *Movement and Anti-persecution Gazette*, February 10, 1844, 70.

18 W. D. Christie, *John Stuart Mill and Mr. Abraham Hayward, Q.C.* (London: Henry S. King & Co, 1873), 11. See also "On the Claims of Women to Political Power," *The Anthropological Review* 7 (1869): xlviii.

19 "Dangers to Society from Celibacy and Over-Population," *Reasoner*, March 25, 1855, 198.

20 For previous studies of the trials discussed in this section, see Sripati Chandrasekhar, *Reproductive Physiology and Birth Control: The Writings of Charles Knowlton and Annie Besant* (London: Routledge, 2018); Norman E. Himes, "Charles Knowlton's Revolutionary Influence on the English Birth Rate," *New England Journal of Medicine* 199, no. 10 (1928): 461–465; Miller, *Slow Print*, 257–298; Rosanna Ledbetter, *A History of the Malthusian League* (Columbus: Ohio State University Press, 1976), 25–55; Royle, *Radicals, Secularists*, 254–257; Gowan Dawson, *Darwin, Literature, and Victorian Respectability* (Cambridge: Cambridge University Press, 2007), 116–161.

R. v. *Bradlaugh and Besant* (1877), marked a major turning point in the history of birth control in Britain: the first significant step that freethinkers took to align the cause of contraception with the cause of free speech. Politicized as suppressed speech, contraception and other causes related to the body and sexuality quickly took on a central role in Victorian social protest. Although the collapse of these categories served different purposes, the events recounted here illustrate how contraception advocates initially used allegations of censorship as a way of repudiating birth control literature's associations with sexual immorality, distancing it from the pornography trade, and reconciling freethinkers to support for it.

The chain of events began to unfold in the autumn of 1876, when a man named Henry Cook was arrested for selling a copy of Knowlton's *Fruits of Philosophy.* Except for the date and location of the arrest, the story could have been ripped from newspaper reports on the Holywell Street raids of the 1850s. The proprietor of a "Book, Periodical, and Newspaper Depot" in Sims Alley, Bristol, Cook was a long-time seller of sexual material. The single-sheet catalogues and card advertisements that he sent to mail-order customers list the kinds of publications hawked by Holywell Street publishers twenty years earlier: descriptions of cheap medical works like *Aristotle's Masterpiece* and Horace Goss's *Woman: Her Physiology and Functions* jostle with listings for erotic prints, novels, and short stories, bawdy songsters, French letters, and sensational pamphlets, including an obscure title called *Seduction by Chloroform* (c. 1850) first issued by William Dugdale's brother, John Lambert Dugdale.[21]

Cook promoted this material by courting arrest. He openly distributed handbills that framed his Sims Alley depot as the site of "A BOOK REVOLUTION" (Figure 6.1) where anyone could get their hands on "racy gems" and "private somethings."[22] The handbills also suggested that these items were suppressed – or would have been had the local authorities been any good at their jobs. Cook's handbill for *Fanny Hill* excerpts a letter to the editor of the *Bristol Gazette* complaining that the police had done nothing to shut down his "infamous and demoralizing" trade.[23] His handbill for Goss's *Woman: Her Physiology and Functions* claims that the editor of the *Bristol Mirror* condemned the work as a "bad book" that "ought not to be circulated."[24]

[21] See DA 676, box 1, items 18, 19, 40, and 62; box 3, items 67 and 74; box 4, item 61; box 5, items 55 and 83; box 6, item 17; box 7, item 7; and box 8, items 24 and 38, MSCE. See also *Seduction by Chloroform* (London: J. Turner, [1850?]), 12331.ee.45, BL. John Lambert Dugdale published under the name J. Turner at 50 Holywell Street, the address printed on the eighth page of the pamphlet, in the early 1850s. See Sheryl Straight, "William Dugdale: A Bibliographical Sketch of an Erotica Publisher, Bookseller, and Printer," *The Erotica Bibliophile*, accessed February 19, 2024, www.eroticabibliophile.com/.

[22] "A Book Revolution in Sims's Alley!" *Handbill* (Bristol: Henry Cook, n.d.), 1 leaf, DA 676, oversize folder 5, item 83, MSCE.

[23] *A Book Revolution in Sims's Alley!*

[24] "*Woman: Her Physiology and Functions* by Horace Goss, M.D. Surgeon," *Handbill* (Bristol: W.H. Cook, n.d.), 1 leaf, DA 676, box 8, item 38, MSCE.

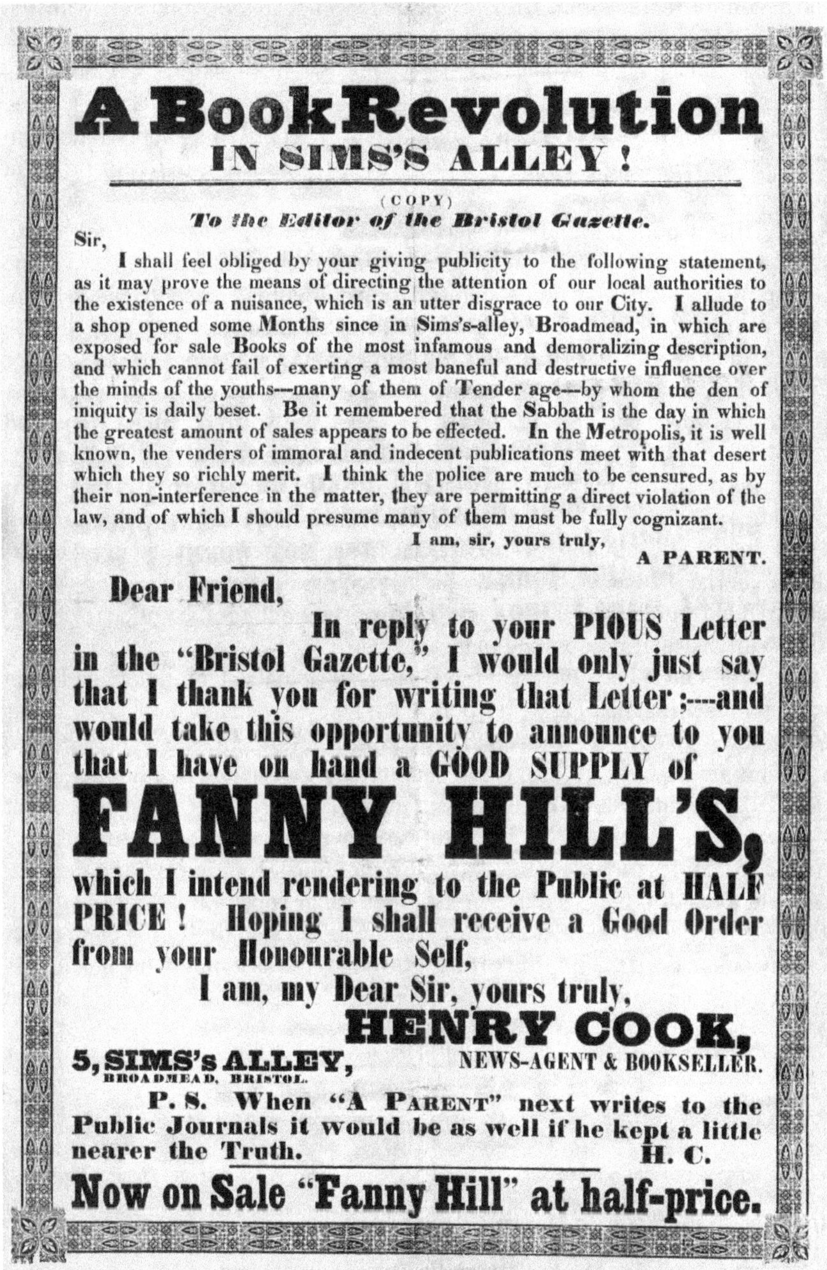

A Book Revolution
IN SIMS'S ALLEY!

(COPY)

To the Editor of the Bristol Gazette.

Sir,

I shall feel obliged by your giving publicity to the following statement, as it may prove the means of directing the attention of our local authorities to the existence of a nuisance, which is an utter disgrace to our City. I allude to a shop opened some Months since in Sims's-alley, Broadmead, in which are exposed for sale Books of the most infamous and demoralizing description, and which cannot fail of exerting a most baneful and destructive influence over the minds of the youths—many of them of Tender age—by whom the den of iniquity is daily beset. Be it remembered that the Sabbath is the day in which the greatest amount of sales appears to be effected. In the Metropolis, it is well known, the venders of immoral and indecent publications meet with that desert which they so richly merit. I think the police are much to be censured, as by their non-interference in the matter, they are permitting a direct violation of the law, and of which I should presume many of them must be fully cognizant.

I am, sir, yours truly,

A PARENT.

Dear Friend,

In reply to your PIOUS Letter in the "Bristol Gazette," I would only just say that I thank you for writing that Letter;—and would take this opportunity to announce to you that I have on hand a GOOD SUPPLY of

FANNY HILL'S,

which I intend rendering to the Public at HALF PRICE! Hoping I shall receive a Good Order from your Honourable Self,

I am, my Dear Sir, yours truly,

HENRY COOK,

5, SIMS'S ALLEY, NEWS-AGENT & BOOKSELLER.
BROADMEAD, BRISTOL.

P. S. When "A PARENT" next writes to the Public Journals it would be as well if he kept a little nearer the Truth. **H. C.**

Now on Sale "Fanny Hill" at half-price.

Figure 6.1 "A Book Revolution in Sims's Alley!" *Handbill* (Bristol: Henry Cook, n.d.), 1 leaf, DA 676, oversize folder 5, item 83, MSCE. Courtesy Lilly Library, Indiana University, Bloomington, Indiana.

His handbills for *Aristotle's Masterpiece* report that the work met with the "opposition of the prejudiced," and that Cook had decided to sell it while "residing in Her Majesty's gaol."[25] As this comment suggests, Cook was well known to the police. Prior to 1876, he had been arrested at least three times: in 1849, for displaying a "stunning spicy letter" in a shop window; in 1862, for selling "filthy books"; and in 1875, for hawking indecent prints at a railway platform.[26]

The Bristol police found themselves under pressure to arrest Cook again when a local upholsterer caught one of his employees with an envelope containing a fistful of Cook's mail-order catalogues. He confiscated them, showed them to local police officers, and urged them to shut Cook's trade down. An undercover officer dutifully visited Cook's shop and asked for several of the works listed in the catalogues. Cook was immediately suspicious. He told the officer that he did not have the items in stock. The officer wandered around Cook's shop and eventually picked up a copy of *Fruits of Philosophy*, which was openly displayed on the shelves. "You can take that book, and read it on the quiet," Cook told him. Cook framed cheap works on reproduction and sexual health as containers of "secret," even suppressed, knowledge in advertising material. However, he clearly did not anticipate that selling *Fruits* would get him into trouble. He was wrong. *Fruits* was enough for the police to charge Cook with distributing obscene material.[27]

That might have been the end of it. Dealers in sexual entertainment had been arrested for selling medical works before, and they would be again. But Cook's connection with Charles Watts, one of the social reformers who printed *Fruits*, turned his arrest into a lit fuse. Cook had gotten interested in freethought in the late 1840s. He intermittently subscribed to and advertised his newspaper depot in several periodicals associated with the movement, and briefly distributed unsolicited copies of Holyoake's *Reasoner* to ministers in the Bristol area. He also sold a handful of "Secular Works," including, apparently, Watts's edition of *Fruits*.[28] It is not clear that the copy Cook was arrested for selling came from Watts. Cook had cut the imprint off the title page (it was thought that he did this so he could charge twenty pence for the pamphlet instead of six pence, as the

25 "The Genuine Edition: *Aristotle, the Famous Philosopher*," *Handbill* (Bristol: Cook, n.d.), 1 leaf, orange, DA 676, box 1, item 19, MSCE.

26 "Friday," *Bristol Times and Mirror*, July 7, 1849, 5; "Bristol Quarter Session," *Bristol Mercury*, October 27, 1849, 3; "Charge of Selling Immoral Publications," *Bristol Mercury*, November 22, 1862, 4; "A Bristol Man in Trouble," *Bristol Mercury*, July 31, 1875, 6.

27 For a detailed account of the events leading up to Cook's arrest, see "Bristol Quarter Session," *Bristol Mercury*, December 30, 1876, 8.

28 See "Imitations," *Reasoner*, August 15, 1849; "Stamp Abolition Subscription," December 8, 1849, 370; "Public Notice," *Reynolds's Weekly News*, May 5, 1850, 8; "Reader," *Reynolds's Newspaper*, August 28, 1853, 13; "Woman: Her Physiology and Functions," *The Western Times*, November 5, 1853, 1; "Mr. Grant's Lectures in Bristol," *Reasoner*, December 7, 1853, 383. "H. Cook, Bookseller," *London Investigator*, May 1854, 32.

publisher intended). His copy also reportedly contained two "obscene pictures," while Watts's edition did not have illustrations.[29] Cook may have added images to the pamphlet. However, it seems more likely that the copy he was arrested for selling was an old Dugdale edition. Dugdale is the publisher of the only known editions to contain two anatomical plates.

Even so, Watts believed that the pamphlet came from his printshop. When he heard of Cook's arrest, he hurried off to Bristol to defend it – and Cook. In court, he testified that *Fruits* was "a legal book used strictly and properly," and emphasized that Cook was merely its seller. *He* was the publisher.[30] Watts's efforts backfired. Cook, who had no legal representation, was imprisoned for two years with hard labour, and the police were forced to arrest Watts and bring him back to London, where he was indicted for publishing *Fruits*.[31] Watts pled guilty and was released on the condition that he destroy his stock of pamphlets and the stereotype plates he had used to make them. He and many of his friends in freethinking circles worried that an obscenity trial in a London court, which would surely attract publicity, would hurt the movement.[32] Others, including Charles Bradlaugh and Annie Besant, a prominent member of Bradlaugh and Watts's National Secular Society, were furious at Watts for not defending his right to publish *Fruits*.[33] Besant devised a plan: she and Bradlaugh would co-publish a 6*d* edition of the pamphlet, updated by Drysdale, with the aim of getting arrested and defending it in court themselves.

The preface to Bradlaugh and Besant's 1877 edition of *Fruits* declares its publication a political act, endorsing all people's "fullest right to free discussion."

> The pamphlet which we now present to the public is one which has lately been prosecuted under Lord Campbell's Act, and which we republish, in order to test the right of publication ... The pamphlet has been withdrawn from circulation in consequence of the prosecution instituted against Mr. Charles Watts, but the question of its legality or illegality has not been tried ... We republish the pamphlet, honestly believing that on all questions affecting the happiness of the people ... fullest right of free discussion ought to be maintained at all hazards. We do not personally indorse [*sic*] all that Dr. Knowlton says ... but since progress can only be made through discussion, and no discussion is possible where differing opinions are suppressed, we claim the right to publish all opinions, so that the public ... may have the materials for forming a sound judgment ... [We are] confident that if we fail the first time, we shall succeed at last, and that the English public will not permit the authorities to stifle a discussion of the most important social question which can influence a nation's welfare.[34]

[29] "Bristol Quarter Session," *Bristol Mercury*, 8.
[30] "Bristol Quarter Session," *Bristol Mercury*, 8.
[31] "The Prosecution of Mr. Charles Watts," *Secular Chronicle*, January 21, 1877, 44.
[32] Royle, *Radicals, Secularists*, 256.
[33] For information about Bradlaugh's earlier interest in contraception, see Robert Jütte, *Contraception: A History* (Cambridge: Polity, 2008), 108.
[34] Charles Knowlton, *Fruits of Philosophy* (London: Freethought Publishing Company, 1877), iii–vi.

On March 23, 1877, Besant and Bradlaugh sent their edition to the local police, the Guildhall, and the solicitor for the City of London along with memorandums advising them when and where they would be selling it the following day. Given the pamphlet's recent history in court, they were sure they would immediately be charged with distributing obscene material.

Nobody came to arrest them. After a few days, members of the Christian Evidence Society, a Christian apologist group that rented the National Secular Society's headquarters for its weekly meetings, visited the Home Secretary and urged him to charge the pair with distributing an obscene book.[35] Still, no warrant was issued for their arrest. Finally, on April 5, more than two weeks after they had begun to sell the pamphlet, the wait was over. Bradlaugh and Besant were summoned to the Guildhall Court, and, on April 17, they were committed to trial at the Old Bailey. Strangely, the identity of the prosecutor remained secret, even to the judge. Given the authorities' obvious lack of enthusiasm for helping Bradlaugh and Besant with their protest, it is tempting to speculate that the secret prosecutor was an ally. Bradlaugh later hinted that it was the Christian Evidence Society. It is plausible that the Society would have done more to assist him: the Christian Evidence Society and the National Secular Society had a friendly relationship and worked together to advance their separate interests, often sparring in public to generate publicity for both organizations.[36] Bradlaugh and Besant were certainly confident that they would be tried. By the morning of April 5, they had raised £390 to cover the defence of a crime that they had not yet been arrested for.[37]

Scholarship on Bradlaugh and Besant's trial has largely focused on their powerful critique of the *Hicklin* test of obscenity. As the pair anticipated, the prosecution conceded that Knowlton's pamphlet was "carefully guarded from any vulgarity of expression," but took issue with its accessibility.[38] A six-penny pamphlet giving "such a minute description of all that has relation to the sexual appetite" could easily fall into the hands of vulnerable youths.[39] Bradlaugh and Besant countered that the concern for vulnerable readers enshrined in the *Hicklin* test was a paper-thin cover for elitism. In practice, they observed, courts destroyed works aimed at lower-middle and working-class audiences as obscene material, while ignoring comparably explicit works aimed at privileged readers,

[35] Ledbetter, *History of the Malthusian League*, 34. For further information about the Christian Evidence Society, see Dale A. Johnson, "Popular Apologetics in Late Victorian England: The Work of the Christian Evidence Society," *Journal of Religious History* 11, no. 4 (1981): 558–577.

[36] See *The Queen v. Charles Bradlaugh and Annie Besant (Specially Reported)* (London: Freethought Publishing Company, 1877), 52–55; Ledbetter, *History of the Malthusian League*, 34; Johnson, "Popular Apologetics," 565. As Johnson notes, the Christian Evidence Society was perennially broke, which does raise the question of where the funds to prosecute Bradlaugh and Besant would have come from.

[37] Royle, *Radicals, Secularists*, 15. [38] *The Queen v. Charles Bradlaugh*, 9.

[39] *The Queen v. Charles Bradlaugh*, 21.

even in cases where they could easily fall into the hands of young people. The *Lancet*, the *Medical Observer*, and the *Obstetrical Journal* were freely sold by news vendors even though they were cheaper than *Fruits* and contained "medical details beside which Knowlton is chaste in extreme."[40] And while it was expensive at ten shillings, the physician William Benjamin Carpenter's *Principles of Human Physiology* (1842), whose vivid descriptions of the adolescent female body Bradlaugh insisted were far more likely to corrupt youths than *Fruits*, was being given out as a prize-book to top pupils in state schools.[41]

As Gowan Dawson has pointed out, Bradlaugh and Besant's focus on *Human Physiology*, which was authored by a respected physician, issued by John Churchill, and widely acclaimed, was deliberately provocative.[42] Their mock indictment of the work was not only intended to demonstrate the elitism of the *Hicklin* definition of obscenity but also to lend support for the second part of their argument: that any legal definition of obscenity needed to take intent into account. Medical men like Carpenter had no practical reason to worry that their publications would be seized and destroyed as obscene material in 1877. Yet, as Bradlaugh went page-by-page through *Human Physiology* in the courtroom, theatrically reading out passages that appeared to demonstrate "the kind of feeling which might be awakened in some minds" by its text, he aimed to raise questions about what would happen if conditions changed.[43] Although works like *Human Physiology* described sexual organs "with the intent of a useful purpose," such works could be presented in ways that could lead to their destruction.[44] *Fruits* was no different save for its price.

If Bradlaugh and Besant hoped to galvanize medical opposition to the *Hicklin* test, they failed utterly. Medical men were aghast at the way they dragged Carpenter's name into the trial. The pair's argument that the *Hicklin* test was flawed because it focused on the contexts of a work's circulation instead of the intentions of its makers also fell flat before medical groups that had embraced the test as a means of cracking down on "obscene quackery," and a wider medical community that was perennially suspicious of authors' and publishers' claims about their intentions. Before the trial ended, campaigning medical journals denounced Bradlaugh and Besant and aggressively distanced *Fruits* from medicine. The *Lancet* deemed the pamphlet different "in no apparent feature from obscene publications circulated under a cloak of excellent purpose, but pandering to the most depraved of tastes."[45] The *Medical Press and Circular* evoked its promiscuous circulation, coyly opining that *Fruits*' "title and contents . . . might almost be compared with those that used to be seen in the windows of the shops of Holywell Street."[46]

40 *The Queen v. Charles Bradlaugh*, 147.
41 Dawson, *Darwin, Literature*, 130–134.
42 Dawson, *Darwin, Literature*, 125–127.
43 Dawson, *Darwin, Literature*, 132–134.
44 *The Queen v. Charles Bradlaugh*, 33.
45 "The Fruits of Philosophy," *Lancet*, June 30, 1877, 947.
46 "The Fruits of Philosophy," *Medical Press and Circular*, July 25, 1877, 74.

Although Bradlaugh and Besant powerfully drew attention to the *Hicklin* test's elitism, the trial was about more than their right to publish *Fruits* or any other work. It was also a publicity stunt aimed at rebranding birth control. As scholars have often pointed out, the pair used the trial as a stage to assert the moral authority of contraception advocacy by framing family planning as a solution to abject poverty that married couples needed to be taught to employ ("It is the advocacy of prudential checks *after* marriage that is now said to be a punishable offence," the pair complained).[47] At the same time, Bradlaugh and Besant used the trial to promote a publishing history for *Fruits* that so successfully implied that it was an exclusive product of freethought that histories of contraception have repeated it for a hundred and fifty years. Promoting this history enabled them to repudiate the pamphlet's associations with the pornography trade, align freethought with contraception advocacy, and suggest that it was not *Fruits*, but freethought and its right to free speech, that was under attack.

Bradlaugh and Besant's preface to *Fruits*, the following piece which Besant read aloud in court, tells readers that the pamphlet was authored by a freethinking American physician in 1832, and introduced to English readers the following year by James Watson, "who came to London and took up Richard Carlile's work, when Carlile was in jail."[48] Watson, it tells us, then

> sold it, unchallenged, for many years, approved it, and recommended it. It was printed and published by Messrs. Holyoake & Co., and found its place, with other works of a similar character, in their "Freethought Directory," of 1853, and was thus identified with freethought literature ... Mr. Austin Holyoake, working in conjunction with Mr. Bradlaugh at the National Reformer office ... printed and published it in his turn ... Mr. Charles Watts, succeeding to Mr. Austin Holyoake's business, continued the sale, and, when Mr. Watson died, in 1875, he bought the plates of the work ... and continued to advertise and to sell it ... *For the last forty years the book has thus been identified with freethought, advertised by leading freethinkers, published under the sanction of their names, and sold in the headquarters of freethought literature.*[49]

This narrative omits Cook, who inconveniently sold sensational and erotic productions as well as "Secular Works." It omits the Holywell Street publishers who had published, advertised, and sold Knowlton's *Fruits of Philosophy* across the country in the 1830s, 1840s, and 1850s. And it omits the new generation of pornographers who sold *Fruits* alongside erotic photographs.

It is extremely doubtful that Bradlaugh and Besant were ignorant of this aspect of *Fruits*' history. Pornographers were regularly advertising the pamphlet in 1877. On the same day Bradlaugh and Besant were arrested, a Birmingham man was indicted

[47] *The Queen v. Charles Bradlaugh*, 1. [48] Knowlton, *Fruits*, 1877, iii.
[49] Knowlton, *Fruits*, 1877, iii–iv. Emphasis added.

for selling *Fruits*, *Fanny Hill*, and large quantities of "extremely spicy" photographs.[50] Moreover, they moved in circles that had connections with the trade. The pair worked closely with Edward Truelove, whose stereotypes of works by Paine and Voltaire had come from William Dugdale's print shop, and Bradlaugh had been a member of the Cannibal Club, a private dining club that included several members who collaborated with pornographers to produce some of the most incendiary erotic literature of the day.[51] They also clearly understood something of the pornography trade's operations. During the trial, Besant drew on her knowledge of the trade to defend *Fruits*, asking the judge why, if the pamphlet was obscene, she and Bradlaugh had not omitted their names from their edition. "I understand that it is the usual thing," she said, "where an obscene book is published, that the printer's and publisher's names are omitted, and they so evade responsibility."[52]

Bradlaugh and Besant erased the pornography trade from *Fruits*' history. By the end of the trial, which culminated in a guilty verdict and then an acquittal on a technicality, a new narrative had been born: the pamphlet was, and always had been, sold by freethinkers as Bradlaugh and Besant defined them (that is, not by men like Dugdale or Cook), and any attack on the pamphlet or any work like it was an attack on freethinkers' free speech. Accomplishing this demanded that Bradlaugh and Besant adopt a position that fell short of endorsing the "fullest right to free discussion" for all, however. Ultimately, the pair called for an alteration to the *Hicklin* test that took "intent for useful purpose" into account. This was more likely to succeed than petitioning for the test's abolishment. However, it was also necessary to avoid defending the other side of Cook's trade. Just as regular practitioners feared that consulting surgeons tainted medicine's public image, freethought's shared texts and histories with the pornography trade threatened to undercut their argument that contraception was respectable. Bradlaugh and Besant protected their cause by framing Cook's sale of the pamphlet as an anomaly best left forgotten, and abandoned free speech where it was put to the purpose of pleasure.

Plausible Deniability

Initially, many freethinkers were furious at Bradlaugh and Besant for engineering the Knowlton trial. "Charles Bradlaugh has dragged the standard of

[50] "Great Seizure of Obscene Prints in Birmingham," *Tamworth Herald*, April 7, 1877, 3; "Great Seizure of Obscene Prints in Birmingham," *Birmingham Daily Gazette*, April 5, 1877, 11.

[51] "Re-issue of Paine's," *The Reasoner*, February 12, 1854, 127; Dane Kennedy, *The Highly Civilized Man: Richard Burton and the Victorian World* (Cambridge, MA: Harvard University Press, 2000), 169–170.

[52] *The Queen v. Charles Bradlaugh*, 57–58.

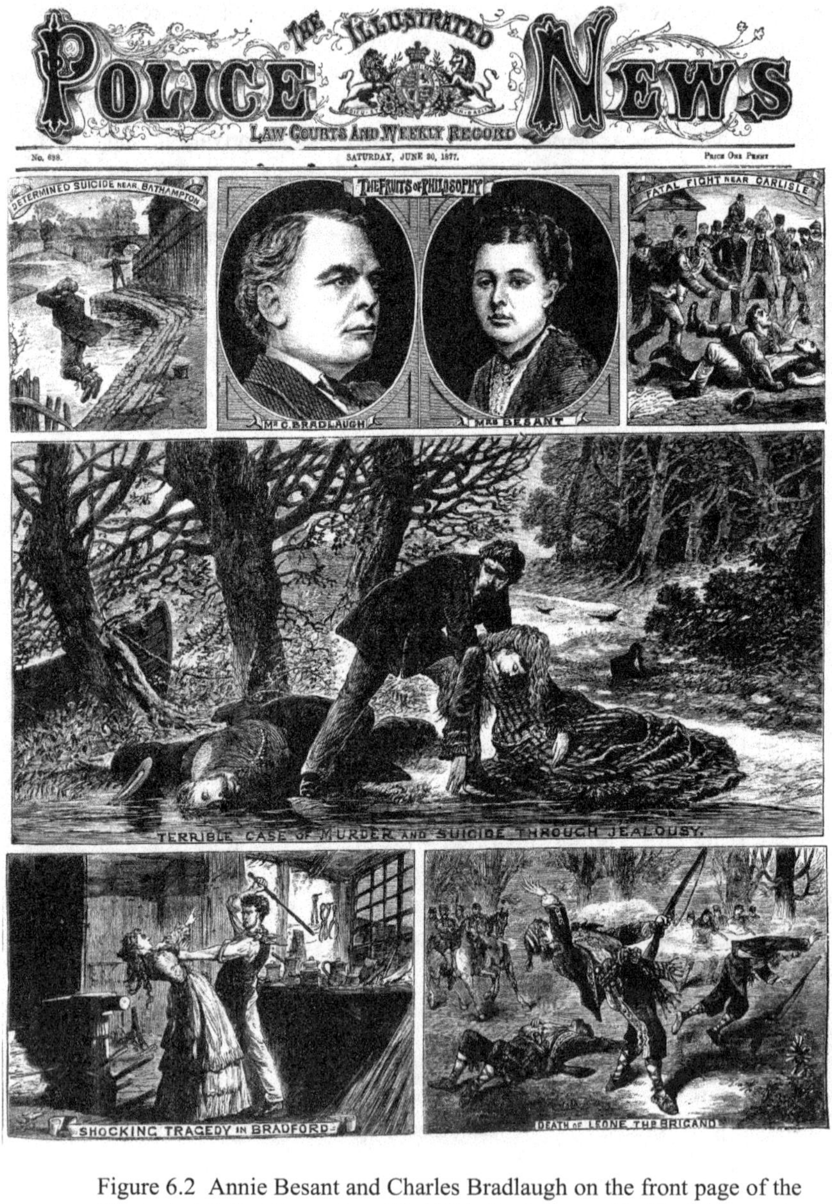

Figure 6.2 Annie Besant and Charles Bradlaugh on the front page of the *Illustrated Police News*, June 30, 1877. Content provided by The British Library Board, with thanks to The British Newspaper Archive

Freethought through the mire of Holywell Street!" one burst out at a meeting, to the horror of Bradlaugh's supporters.[53] In politicizing the acts of publishing and selling contraception manuals, however, the Knowlton trial gave birth to a movement.[54] At the same time, it attracted to that movement a stunning amount of publicity. Reports of the lengthy trial set off rapacious public curiosity about *Fruits*. The market was awash with piracies and imitations before it was over, and Besant and Bradlaugh's edition reportedly sold more than 50,000 copies the following year.[55] Examining the activities of the Malthusian League, the organization that Bradlaugh, Besant, and their allies set up to advocate contraception in the trial's wake, offers an instructive look at how birth control advocates continued to represent contraception literature as suppressed speech even as they played an important role in expanding trade in it.

The League's mission statement oriented the organization around two causes that the trial had effectively collapsed: free speech and public education on "Malthusian principles" – roughly, economic arguments against overpopulation propounded by Thomas Robert Malthus and the philosopher John Stuart Mill:

1. To agitate for the abolition of all penalties on the public discussion of the Population Question, and to obtain such a statutory definition as shall render it impossible, in the future, to bring such discussions within the scope of the common law as a misdemeanour.
2. To spread among the people, by all practicable means, a knowledge of the laws of population, of its consequences, and of its bearing upon human conduct and morals.[56]

The League rapidly developed infrastructure to recruit new members and spread its message. It held public meetings in several cities, published a monthly magazine, *The Malthusian*, and issued a series of pamphlets, the Malthusian Tracts, out of Besant's Freethought Publishing Company at 28, Stonecutter Street, London. From the standpoint of price alone, these publications were extremely accessible.[57] However, their appeal, and the appeal of membership

[53] Quoted in Charles R. Mackay, *Life of Charles Bradlaugh, M.P.* (London: D.J. Gunn & Co., 1888), 420.
[54] Stopes, *Early Days of Birth Control*, 22.
[55] "Fruits of Philosophy," *Sporting Times*, June 16, 1877, 1; Annie Besant, "The Law of Population," in *Autobiographical Sketches*, ed. Carol Hanbery MacKay (Peterborough: Broadview, 2009), 352. See also Angus McLaren, *Birth Control in Nineteenth-Century England* (London: Croom Helm, 1978), 109; Richard A. Soloway, *Birth Control and the Population Question in England, 1877–1930* (Durham: University of North Carolina Press, 1982), 57. As Claire L. Jones emphasizes in *The Business of Birth Control: Contraception and Commerce in Britain before the Sexual Revolution* (Manchester: Manchester University Press, 2020), 106, sales numbers for contraception manuals did not necessarily correlate with contraception use.
[56] Quoted in Ledbetter, *History of the Malthusian League*, xiii.
[57] See notes on pricing in Malthusian Tract no. 2, Charles R. Drysdale, *The Struggle for Enjoyable Existence* ([London]: [Malthusian League], 1878), including an allusion to the fact that League members routinely gave the tracts away for free.

in the League by association, was awfully limited. The tracts mostly consist of dry summaries of Malthus and Mill's economic arguments, and provide no practical information about how to prevent conception.[58] *The Malthusian* and the Malthusian League's public lectures were just as bereft of practical instruction.

As the phrasing of the League's second official aim, to spread knowledge of the laws of population through "all *practicable* means," suggests, the League framed the omission of practical information from its publications as a necessity in the wake of the judgement against Bradlaugh and Besant and two actions against Edward Truelove for distributing Owen's *Moral Physiology* (1830) and John Henry Palmer's *Individual, Family, and National Poverty* (1875) in May 1877, and *Fruits of Philosophy* in 1878.[59] These actions were brought by Charles Hastings Collette on behalf of the Society for the Suppression of Vice.[60] Collette claimed that the Society aimed to prevent booksellers from profiting from *Fruits*' notoriety in the wake of the Knowlton trial. Truelove's solicitor claimed that Collette was aiming to profit from the Knowlton trial himself, attempting to generate publicity for his struggling organization by replicating it.[61] Either way, the elderly Truelove was fined fifty pounds and forced to serve four months in prison.

During the late 1870s and early 1880s Malthusians were justifiably worried that other prosecutions would follow Truelove's. Early issues of the *Malthusian* rail against the Society for the Suppression of Vice, which the League framed as "one of the consequences of . . . failure in the organisation of English Criminal Law."[62] When, in 1879, Collette was sued for embezzling from a young couple who had trusted him to invest their life savings, the *Malthusian* reported on the proceedings with palpable *schadenfreude*.[63] Its editors continued to monitor the Society's activities, and lobbied members of Parliament to legislate a new definition of obscenity that took the intentions of authors, publishers, and distributors into consideration.[64] Additionally, the

[58] See Drysdale, *Struggle*; Malthusian Tract no. 1, Charles R. Drysdale, *The Principles of Population* ([London]: [Malthusian League], [1878]); and Malthusian Tract no. 3, *The Limitation of Families* (London: Malthusian League, [1878]); The focus on maternal health in Malthusian Tract no. 4, Henry Arthur Allbutt 's *Evils Produced by Over-Childbearing and Excessive Lactation* ([London]: [Malthusian League], [1878]), is a refreshing change.

[59] *Truelove*, 1878. Old Bailey Proceedings Online (t18780506-511).

[60] *The Queen v. Edward Truelove, for Publishing the Hon. Robert Dale Owen's "Moral Physiology," and a Pamphlet, Entitled "Individual, Family, and National Poverty." (Specially reported)* (London: Edward Truelove, 1878), 38.

[61] *The Queen v. Edward Truelove*, 35.

[62] "The Malthusian Prosecutions of 1877 and 1878," *Malthusian*, June 1879, 36–37.

[63] "The Charge against Mr. C.H. Collette," *Daily News*, December 12, 1879, 2; "A Charge against Mr. Collette," *Malthusian*, January 1880, 91.

[64] For example, see "Official Notices," *Malthusian*, June 1879, 36 and "Current Topics," *Malthusian*, July 1879, 47.

Malthusian League's leaders baked caution into its policies. Until 1913, the League not only prohibited the publication of practical details about contraception in its own publications but also officially advised its members not to publish or sell instruction manuals of their own. Correspondents often urged the League to abandon these policies. However, its leaders insisted that it was "illegal to publish" practical advice.[65]

There was, however, a marked and ever-increasing disjuncture between the League's official stance on distributing practical advice on contraception and its unofficial activities. From its establishment, the League informally sponsored a variety of works that contained practical information about contraception; promoted them within and outside its official publications; and advertised contraceptive devices. Initially, this activity was modest. During the late 1870s and early 1880s, when concern about prosecution was at its height among the League's leadership, it confined itself to endorsing and advertising two works that provided such information in the *Malthusian* and the Malthusian Tracts: a version of Drysdale's *Physical, Sexual, and Natural Religion*, now sporting the euphemistic title *Elements of Social Science*, and Besant's pamphlet *The Law of Population* (1878). These works were not officially League publications but they were so tightly associated with the League that they might as well have been. Their authors and publisher were founding members of the League, and they were printed at the same London address as the *Malthusian* and the Malthusian Tracts, 28, Stonecutter Street.

Expanded prior to its publication under a new title, Drysdale's four-part *Elements* frames sexual abstinence as physically and psychologically unhealthy. After presenting readers with a catalogue of blights supposedly caused by suppressed sexual desire, Drysdale proposes condoms and vaginal sponges as solutions to these problems, enabling people to express their desires within and outside marriage while avoiding venereal disease and unplanned pregnancies. Ideologically, Drysdale's book was radical even by radical standards. For this reason, it did not carry his name until after he died. However, *Elements* was not designed to function as an instruction manual, and it was not an especially accessible alternative to one. Costing either two shillings and sixpence or three shillings, depending on its binding, it was also much more expensive than Besant and Bradlaugh's *Fruits*. Although the Malthusian League promoted *Elements* in its publications for years and Truelove reportedly sold thousands of copies through his bookshop, it does not appear to have approached *Fruits*' commercial success.[66]

[65] Quoted in F. D'Arcy, "The Malthusian League and the Resistance to Birth Control Propaganda in Late Victorian Britain," *Population Studies* 31, no. 3 (1977): 433.

[66] See sales estimates in David Victor Glass, *Population Policies and Movements in Europe*, 2nd ed. (London: A.M. Kelly, 1967), 40 and Mason, *Victorian Sexual Attitudes*, 196.

Issued by the same publisher and sold by post for the same price as *Fruits*, sixpence, Besant's *Law of Population* was arguably the more daring work. It is more socially conservative than Drysdale's book, and most of its text is given over to the same dry economic theory that suffused the *Malthusian* and Malthusian Tracts. However, it also provides readers with an accessible introduction to contraceptive techniques. In one discrete section, the pamphlet offers a detailed description of the mechanics of conception, and discusses virtually all methods of limiting births known at the time: sponges, pessaries, and diaphragms of various types; douching with spermicidal agents; sheaths or condoms; withdrawal; the "safe period" or rhythm method; extended breastfeeding; and abortion.[67] It also provides readers with brief evaluations of each technique. Besant did not recommend withdrawal, extended breastfeeding, or abortion as methods of controlling reproduction, on the grounds that they were ineffective, unhealthy, and immoral, respectively, and she was skeptical about the condom's reliability.[68] In her opinion, vaginal pessaries provided the most reliable check against conception, and (echoing Richard Carlile's reasoning for advocating the contraceptive sponge) had "the enormous advantage of being entirely in the hands of the woman."[69] By Besant's account, this approach was successful: she reported that she sold more than 40,000 copies of *Law of Population* within three years of its publication.[70]

Sellers of these works met with no discernible opposition, and, after a few years, the Malthusian League grew more daring. The early 1880s witnessed a rapid expansion in the production of contraceptive devices, partly as a result of the rubber industry's growth following improvements to moulding and vulcanization processes, and partly, some scholars have argued, as a result of the attention that Bradlaugh and Besant's trial drew to contraception.[71] By 1883, as Claire Jones has demonstrated, at least eight manufacturers of condoms, syringes, cervical caps, and rubber pessaries were operating out of Hackney Wick and Dalston in London's East End, including James George Ingram, John George Franklin, and Edward Lambert and Son.[72] Beginning in 1885, endorsements of and advertisements for contraceptive devices made by

67 Annie Besant, *The Law of Population: Its Consequences, and Its Bearing upon Human Conduct and Morals* (London: Freethought Publishing Company, [1878]), 31–37.

68 Besant, *The Law of Population* [1878], 33–37.

69 Annie Besant, *The Law of Population: Its Consequences, and Its Bearing upon Human Conduct and Morals* (London: Freethought Publishing Company, 1887), 32.

70 Chandrasekhar, *Reproductive Physiology*, 57. Besant further reported in *Autobiographical Sketches*, 290, that by 1885, the pamphlet had been translated into Swedish, Danish, Dutch, French, German, and Italian, and sold more than 110,000 copies in the United States.

71 Jones, *Business of Birth Control*, 33–34.

72 Jones, *Business of Birth Control*, 34. Like many consulting surgeons, many of these manufacturers were Jewish. I have no evidence to support this theory, but alongside their owners' shared ethnicity, the timing of this proliferation of contraceptive manufacturers, and the fact that Lambert shared Joseph Lambert's name, raises the possibility that some of these manufacturers built their businesses on the infrastructure of declining consulting surgeon firms.

several of these manufacturers, including the self-identified Malthusian W. J. Rendell, became tightly integrated into the Malthusian League's unofficial publications, and, more discreetly, into its official ones.

Besant worked endorsements for contraceptive devices into a revised edition of *The Law of Population*, recommending soluble pessaries containing spermicidal agents from Rendell and India-rubber pessaries from Lambert and Son in the pamphlet's chapter on contraceptive techniques. Her revised edition also directs readers to full-page advertisements at the back of the pamphlet, which provide these manufacturers' addresses, further information about their products, and how to order them (Figure 6.3).[73] These pages considerably expanded *Law of Population*'s utility, essentially turning it into a less salacious version of William Dugdale's earlier pamphlet *On the Use of Night Caps*: an expert-endorsed catalogue for those interested in acquiring and learning how to use contraceptive devices. Indeed, John Peel has argued that the advertisements were "probably the most widely-read part" of such pamphlets.[74]

The *Malthusian* followed suit, publishing letters from members endorsing various contraceptive devices as well as advertisements: first for a contraceptives retailer, a Mr. Page of Bethnal Green, and then for a manufacturer, Lambert and Son. Lambert's advertisements in the *Malthusian* highlight devices endorsed in *The Law of Population* and cite Besant's endorsement.[75] Together, these publications effectively created a promotional feedback loop in which an activist organization and a manufacturer reinforced trust in each other's aims and expertise, and always brought readers back to the same techniques and products. As with Besant's *Law of Population*, many people probably read the *Malthusian* for the advertisements. By the end of the nineteenth century, the League's membership had hardly cracked 1,000 individuals. However, editors for the *Malthusian* reported receiving 2,000 requests monthly for information about devices advertised in the periodical.[76] In practice, the periodical mainly functioned as a catalogue.

1886 witnessed the publication of a third League-supported work on contraception, *The Wife's Handbook*, written by the physician and founding League member Henry Arthur Allbutt. This work further extended the unofficial partnership between the Malthusian League and contraceptive manufacturers. Like *The Law of Population* and *Elements*, *The Wife's Handbook* was initially printed at Stonecutter Street and promoted in the *Malthusian* and Malthusian Tracts.

[73] Besant, *Law of Population*, 1887, 32–33; 37–38.

[74] John Peel, "The Manufacture and Retailing of Contraceptives in England," *Population Studies* 17, no. 2 (1963): 117.

[75] Amicus, "A Recommendation," *The Malthusian*, March 1886, 21; A. Allbutt, "A Recommendation," *Malthusian*, April 1886, 30; "Malthusian Appliances," *Malthusian*, June 1887, 47; "The New Vertical and Reverse Current Syringe," *Malthusian*, January 1889, 7.

[76] Soloway, *Birth Control*, 64.

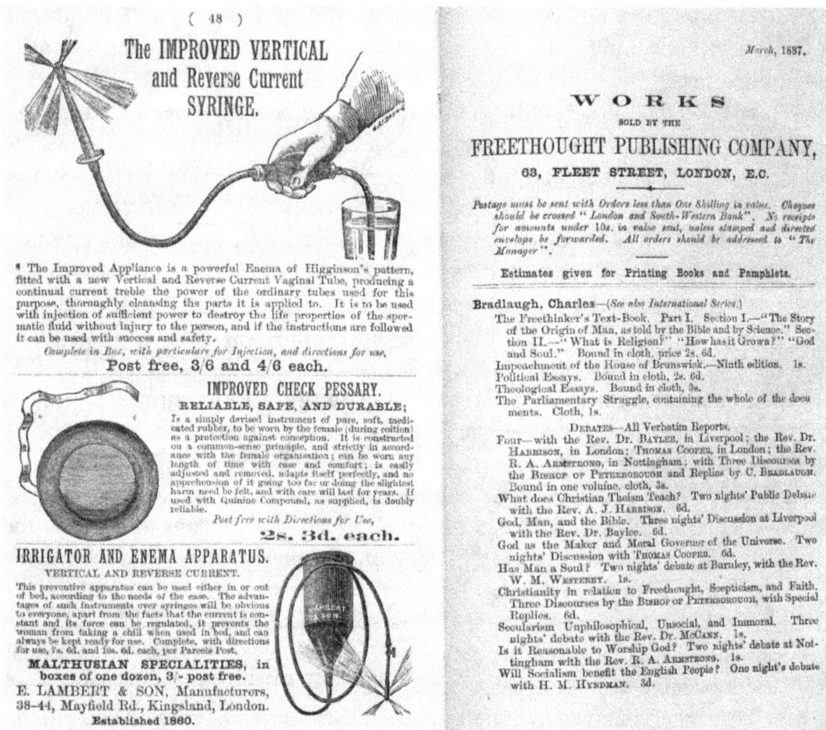

Figure 6.3 Advertisements for contraceptive devices and freethought literature in Annie Besant, *The Law of Population: Its Consequences and Its Bearing upon Human Conduct and Morals* (London: Freethought Publishing Company, 1887), HB875.B47 1887, Robarts Library, University of Toronto. By courtesy of The University of Toronto Libraries.

However, its focus is quite different. As suggested by the unwieldy working title that Allbutt gave the manuscript, *How a Woman should order herself during Pregnancy, in the Lying-in Room, and after Delivery; with Hints on the Management of the Baby, and on other matters of importance necessary to be known by Married Women*, Allbutt was primarily interested in contraception's efficacy as a preventive for maternal mortality, and had absolutely no interest in marching his readers through a tour of economic theory.[77] *The Wife's Handbook* is therefore focused on maternal health, outlining the processes of pregnancy, antenatal care, labour and delivery, post-natal recovery, menstruation, and menopause.[78] Contraception, covered between chapters on post-natal recovery

[77] "Correspondence: Practical Malthusianism" *Malthusian*, February 1885, 583.
[78] See *Malthusian Tracts*, nos. 4, 3.

and menstruation, is framed as a crucial aspect of healthcare for married women, one that ensures that they have the strength to care for their families.

The Wife's Handbook also has a stronger commercial flavour than previous League-supported publications. Early editions endorsed and advertised a wide variety of contraceptive devices, including condoms sold by Constantine and Jackson of Wych Street, London; a vaginal syringe manufactured by Lambert; Rendell's pessaries; and the Mensinga pessary, sold by R. Vaughn out of Caledonian Road, Leeds.[79] They also advertised a panorama of domestic products, such as Redhead's Celebrated Household Salve, that had nothing to do with the work's mission, but were aimed at its target audience. The appearance of both kinds of advertisements in the manual reflects Allbutt's interest in making a meaningful income from it. He developed a particularly close advertising partnership with Rendell, whose pessaries, branded "Wife's Friend," mimicked the *Handbook*'s title. After 1891, following Rendell's death and an exclusive advertising deal struck between Allbutt and the firm's new owners, as Jones has argued, the *Handbook* became "little more than a promotional tool" for Rendell.[80]

The first serious blow to this publishing activity arrived later in 1886, when Joseph Williamson, a wandering minstrel, was arrested by local authorities first in Gainsborough and then in the nearby town Goole under the 1824 Vagrancy Act for selling copies of *The Wife's Handbook* on the street.[81] He was fined and quickly released, but the secretary of a local social purity group got wind of the arrest and complained to the General Medical Council. The Council investigated, charged Allbutt with "conduct unbecoming of a physician," and struck him from the Medical Register. These events are examined in the next section. In terms of the League's involvement in the distribution of practical information on contraception, however, it is important to note that neither Williamson's arrest nor Allbutt's ejection from the Medical Register put an end to the League's support for these kinds of works. In fact, it doubled down on its support. In the wake of Williamson's arrest, the League not only sent its official literature to all of Gainsborough's and Goole's rate-payers but also launched a five-year campaign to promote *The Wife's Handbook* and *The Law of Population* across the country in local newspapers.[82]

Paid for by the League but placed in the name of the publisher and League member W. H. Reynolds, these newspaper advertisements were fairly discreet:

79 *The Wife's Handbook*, 7th ed. (London: R. Forder, 1888), 47–51.
80 Jones, *Business of Birth Control*, 64.
81 Ledbetter, *History of the Malthusian League*, 75–76.
82 Both efforts were funded through a special fund controlled by the national League office reserved for sending Malthusian literature to new districts. See "Special Fund," *Malthusian*, November 1886, 86 and "Special Fund for Sending Malthusuan Literature into New Districts," *Malthusian*, January 1887, 7. Several branches of the League advertised *The Law of Population* independently in local newspapers. The Edinburgh branch, for instance, posted "Advertisement," *Edinburgh Evening News*, September 21, 1881, 1.

they simply urged readers to "READ 'The Wife's Handbook' by Dr. ALLBUTT (Leeds), a work designed to induce married people to limit their family within the means of subsistence," and to write to Reynolds to purchase a copy.[83] Nevertheless, they were reportedly effective: in 1889, Reynolds claimed that he received 3,000 responses monthly.[84] The League continued to fund advertising for *The Wife's Handbook* in the 1890s, and supported the publication of *The Malthusian Handbook* (1893), conceived as a successor to *The Law of Population* after Besant converted to the esoteric religion Theosophy, abandoned Malthusianism, and stopped publishing her pamphlet in 1891.[85] Like *The Law of Population*, *The Malthusian Handbook* was not an official League publication, but it sure looked like one. It was written by League members; it cost sixpence; it describes contraceptive devices and how to use them; it advertises "a complete List of Malthusian Appliances, with prices" that readers could send for by post; and Reynolds promoted it on the League's behalf.[86] Notably, the pamphlet also contains a lengthy history of Malthusianism in which League members are prominently featured, and two pages that identify the League's executive members and describe the organization's aims and rules.

The Malthusian League's claim that it did not distribute practical information about contraception was deliberately misleading. The organization devoted increasing and by the late 1880s substantial resources to promoting publications written by its own leaders that offered people practical instruction in contraceptive techniques. Endorsements for contraceptives manufacturers were increasingly integrated into these works and into the League's official publications, as were manufacturers' advertisements. These methods of disseminating information about birth control were beneficial to the League financially, promotionally, and politically. Carrying advertisements for manufacturers underwrote the costs of publishing and promoting the League's official literature, made it more desirable to readers who had little appetite for economic theory, and, because the manufacturers endorsed them, probably increased the sale of practical works unofficially associated with the League: Besant had reportedly sold 175,000 copies of *The Law of Population* in Britain alone by 1891, while Allbutt had sold 250,000 copies of *The Wife's Handbook* by 1900.[87] All the

[83] For examples of these advertisements, see *Leeds Times*, June 4, 1887, 1 and *Northampton Mercury*, April 1, 1892, 1. The text of Reynolds's advertisements for *The Law of Population* is almost identical. For example, see *Western Mail*, July 6, 1891, 1.

[84] Ledbetter, *History of the Malthusian League*, 63.

[85] Ledbetter, *History of the Malthusian League*, 69.

[86] *The Malthusian Handbook: Designed to Induce Married People to Limit Their Families within Their Means* (London: W.H. Reynolds, 1898), unpaginated final page. For an example of Reynolds's advertisements, see "READ 'The Malthusian Handbook'," *North Wales Chronicle*, December 9, 1893, 4.

[87] Chandrasekhar, *Reproductive Physiology*, 57; Jones, *Business of Birth Control*, 67.

while, the League could claim that it did not offer practical advice on contraceptive techniques.

Rendell and Lambert benefitted from the League's promotional work too. As Jones has shown, these and other contraceptives manufacturers quickly aligned themselves with the organization – not just by name-dropping its unofficial publications but also by choosing trade names for their products that echoed key words in its official literature. Lambert's brand name for its condoms, for instance, was "Malthusian."[88] This web of affiliation made it increasingly difficult to distinguish where Malthusian activism ended and the contraceptive devices trade began. Lambert and Son published its own company pamphlets on the "Population Question," representing itself as a medical bookseller, and even set up a lending library for works on family planning.[89] Eventually, the company supplied birth control clinics run by the Malthusian League, Marie Stopes, and the National Birth Control Association/Family Planning Association.[90]

A Risky Business?

The Malthusian League and the manufacturers it worked with were far from isolated in their production, advertisement, and distribution of practical information about contraception. In the wake of the Knowlton trial, a wide variety of social protestors embraced the cause. Birth control manuals and contraceptive devices were advertised by and endorsed in radical periodicals that were not specifically Malthusian publications.[91] Some of these devices were manufactured by self-identified Malthusians, including J. Greevz Fyssher of Leeds and J. R. Holmes of Wantage, but the birth control manuals were increasingly issued by people who were affiliated with radical politics but not – to its leaders' consternation – with the Malthusian League.[92] Two of these pamphlets, *A Book for Married Women* (1894), by Thomas Richard Allinson, an anti-vaccinationist doctor and vegetarian, and *A True Remedy for Poverty!* (1895), by W. J. Douse, a member of the left-wing Nottingham Society, were advertised heavily in the press. In the early 1890s, the activist Ernest May established a new periodical dedicated to promoting Malthusianism, *The Malthusian Herald* (1891).[93]

After just one issue, *The Malthusian Herald* was rebranded the *Hygienic Advertiser* to describe the content it ended up containing more accurately. One

88 Jones, *Business of Birth Control*, 65. 89 Jones, *Business of Birth Control*, 65.

90 Jones, *Business of Birth Control*, 56, 70–71. 91 Royle, *Radicals, Secularists*, 258–259.

92 Lesley Hall, "Malthusian Mutations: The Changing Politics and Moral Meanings of Birth Control in Britain," in *Malthus, Medicine, and Morality: "Malthusianism" after 1798*. ed. Brian Dolan (London: Clio Medica, 2000), 148.

93 *The Malthusian Herald*, vol. 1 (London: New Fellowship Press, 1891), 1866.a.10.(10.). BL.

of the corollaries of birth control's rapid upswing in popularity in radical circles was that its promotion was increasingly entangled with the promotion of many alternative lifestyles and medical perspectives, including anti-vaccination, vegetarianism, teetotalism, and hydropathy, and various products to support them. *The Malthusian Herald* advertised birth control manuals, condoms, pessaries, and spermicidal syringes, for example, alongside the Ida Nut Grinder, a device for "grinding all kinds of Nuts, Dried Bread, Vegetables," India-rubber-tipped laundry gloves, and other domestic items.[94] May was the inventor of many of these products, and endorsed them throughout the *Herald*'s main text. As well as helping May promote his inventions, advertisements for these items helped promote medical perspectives that May supported alongside Malthusianism. For instance, the Nut Grinder, a tool designed to facilitate a vegetarian diet, supported a theory of health promoted by Allinson's Natural Living Society, which the *Herald* also endorsed.[95]

Trade in advice on how to practise contraception also flourished apart from radical circles. Manufacturers that were not associated with any radical group advertised widely in the press, instructing "persons who cannot afford to keep a large family" to send away for their own manuals on the "population question."[96] Booksellers with no evident connections with radical politics sold manuals written by Malthusian activists alongside older works on contraception, midwifery, and sexual health.[97] As they did prior to the Knowlton trial, birth control manuals and contraceptive devices also circulated through the pornography trade, though they were now less tightly associated with it in the public imagination. C. J. Wilcox, "late of Holywell Street," advertised contraceptive pessaries for sale alongside nude photographs in the *Illustrated Police News* throughout the 1880s, while G. Birt sold contraception manuals, including (likely pirated) editions of Besant's *Law of Population*, alongside pornographic novels in the 1890s.[98]

94 *Malthusian Herald*, 8, 10, 18, 22. For more on the periodical, see James Gregory, *On Victorians and Vegetarians: The Vegetarian Movement in Nineteenth-Century Britain* (London: Taurus Academic Studies, 2007), 146–148.

95 Gregory, *Vegetarians*, 147, 80.

96 McLaren, *Birth Control*, 255; Jones, *Business of Birth Control*, 101–102. Jones argues that birth-control manuals enabled these companies to develop "invaluable . . . impersonal relationships with customers over vast distances," allowing "rubber goods manufacturers to promote their products across 10–60 pages." See Claire Jones, "Under the Covers? Commerce, Contraceptives, and Consumers in England and Wales, 1880–1960," *Social History of Medicine* 29, no. 4 (2015): 740. See also Jütte, *Contraception*, 117–134.

97 *Berrow's Worcester Journal*, January 5, 1889, 1; *Hull Daily Mail*, April 29, 1891, 1; *Western Gazette*; March 22, 1895, 1; *Reynolds's Newspaper*, November 15, 1896, 4.

98 "To Those About To Marry," *Illustrated Police News*, November 6, 1897, 11; "Curious Books," *Illustrated Police News*, May 22, 1886, 4. For further information, see Jones, *Business of Birth Control*, 43–44, 102–105.

In other words, trade in contraception manuals and devices was booming in the late-nineteenth century, and their promotion was often treated with the same (lack of) reverence as the promotion of laundry gloves. Yet, birth controllers continuously suggested that it was risky to sell them. A full-page advertisement for Truelove's pamphlet on his 1878 trial, *The Queen v. E. Truelove*, printed on the back cover of his 1881 edition of Drysdale's *Elements of Social Science*, frames Drysdale's work as jeopardized by censorious forces: ". . . the fair and legitimate liberty of the Press has been imperilled by the attempt of the 'Society for the Suppression of Vice' to bring such a work as the 'Moral Physiology' of R.D. Owen . . . within the scope of Lord Campbell's Act and English Common Law," it reads.[99] This copy of *Elements* was issued only a handful of years after Truelove's imprisonment for distributing birth control pamphlets, but more than a decade later radicals were still framing contraception literature as censored, or liable to be censored. Allinson's 1895–6 advertisements for *A Book for Married Women* imply that he anticipated opposition, claiming "No book is written which goes so thoroughly into matters relating to married women. Some may think too much is told."[100] In 1897 advertisements for *A True Remedy for Poverty!*, Douse announced that he "invite[d] criticism and def[ied] prosecution": "The truth shall be known!" his advertisements cried.[101]

Published in 1893, *The Malthusian Handbook* portrays contraception as a cause blighted with legal struggle. Twenty-four pages of the pamphlet – a major portion of the work, which only runs to forty-six – furnish readers with an account of the opposition that Malthusians had encountered. Incorporating drawn-out excerpts from court reports and other documents, this section recounts Bradlaugh and Besant's arrest and trial for selling *Fruits*, framing it as the immediate act of a censorious government; Truelove's imprisonment; Allbutt's clash with the General Medical Council over *The Wife's Handbook*; and two other obscenity trials (one in Australia) involving birth control manuals. It also surveys reports of opposition to Malthusianism around the world, in countries as diverse as India, France, Germany, and the Netherlands. "Hence the task of the pioneers of the movement is rendered excessively difficult," an 1898 edition of the pamphlet concludes, "but from the very inception of the Malthusian League, the work of propaganda has been carried forward with unfailing devotion and singleness of purpose."[102]

99 A Doctor of Medicine [George Drysdale], *The Elements of Social Science, or, Physical, Sexual, and Natural Religion*, 20th ed. (London: Edward Truelove, 1881), back cover.

100 "A Book for Married Women," *Manchester Weekly Times*, December 13, 1895, 8. Allinson used the same line in shorter advertisements. See "A Book For Ladies," *Pick-Me-Up*, September 16, 1896, 415.

101 "A True Remedy for Poverty!," *Leeds Times*, September 24, 1897, 1.

102 *Malthusian Handbook*, 28.

In advertisements, in and on their publications, and in the radical press, Malthusians thus suggested that their plight was the same as their counterparts in the United States, who were zealously pursued for purveying obscene material in the late-nineteenth century.[103] Founded in 1873, the New York Society for the Suppression of Vice (NYSSV) crusaded against information on contraception, contraceptive devices, and abortion paraphernalia alongside other forms of "indecent" literature. Its success in lobbying for new laws against trade in indecent articles – and its tight alignment with law enforcement – facilitated these efforts. The same year in which it was founded, Anthony Comstock, the NYSSV's secretary and the face of the American anti-vice movement, was made the United States Postmaster General.[104] By 1880, Comstock had had ninety-seven people arrested under federal laws for advertising or selling abortifacients or "indecent rubber articles" through the mail, and more for distributing books and pamphlets on contraception.[105] Under the Comstock Law, which prohibited distributing obscene material through the mail, sellers faced harsh penalties of up to 5,000 dollars in fines and prison terms of up to ten years.[106]

Yet, prosecutions for distributing works on contraception were much rarer in Britain. The Home Office was concerned about freethought's political influence, and laws against blasphemy were used against freethinkers with increasing frequency in the 1880s and 1890s.[107] However, between 1879 and 1901, less than a dozen people were charged for selling works on contraception under obscenity laws.[108] Many of those people were itinerant booksellers, arrested in provincial towns by local authorities under the 1824 Vagrancy Act following complaints that they were hawking indecent works in public spaces. Most received small fines or spent a day in gaol. Accounting for people who sold contraception literature alongside erotic photographs and were arrested for selling both could as much as triple this number. However, police records emphasize that, like Cook, these dealers were targeted because they sold pornography.[109] The Knowlton trial made contraception literature notorious and opposition to trade in it does seem to have increased, especially in the

[103] For further details, see Amy Werbel, *Lust on Trial: Censorship and the Rise of American Obscenity in the Age of Anthony Comstock* (New York: Columbia University Press, 2018); Andrea Tone, *Devices and Desires: A History of Contraceptives in America* (New York: Hill and Wang, 2001); Nicola Kay Baisel, *Imperiled Innocents: Anthony Comstock and Family Reproduction in Victorian America* (Princeton, NJ: Princeton University Press, 1998); Janice Ruth Wood, *The Struggle for Free Speech in the United States, 1872–1915: Edward Bliss Foote, Edward Bond Foot, and Anti-Comstock Operations* (London: Routledge, 2008).

[104] Werbel, *Lust on Trial*, 130. [105] Baisel, *Imperilled Innocents*, 45.

[106] Wood, *Struggle for Free Speech*, 3. [107] Marsh, *Word Crimes*, 204–268.

[108] For a description of these cases, see Edward Royle, *Radicals, Secularists*, 276, 291–292. I have found records of just three other cases. "Phrenologists in Court," *Morpeth Herald*, January 2, 1892, 6 and the Lambert and Smith-White cases, cited below, which were quickly thrown out.

[109] For instance, see HO 45/23588, TNA.

provinces. However, the scattered nature of the prosecutions and the absence of any records documenting organized efforts to suppress trade in contraception literature suggest that opposition to it was much weaker than Malthusians made it out to be.

Home Office records suggest that British authorities were reluctant to charge distributors of contraception literature even when complaints were made about them. The publicity that the Knowlton trial generated seems to have made them wary of being targets of another publicity stunt. They typically discouraged complainants from prosecuting distributors of medical material on the basis that a trial would simply publicize the works at issue. Officials also did not want to recommend – much less bring – prosecutions if they scented any risk of failure.[110] They had their own credibility to protect. Although some magistrates had supported actions against irregular practitioners under obscenity laws in the 1870s, government officials often had doubts that prosecutions involving medical material would be successful and advised against them on this basis too. In 1896, a group of medical practitioners seeking obscenity charges against Allinson for distributing his pamphlet *A Book for Married Women* received this response from an official:

> The conclusion arrived at in respect of prosecutions of this nature has been generally against the expediency of prosecuting, both as a matter of public policy, prosecutions resulting in giving a wide publicity to the publication and on account of the difficulty of determining the question of fact. . . . I have not seen the book, but unless it is something more than a popularised medical work and contains matter which is on the face of it obscene for the sake of obscenity and intended to gratify the base passions, a prosecution . . . would be neither expedient nor successful.[111]

The outcome of an 1898 case against Lambert and Son for selling a copy of its manual *The Wife's Medical Advertiser*, a contraceptive device, and an illustrated price list affirmed this official's doubts. The magistrate threw the Lambert case out on the grounds that if works advocating contraception could be sold widely, information about how to practise it could not be suppressed.[112]

Anti-vice societies also mounted little opposition to trade in contraception literature. Apart from the actions against Truelove in 1877 and 1878, the Society for the Suppression of Vice did not prosecute distributors unless they sold

[110] For instance, see HO 144/238/A525391 and HO 144/233 A52539/2, TNA, which also document concerns that failed prosecutions involving medical material could hamper separate efforts to regulate the drug trade. See Lisa Z. Sigel, "Censorship in Inter-War Britain: Obscenity, Spectacle, and the Workings of the Liberal State," *Journal of Social History* 45, no. 1 (2011): 68–70 for a discussion of similar concerns among Home Office officials in the twentieth century.

[111] "The Legal Aspects of Obscene Advertising," *Medical Press and Circular*, June 3, 1896, 584.

[112] Ledbetter, *History of the Malthusian League*, 157. Two similar cases yielded the same conclusion. See *Newbold*, 1892 (t18920725-695) and *Smith, Henry, and White*, 1892 (t18920725-696) in Old Bailey Proceedings Online.

pornography. The Society also did not survive for very long after Truelove's trial: the bad publicity generated by Collette's embezzlement case brought about the organization's unofficial collapse in 1880.[113] The National Vigilance Association (1885–1953), often seen as a successor to the Society, was not especially interested in trying to suppress contraception literature, either. Like other late nineteenth-century social purity groups, it focused its efforts on combating prostitution, child abuse, and sexual assault. Although the Association joined medical practitioners in championing the Indecent Advertisements Act (1889), no discussion of contraception literature or other medical material appears in minutes from its meetings.[114] The Association's few actions to suppress obscene material, clustered in the years immediately following its establishment, focused on literary works, photographs, and artworks.[115] These actions were led by its secretary, William Coote, the mercurial journalist W. T. Stead, and Charles Hastings Collette, all of whom were eager to make (or, in Collette's case, re-make) their names as moral crusaders – and make some money – under the Association's banner.[116]

Prosecution was not a priority for medical groups, either. Many regular practitioners thought that practising contraception was immoral. However, they were far more concerned about trade in abortifacients. Abortion remained a common method of controlling fertility in the late-nineteenth century, but it was illegal; methods to self-induce it were dangerous and unreliable; and abortions performed in secret by trained surgeons could be prohibitively expensive. William Hitchman, a Liverpool-based physician, reported in 1883 that prices ranged from three to thirty pounds.[117] This maintained a flourishing market for (sometimes deliberately fraudulent) patent medicines that promised

113 See Katherine Mullin, "Poison More Deadly than Prussic Acid: Defining Obscenity after the 1857 Obscene Publications Act (1850–1885)," in *Prudes on the Prowl: Fiction and Obscenity in England, 1857 to the Present Day*, ed. David Bradshaw and Rachel Potter (Oxford: Oxford University Press, 2013), 28.

114 Anat Rosenberg, *The Rise of Mass Advertising: Law, Enchantment, and the Cultural Boundaries of British Modernity* (Oxford: Oxford University Press, 2022), 291; National Vigilance Association Meeting Minutes, 1885–1969, Woman's Library Archives, GB 106 4NVA, LSE. This may have changed in the twentieth century. Because of the volume of the material, I limited my investigation of the NVA's records to 1885–1901.

115 See Katherine Mullin, *James Joyce, Sexuality, and Social Purity* (Cambridge: Cambridge University Press, 2003), 6–10; Lesley A. Hall, *Sex, Gender and Social Change in Britain since 1880*, 2nd ed. (London: Bloomsbury, 2017), 46, 68 for accounts of some of these actions. For further accounts, see "Occasional Notes," *Pall Mall Gazette*, April 26, 1886, 3; "Fourth Edition," *Pall Mall Gazette*, December 18, 1886, 9; "Alleged Indecent Pictures," *Bristol Mercury*, October 31, 1888, 3; "The Charge of Selling Indecent Prints," *Reynolds's Newspaper*, March 2, 1890, 8.

116 Christopher Hilliard, *A Matter of Obscenity: The Politics of Censorship in Modern England* (Princeton, NJ: Princeton University Press, 2021), 26–27.

117 MacLaren, *Birth Control*, 117–120; Patricia Knight, "Women and Abortion in Victorian and Edwardian England," *History Workshop* 4, no. 1 (1977): 57–68; Angus McLaren, "Abortion in England, 1890–1914," *Victorian Studies* 20, no. 4 (1977): 379–400; William Hitchman, "Popular Abortion and Infanticide," *The Malthusian*, September 1883, 441.

safe, effective abortions.[118] Medical journalists railed at advertisements for these medicines, and, as we have seen, lobbied the government to crack down on them alongside advertisements for treatments for venereal disease. Trade in contraception literature did not command nearly the same level of opposition. This seems be partly because medical practitioners did not see contraception advocacy as a threat to public health, and partly because they had long argued that controlling fertility was not a medical issue.[119] Although the latter view began to change in the 1870s, medical men do not seem to have considered trade in advice on contraception a threat to their profession.

Medical opposition to Allbutt's and Allinson's publications had more to do with their style of medical practice than the fact that they sold contraception literature. As Ann Stuart has shown, the General Medical Council's decision to strike Allbutt from the Medical Register for publishing *The Wife's Handbook* was strongly influenced by its concern about the wide variety of "advertisements bound up with the book."[120] Allbutt claimed that the advertisements' main purpose was to cover the cost of printing, and not to generate "monetary profit or with the view of attracting patients to himself."[121] However, the sheer number of advertisements in the *Handbook*, and Allbutt's endorsement of so many of the products they featured in its text, made this claim very dubious. As Stuart points out, the question that the committee set up to investigate Allbutt's pamphlet ultimately asked the Council to rule on was "whether the book was a fair medical treatise or an indecent advertisement, and was it a book so injurious to the public in point of health as well as morals, and so evil in its tendency as regards to the profession, that its publication would be considered to be 'infamous conduct in a professional respect'."[122] We see, yet again, a conflation of indecency and quackery in this question: concerns about the effect that Allbutt's commercialism could have on the profession's reputation were collapsed with concerns about the *Handbook*'s moral effects.

The General Medical Council did not seek to censure Allbutt. However, after it was compelled to investigate *The Wife's Handbook*, it seized the opportunity to make an example of a practitioner who not only advocated a practice that many medical men considered immoral but was also embracing partnerships with companies that sold drugs and medical devices during a period in which

118 McLaren, "Abortion in England," 388–389. For examples of advertisements, see "Nurse Lilley's Royal Female Pills," *Englishwoman's Domestic Magazine*, October 1, 1875, 10; "An Honest Medicine," *Myra's Journal of Dress and Fashion*, September 1, 1897, 26; "Mrs. Lebet's Female Pills," *The World of Fashion and Continental Feuilletons*, January 1, 1890, Advertisement Sheet; *Judy*, January 1, 1896, Advertisement Sheet.

119 See McLaren, "Abortion in England," 394.

120 Ann Elisabeth F. Stuart, "The Case of Dr. Allbutt." (M.Phil diss., University of Cambridge, 2000); "Meeting of the General Medical Council," *Lancet*, November 26, 1887, 1085.

121 "General Medical Council," *Lancet*, 1085.

122 "General Medical Council," *Lancet*, 1085.

the Council was beginning to see this as a major problem for the profession. Many medical men took money from drug and medical device companies to endorse products in their own publications, in trade catalogues, and in company-produced pamphlets, handbills, and advertisements during the 1880s.[123] These arrangements represented a welcome stream of revenue for medical practitioners. However, as Jones has shown, leading medical men considered them dangerous to patients, to medical careers, and to the medical profession. Endorsements for commercial products could "damage an individual practitioner's career should the product prove to be useless or dangerous . . . by bringing their knowledge and expertise into question," and they could arouse doubt in the medical profession's commitment to health over profit.[124] Opposition to endorsement deals mounted rapidly. By 1900, the General Medical Council had struck around thirty practitioners from its register for endorsing medical products in print.[125]

Efforts to get Allinson charged for selling *A Book for Married Women* throughout the last half of 1890s further suggest that it was not opposition to contraception but concern about defining medicine's relationship with commerce that drove rare medical attempts to get practitioners in trouble with the law for distributing birth control literature. In 1892, Allinson was struck from the Medical Register for "systematically seeking to attract practice by a system of extensive public advertisements" which contained "his name, address, and qualifications, and invitations to persons in need of medical aid to consult him professionally."[126] Allinson refused to stop practising under the title Licentiate of the Royal College of Surgeons after his expulsion. Multiple actions against him for violating the Medical Act were ineffectual. In 1896, two years after *A Book for Married Women* was published, his former colleagues changed course and began to hound the authorities to charge Allinson with distributing obscene material.[127] In 1901, these efforts finally succeeded: a police officer posing as a seventeen-year-old girl obtained one of Allinson's pamphlets through the post, and charged him with distributing obscene material.[128] Allinson was fined £250 and his stock was destroyed. However, the episode

[123] Claire L. Jones, *The Medical Trade Catalogue in Britain, 1870–1914* (London: Routledge, 2016), 4.

[124] Jones, *Medical Trade Catalogue*, 143. [125] Jones, *Medical Trade Catalogue*, 4.

[126] "Medico-Legal and Medico-Ethical," *BMJ*, August 6, 1892, 331. See also "The Case of Mr. T. R. Allinson," *BMJ*, June 4, 1892, 1203; "Medico-Legal and Medico-Ethical," *BMJ*, June 11, 1892, 1277; "Medico-Legal and Medico-Ethical," *BMJ*, July 1, 1893, 42–43; "In the Matter of Mr. T.R. Allinson," *Lancet*, July 6, 1895, 1656.

[127] "Allinson v. the General Medical Council," *Lancet*, July 8, 1893, 99; "In the Matter of Mr. T.R. Allinson," *Lancet*, July 6, 1895, 57; "The Use of Medical Titles after Erasure from the Medical Register," *BMJ*, July 13, 1895, 93. "Association of Fellows R.C.S," *BMJ*, November 25, 1895, 1319; "Prosecution under the Medical Acts," *BMJ*, April 22, 1899, 1007.

[128] "The Prosecution of T.R. Allinson," *Lancet*, April 13, 1901, 1095; "Medico-Legal and Medico-ethical," *BMJ*, April 13, 1901, 931.

did not, as writers for the *Lancet* had hoped, stop Allinson from practising medicine.[129]

Malthusians presented the *Hicklin* test as a danger to free speech. However, its impact on the publication and distribution of works on contraception was largely indirect. In a context in which authorities had little interest in suppressing trade in contraception literature, the test's influence is clearest in how it was used to authorize contraception advocacy. The fact that sellers of contraception literature could be charged with distributing obscene material does seem to have genuinely worried birth controllers, at least for a time. The Malthusian League's publishing strategies, which maintained a kind of plausible deniability by keeping trade in practical information about contraception at arm's length from the organization, evince careful thinking about how to protect the League during a period in which obscenity laws were applied creatively and haphazardly, and the risks of selling practical literature on contraception could be hard to gauge. However, the League's integration of language that alluded to the test in its mission statement, and social protestors' tireless framing of contraception pamphlets as illegal amid the massive expansion of the contraceptive devices industry and a booming trade in practical works on how to control reproduction, emphasize its powerful function as a framing device.

In 1877, it was a device that enabled Bradlaugh and Besant to distance contraception from the pornography trade, align it with a cause around which most social protestors could rally, and attract enormous publicity to the cause. During the 1880s and 1890s, it operated as a device that helped birth-controllers and contraceptives manufacturers frame themselves as different from the other medical entrepreneurs: they were not self-seekers, but visionaries, working tirelessly in the shadow of "the spirit of persecution" to save people from poverty and misery.[130] Malthusians were ultimately unable to fully distance contraception from its associations with sexual immorality. As historians have often noted, their literature was never popular with working-class readers for this reason, and condoms seem to have retained their seedy reputation. Marie Stopes opined that Bradlaugh and Besant's emphasis on birth-control pamphlets' vulnerability to destruction under obscenity laws actually strengthened these associations and nearly "killed" the movement.[131] However, framing information about contraception as suppressed speech undeniably attracted support and publicity too.

Sexual scientists, whose circles overlapped with those of Malthusians and other sex radicals in the 1890s, faced a more difficult task than Bradlaugh and Besant had as they sought to establish sexuality in general and same-sex desire

[129] "Unregistered Practitioners and the Notification of Diseases Act," *BMJ*, July 6, 1902, 295; "The Coroner and Unregistered Medical Men," *Lancet*, July 4, 1903, 69.

[130] *Malthusian Handbook*, 30. [131] Stopes, *Early Days of Birth Control*, 23.

in particular as respectable foci of medical and scientific enquiry, to win the support of the public, and to galvanize social and legal change. The same concerns about damaging print associations that had plagued birth controllers and regular medical practitioners plagued sexual scientists, whose work was promoted, reprinted, compiled, and imitated by publishers who they worked with and often shared values with, but feared would imperil their ambitions. Sexual scientists took strategies for defining publications and causes examined in this and the previous chapters and adapted them for their own purposes.

7 Be Careful about the Publisher

R. v. *Bedborough*, the 1898 trial in which Britain's first textbook on homosexuality, Havelock Ellis and John Addington Symonds's *Sexual Inversion* (1897), was labelled an obscene book, is one of the most famous obscenity trials in British history. Like Bradlaugh and Besant's 1877 trial, it became a potent touchstone in critiques of Victorian morality that framed not the free circulation of sexual knowledge but its suppression as indecent. In the eyes of its supporters, the emergent field of sexology fulfilled modern scientists' duty to develop rational understandings of all aspects of human experience. In its indictment of *Sexual Inversion*, the Bedborough trial seemed to expose censorship as a formidable roadblock to this work. By the 1920s, sexology was tightly linked with opposition to restrictions on free sexual discussion by means of the law, institutional policies, and public opinion. As Kate Fisher and Jana Funke have noted, an entire section of the programme for the 1929 London Congress of the World League for Sexual Reform was devoted to the issue.[1]

Sexology certainly operated at the edges of respectable scientific enquiry. Yet, as in the Malthusian context, its supporters' public positions on censorship can give an exaggerated impression of the role that the law played in mediating the distribution of its literature. It was unusual for distributors to be arrested during the late nineteenth and early twentieth centuries, and those who were arrested were typically involved in activities that the state was more invested in combating: pornography trafficking and fraud.[2] Even the Bedborough trial was driven

[1] Kate Fisher and Jana Funke, "'Are We to Treat Human Nature as the Early Victorian Lady Treated Telegrams?' British and German Sexual Science, Investigations of Nature and the Fight against Censorship, ca. 1890–1940," *Journal of the History of Sexuality* 32, no. 1 (2024): 91.

[2] For the most detailed work on this topic to date, see Phillip Kuhn, "The Sexual Life of Our Time: Medical Censorship in Early-20th-Century England," *History of Psychology* 23, no. 1 (2020): 40–61. See Harry G. Cocks, "Saucy Stories: Pornography, Sexology and the Marketing of Sexual Knowledge in Britain, c. 1918–70," *Social History* 29, no. 4 (2004): 479 for a discussion of cases in 1934 and 1937 involving sexological works in shops that sold pornographic and pulp material. In some cases, officials considered prosecuting publishers or distributors of sexual-scientific material after they received complaints about it, but decided against prosecuting them on the basis that prosecution would only lend this material publicity. For example, see HO 144/1043/183472, TNA, which documents officials' debates about how to respond to a 1910 complaint about Edward Carpenter's *Homogenic Love* (1894).

not by state concern about *Sexual Inversion*'s effects on readers' morals but by state interest in breaking up a group that Scotland Yard was convinced was a front for anarchist organizing. If the trial illustrated urgent problems for sexology's establishment as a scientific field, those problems lay less with state censorship of its literature than with its queer disciplinary position. Perhaps even more than medicine in the early decades of the Victorian period, and more than Malthusianism in the 1870s, sexology had an identity problem.

At the *fin de siècle*, sexological research was awkwardly situated at the edges of medical and social-scientific enquiry, radical activism, humanist scholarship, literary expression, and erotic print culture.[3] In Britain, and around the world, it was taken up by people with commitments to progressive politics, people who advocated interdisciplinary approaches to research on sexuality, and people who had marginal, or no, training in medicine or science. Sexual-scientific works often drew on literary, artistic, historical, and (auto)biographical sources, and circulated far beyond the medical context, through networks of homophiles, socialists, anarchists, and free-lovers. The pornography trade began to emerge as a fixture in the distribution and, in some cases, production of sexual-scientific literature, and also became imbricated in these networks. Taking *Sexual Inversion*'s vexed publication history as its starting point, this chapter examines sexological literature's unruly circuits of production and distribution and how they destabilized Ellis's initial attempts to frame *Sexual Inversion* as a medical book. It also examines how allegations of obscenity and censorship on the grounds of obscenity emerged as instruments that sexologists and their allies used to define an identity for their emergent field and make a case for sex research.

The case of sexology is a fitting end point for this book because it illustrates how different frameworks for guiding understandings of books, people, and collectives, whose development was explored in earlier chapters, interacted and extended in the Victorian period's twilight years. Ellis sought to frame *Sexual Inversion* as a medical book by adhering to various conventions for writing, publishing, and advertising professional medical literature, whose increasing crystallization was plotted in Chapter 5. Yet, in seeking to make the work accessible to non-medical readers, he followed these conventions imperfectly. This undermined *Sexual Inversion*'s credibility in the eyes of many medical practitioners. Its credibility was further undermined by an

[3] For more on the interdisciplinary character of early sexology, see Kate Fisher and Jana Funke, "'Let Us Leave the Hospital; Let Us Go on a Journey around the World': British and German Sexual Science and the Global Search for Sexual Variation," in *A Global History of Sexual Science, 1880–1960*, ed. Veronika Fuechtner, Douglas E. Haynes, and Ryan M. Jones (Berkeley: University of California Press, 2017), 51–69. For a different view, see Ivan Crozier and Heike Bauer, "Sexology, Historiography, Citation, Embodiment: A Review and (Frank) Exchange," *Book Reviews* (blog), *History of the Human Sciences*, June 27, 2017, www.histhum.com/category/book-reviews/.

issue that presented a persistent problem in the history this book has traced: the cocirculation of medical, radical, and pornographic material. Building on strategies examined in Chapter 6, Ellis and his allies turned to a different method of making sex research respectable. They portrayed sexology as a progressive scientific field unjustly censored by ignorant authorities, and decried pornography as its opposite: the "unnatural" and "inaccurate" product of a culture deprived of the scientific truth about sex.

It is here that we see a myth emerge that would define how people understood the modern history of sexual knowledge through the first half of the twentieth century: the myth of Victorian sexual ignorance. Historians have shown that this myth functioned as a powerful means through which twentieth century sexologists and sex educators authorized their expertise.[4] Accounts of the Victorian "repression," "censorship," and "silencing" of sexual discussion enabled a new generation of self-appointed experts to "disqualify existing practices and knowledge" and frame their own work as scientific, modern, and progressive.[5] Setting this myth's emergence within the longer, wider context of Victorian debates about medical obscenity makes its origins more legible, showing that it reflected a longer pattern of contesting and producing authority by framing sexual knowledge as censored that stretched back to the Victorian period itself. It also emphasizes that the emergence of Victorian sexual ignorance as a framework for understanding the modern history of sexual knowledge was not inevitable. While it certainly owed something to chafing at changes in attitudes toward sex over the course of the nineteenth century, it also owed a great deal to the haphazard ways in which obscenity laws were employed and sexual-scientific authority was contested, and the unruly commercial conditions that influenced them. The myth of Victorian ignorance would blot these conditions from memory.

Making and Unmaking a Medical Book

Although historians are increasingly viewing the development of sexology through a global lens, most histories trace its roots to Continental Europe, where, from the 1860s, psychiatrists sought to investigate sexual aberrations alongside a host of anti-social and criminal practices.[6] Same-sex desire was both the earliest and the largest focus of these investigations, which

[4] Harry Cocks, "Review: The Growing Pains of the History of Sexuality," *Journal of Contemporary History* 39, no. 4 (2004): 661. See also Simon Szreter and Kate Fisher, *Sex before the Sexual Revolution: Intimate Life in England 1918–1963* (Cambridge: Cambridge University Press, 2010), 66, 384.

[5] Cocks, "Review," 661.

[6] For information about sexology in its broader geographic and disciplinary contexts, see Veronika Fuechtner, Donald E. Haynes, and Ryan M. Jones, eds., *A Global History of Sexual Science, 1880–1960* (Berkeley: University of California Press, 2017) and Heike Bauer, ed.,

increasingly framed what the German journalist Karl-Maria Kertbeny coined "homosexuality" in 1868 as either a congenital or a socially acquired perversion of normal sexuality.[7] Britain developed a tradition of writing on sexuality more slowly, but by the 1890s a small body of work had emerged. Some of this work built on Charles Darwin's theory of sexual selection and primarily focused on reproductive, heterosexual sex,[8] but another strand of British sexual science focused on variant sexualities. Much of this work was overtly interdisciplinary, and deeply influenced by socialist, feminist, and homophile perspectives. It fit into the mould of recognized models of medical enquiry almost as uncomfortably as sexual inverts (a term often used for those who experienced same-sex desire) felt they fit into a culture gripped with anxiety about same-sex sex.

This is evident in the qualifications of those who wrote this work and in how they published it. Authors of influential British works on same-sex desire, including Edward Carpenter, John Addington Symonds, and Richard Burton, made their livings as poets, critics, and translators, not as medical practitioners; and those works, including Burton's 1886 "Terminal Essay" to his translation of the *Arabian Nights*, Symonds's *A Problem of Greek Ethics* (1883) and *A Problem of Modern Ethics* (1891), and Carpenter's *Homogenic Love* (1894), were not issued by medical publishers. Instead, their authors had them privately printed in limited numbers under obscure imprints, such as that of the Kama Shastra Society, an outfit primarily set up to issue translations of South Asian and Middle Eastern literature on sexual matters, or no imprint at all.[9] This form of publication enabled discreet exchanges of ideas between small groups of like-minded and often wealthy thinkers. However, it also limited their influence. Private publication severely narrowed the audience of the works involved. It also differentiated them from mainstream medico-scientific publications and the growing cultural authority of the fields with which they were associated.

Havelock Ellis and John Addington Symonds broke with this tradition when they sought to openly publish a study of sexual inversion. While their goal was not to make a political statement about their right to publish such a book, their motivation for publishing it openly was political: they sought to galvanize opposition to the 1885 Criminal Law Amendment Act, which had made gross

Sexology and Translation: Cultural and Scientific Encounters across the Modern World (Philadelphia, PA: Temple University Press, 2015).

7 Judit Takács, "The Double Life of Kertbeny," in *The Past and Present of Radical Sexual Politics: Working Papers: Fifth Meeting of the Seminar "Socialism and Sexuality," Amsterdam, October 3–4, 2003*, ed. G. Hekma (Amsterdam: Mosse Foundation, 2004), 51–62.

8 Kimberly A. Hamblin, *From Eve to Evolution: Darwin, Science, and Women's Rights in Gilded Age America* (Chicago: University of Chicago Press, 2014).

9 Sean Brady, *John Addington Symonds and Homosexuality: A Critical Edition of Sources* (Basingstoke: Palgrave Macmillan, 2012).

indecency – an ambiguous term that was interpreted as including any sexual activity between men, in public or private – punishable by imprisonment for up to two years.[10] Ellis, a social reformer, writer, and trained physician, and Symonds, a literary critic, cultural historian, and self-described invert, were horrified that private, consensual sex between men had been made illegal. In *Sexual Inversion*, they sought to outline a model of sexual behaviour that situated same-sex desire as natural, and therefore defensible. They hoped that the book, which was based on a theoretical model of sexuality developed by Ellis and supplemented with literary and historical evidence from Symonds's scholarship, would persuade medical experts and lay readers alike that the law should be reformed.

The prospect of publishing *Sexual Inversion* made both men nervous. The first editions of *A Problem of Greek Ethics* and *A Problem of Modern Ethics* had comprised only ten and fifty copies, giving Symonds considerable control over his audience. Ellis had prior experience with publishing sexually detailed works for the open market. However, he was keenly aware that it could go awry. In 1888, while Ellis was editing unexpurgated editions of Elizabethan dramas for the publisher Henry Vizetelly, Vizetelly was prosecuted by Charles Hastings Collette under the banner of the National Vigilance Association for issuing five- and six-shilling translations of Émile Zola's novels *La Terre* (1887), *Nana* (1880), and *Pot-Bouille* (1883).[11] Vizetelly shrugged off the fine that resulted, and reissued new Zola translations the following year. He was prosecuted again, and saddled with a larger fine and a three-month prison sentence. In the wake of these trials, Ellis translated an unexpurgated edition of Zola's novel *Germinal* (1885) for Leonard Smithers, a publisher equally well known for issuing avant-garde literature and expensive pornography.[12] Ellis was more than willing to write on controversial topics and produce risqué books for others. However, he did not want *Sexual Inversion* to share *La Terre*'s fate.

Some historians have speculated that Ellis earned a medical degree from St. Thomas's Hospital Medical School in 1889 to furnish his writing on sexual matters with the stamp of scientific legitimacy.[13] If this was his aim, it was the

[10] Matt Cook, *London and the Culture of Homosexuality, 1885–1914* (Cambridge: Cambridge University Press, 2003), 42.

[11] Denise Merkle, "When Expurgation Constitutes Ineffective Censorship: The Case of Three Vizetelly Translations of Zola," in *Proceedings of the Maastricht Session of the 3rd International Maastricht-Lodz Duo Colloquium*, ed. B. Lewandowska-Tomaszczyk and M. Thelen (Maastricht: Hogeschool Maastricht, 2001), 285–293. For details about Collette's involvement, see "The Police Courts," *Daily News*, August 11, 1888, 6.

[12] Denise Merkle, "The Lutetian Society," *TTR: traduction, terminologie, redaction* 16, no. 2 (2003): 73–101.

[13] Ivan Crozier, "Pillow Talk: Credibility, Trust, and the Sexological Case History," *History of Science* 46, no. 4 (2008): 391.

first in a series of steps that he, and to a lesser extent Symonds, took to try to ensure that *Sexual Inversion* would be received as a serious medical book by adhering to writing, publishing, and advertising conventions that, by the 1890s, marked a book as a legitimate medical intervention. Although they each contributed to it, the co-authors agreed that Ellis's name would appear first on the title page, emphasizing the contribution of a qualified medical practitioner. As Ivan Crozier has shown, the content was also developed to appear as "scientific" as possible. Unlike either author's previous publications, *Sexual Inversion* is centred on a series of case studies, based on questionnaires that Ellis and Symonds asked friends and friends of friends to fill out. Ellis steered the book more deeply into medico-scientific territory by persuading Symonds to reduce its literary content. After Symonds died in 1893, Ellis edited the manuscript, further marginalizing Symonds's humanist contributions to emphasize the book's focus on "scientific facts" about sexual inversion.[14]

Ellis also seriously considered the effect that the book's publisher, price, and advertisement would have on its medical reception. Symonds proposed publishing *Sexual Inversion* in the Walter Scott Publishing Company's middlebrow Contemporary Science Series, which Ellis edited.[15] At first glance, the series was a good fit. Its mandate was progressive: to publish books that addressed "questions of modern life – the various social and political economical problems of to-day, the most recent researches in the knowledge of man, the past and present experiences of the race, and the nature of the environment."[16] Moreover, several sexual-scientific works on sexuality – works in the tradition that had developed in response to Darwin's theories – had already been published in it. However, Ellis told Symonds that Walter Scott did not want the book (there was "too much at stake to involve the series in any really pioneering experiment") and that, in any case, he worried that some of the books in the series would compromise *Sexual Inversion*'s reception. "Several of the volumes approach various forbidden topics as nearly as is possible," Ellis argued. "From the point of view of the book, alas, I doubt if it would be the wisest mode of publication."[17]

Ellis may have had Patrick Geddes and J. Arthur Thomson's *The Evolution of Sex* (1889) in mind, which naturalized traditional gender roles by linking them with binary biological processes and recommended contraception as

[14] Ivan Crozier, "Introduction: Havelock Ellis, John Addington Symonds and the Construction of Sexual Inversion" in *Sexual Inversion: A Critical Edition*, ed. Ivan Crozier (Basingstoke: Palgrave Macmillan, 2008), 58–60.

[15] For further information about this series, see Bernard Lightman, *Victorian Popularizers of Science: Designing Nature for New Audiences* (Chicago: University of Chicago Press, 2009), 30.

[16] "The Contemporary Science Series," *Journal of Mental Science* 36, no. 153 (1890): 265.

[17] Havelock Ellis to John Addington Symonds, July 1, 1892, Havelock Ellis Collection, 1875–1955, HRC.

a means of shaping evolution. The book was never framed as indecent in medical circles, but it was controversial, and not reviewed in many medical journals until after the medical publisher H. K. Lewis issued a new edition. Ellis was convinced that a publisher "who is both medical and scientific and general," like Macmillan or Smith Elder, would serve their ambitions better.[18] He thought that such a publisher could distribute *Sexual Inversion* beyond medical circles – a key commitment for both authors – even as it lent the book the authority of a house known for issuing conventional medical writing. Unfortunately, Ellis could not get Macmillan, Smith Elder, or a similar publisher interested in *Sexual Inversion.*[19] The medical publisher F. J. Rebman had issued English translations of Continental studies of variant sexualities in 1893 and 1895, and encountered no discernible opposition.[20] In the wake of Oscar Wilde's headline-making trial for "gross indecency" in 1895, however, general publishers apparently did not want to touch a work on same-sex desire aimed at a broader audience.

Ellis published chunks of *Sexual Inversion* in the progressive American medical journal *Alienist and Neurologist*, and then the book itself in German, in 1896, to "pave the way for English publication."[21] The following year, *Sexual Inversion* was finally published in England under the imprint Wilson & Macmillan. Infamously, this was not an imprint of Macmillan, but of the University Press, an outfit run by the radical campaigner and free-love advocate Georg Ferdinand Springmühl von Weissenfeld under the name George Astor Singer.[22] Weissenfeld moved in activist circles that overlapped with Ellis and Symonds's, and would become a notable, if short-lived, publisher of sexual-scientific literature. At the time, though, his was far from the kind of press that Ellis had hoped for – but at least it was a press. At the request of his family, Symonds's literary executor immediately bought up the first English edition of *Sexual Inversion* in exchange for an agreement with Weissenfeld that any new editions omit Symonds's name.[23] A new, revised edition, issued by Weissenfeld

[18] Havelock Ellis to John Addington Symonds, December 21, 1892, Havelock Ellis Collection, 1875–1955, HRC.

[19] Havelock Ellis, "'The Question of Indecent Literature' (Letters to the Editor)," *Lancet*, November 19, 1898, 1344. Unfortunately, I have been unable to find any correspondence between Ellis and these publishers.

[20] Richard von Krafft Ebing, *Psychopathia Sexualis, with Especial Reference to Contrary Sexual Instinct: A Medico-Legal Study*, trans. Charles Gilbert Chaddock (London: F. J. Rebman, 1893); Albert von Schrenck-Notzing, *Therapeutic Suggestion in Psychopathia Sexualis (Pathological Manifestations of the Sexual Sense), with Especial Reference to Contrary Sexual Instinct*, trans. Charles Gilbert Chaddock (London: F. J. Rebman, 1895).

[21] Quoted in Kirsten Leng, *Sexual Politics and Feminist Science: Women Sexologists in Germany, 1900–1933* (Ithaca, NY: Cornell University Press, 2018), 43.

[22] Ellis was introduced to Weissenfeld through a mutual friend. See Havelock Ellis, *My Life: The Autobiography of Havelock Ellis* (Boston, MA: Houghton Mifflin, 1939), 351–353.

[23] Crozier, "Introduction," 56.

under a different imprint, the University Press of Watford, appeared in 1898. The book's high price, at ten shillings, and its limited (though not, as Ellis claimed, nonexistent) advertisement outside medical venues were pitched to evade any charge that *Sexual Inversion* was not a serious medical intervention.[24]

The choice of publisher proved to be a mistake.

Between 1899 and 1902, it gradually came to the attention of the police, and then to the public, that Weissenfeld was a convicted forger and active operator of several swindling schemes; that the University Press was not connected with a university; and that the signatories on its memorandum of association were all aliases of Weissenfeld's.[25] He died in 1902, reportedly of apoplexy, in Cambridge following a raid on his home that unearthed 30,000 allegedly obscene works, most of which appear to have been publications advocating free love and copies of Ellis's books. It was not Weissenfeld's shady business practices, however, but his use of his activist networks to distribute *Sexual Inversion* that brought the book into court in 1898. That year, George Bedborough, the secretary of an organization called the Legitimation League and the editor of its periodical, *The Adult: The Journal of Sex*, which Weissenfeld published, was arrested and charged with eleven counts of distributing obscene material: one for *Sexual Inversion*, one for the writer Orford Northcote's pamphlet "The Outcome of Legitimation," and nine for material in the *Adult*.

Bedborough's arrest had little to do with these works. Just as medical groups prosecuted doctors under obscenity laws with the aim of suppressing "quackery," the police charged Bedborough with the aim of suppressing anarchism. The Legitimation League, formed in 1893 to advocate for the inheritance rights of children born to unmarried parents, had a diverse membership. By 1898, its members included activists connected with the anarchist movement, and Scotland Yard thought it had "good reason to believe that Anarchistic proselytising took place over and over again in connection with [the League's] meetings."[26] One of its detectives, John Sweeney, went undercover to surveil the meetings. He reported that lectures at the meetings were "often of an

[24] Ellis, "The Question of Indecent Literature," 1344. Weissenfeld advertised *Sexual Inversion* in *Academy*, December 4, 1897, 470; *Bookseller*, November 4, 1897, 1157; and *Adult*, April 1898, 3.

[25] Accounts of Weissenfeld's activities, arrest, and death vary slightly. See Phyllis Grosskurth, *Havelock Ellis: A Biography* (New York: Knopf, 1960), 203; John Sweeney, *At Scotland Yard: Being the Experiences during Twenty-Seven Years Service* (London: Grant Richards, 1904), 195–196; Arthur Calder-Marshall, *Havelock Ellis: A Biography* (London: Hart-Davis, 1959), 157–172; Vincent Brome, *Havelock Ellis: Philosopher of Sex: A Biography* (London: Routledge, 1979), 96–108; Ellis, *My Life*, 370.

[26] Sweeney, *At Scotland Yard*, 178–179. See Edward Royle, *Radicals, Secularists, and Republicans: Popular Freethought in Britain, 1866–1915* (Manchester: Manchester University Press, 1980), 253 for further information about anarchists in the Legitimation League.

entirely innocent and even elevating nature . . . [but] the public discussions after the lecture were mainly supported by Anarchists, and some speeches of a highly incendiary character were occasionally delivered."[27] Convinced that these speeches concealed more robust anarchist organizing, Scotland Yard went looking for ways to break up the League.

According to Sweeney, the police asked a public prosecutor to charge Bedborough with distributing obscene material on the basis that the *Adult* was obscene. Although their language was "carefully chosen," its articles could be interpreted as a threat to public morals.[28] The prosecutor refused, arguing that targeting the periodical would give rise to claims that the state was censoring the press. Allegedly, a more acceptable route to prosecuting Bedborough presented itself when a young Liverpool man ordered a pamphlet from the Legitimation League only to be sent a copy of *Sexual Inversion* by mistake, and his parents complained to the police. Sweeney purchased a copy, used it as the basis for a warrant to raid Bedborough's home and office, and arrested him for selling it alongside the other publications.[29]

Debate about *Sexual Inversion* played a prominent role in the trial, where its distribution through Bedborough's office and its publication by a non-medical press were used to justify charges that it was an obscene book. Taking the stand as a witness, Sweeney pondered why, if "his book could be defended," Ellis had not published it with "one of the many high-class publishers of medico-scientific literature," and concluded, "there is nothing whatever in its mode of publication to suggest that it deserved a better fate."[30] The prosecutor followed the same line of reasoning, linking *Sexual Inversion*'s potential effects on readers with how it had been published and distributed: a "medical man might be the author of such a book without it being considered wrong," he argued, "but it was different for another man to publish such a work amongst all sorts of people."[31] In other words – following the logic of the *Hicklin* test – the fact that *Sexual Inversion* had been issued by a press that was not known for issuing medical works and distributed to readers who had no professional qualifications to study sexual inversion made what might otherwise be an acceptable medical publication a threat to public morals.

Ellis was horrified. *A Note on the Bedborough Trial*, the pamphlet that he published with Weissenfeld after a panicked Bedborough pled guilty to the charges, cries that "if the sale of [*Sexual Inversion*] could be regarded as improper under such circumstances, there were practically no circumstances under which it could be regarded as proper."[32] The application of obscenity law

[27] Sweeney, *At Scotland Yard*, 179. [28] Sweeney, *At Scotland Yard*, 179, 182.
[29] Sweeney, *At Scotland Yard*, 179–182. [30] Sweeney, *At Scotland Yard*, 185.
[31] "Charge against a Publisher: Alleged Improper Books," *Daily News*, June 8, 1898. n.p.
[32] Havelock Ellis, *A Note on the Bedborough Trial* (London: University Press, 1898), 5–6. Add. MS.70524.ff.165–177, BL.

to the distributor of a work like *Sexual Inversion*, Ellis claimed, clearly illustrated that the law needed to be changed in the interest of scientific progress. "The mere expectation of such a prosecution is fatal," he opined. "In submitting to these conditions an author puts his publisher and printer and their agents into an unmerited position of danger; he risks the distortion of his own work while it is in progress; and when he has written a book which is approved by the severest and most competent judges he is tempted to adapt it to the vulgar tastes of the policeman."[33] Like Bradlaugh and Besant in 1877, Ellis suggested that his book's fate was one that might meet any respectable medical work. British medical practitioners did not agree: to the surprise of some of their foreign counterparts, not one major medical figure came out to defend *Sexual Inversion*. In sexual matters, the American physician James Kiernan concluded, "the cant element is stronger in Great Britain than it is in the United States."[34]

Kiernan was right. When it engaged with works on variant sexualities at all, the British medical press was extraordinarily cautious and, their supporters thought, all too eager to find fault with them.[35] In the medical journals that did review *Sexual Inversion* – and many did not – writers frequently objected to its inclusion of literary and historical evidence and the fact that it relied on theories formulated by people who were not medical practitioners, such as the German jurist and self-described *urning* (homosexual) Karl Heinrich Ulrichs. What the medical press took issue with most, though, was Ellis's decision to publish *Sexual Inversion* with the University Press. The *Lancet*'s editors reported that even though the book had "proper claims for discussion" and was written in a "purely dispassionate and scientific style," they decided not to review it because of its "method of publication." Since it was not "published through a house able to take proper measures for introducing it as a scientific book to a scientific audience," the *Lancet* "considered the circumstances attendant on its issue suspicious."[36] "The moral of the story for scientific writers, who must often publish what would be obscene if appearing in doubtful channels or confided to dirty hands, is obvious," the journal concluded. "It is – be careful about the publisher."[37]

It is often suggested that the *Lancet*'s stance illustrates "the conservative and prurient attitude of the official British scientific community in dealing with sexual matters."[38] Homophobia was certainly a major factor in the medical

[33] Ellis, *Note on the Bedborough Trial*, 13.

[34] Quoted in Chiara Beccalossi, *Female Sexual Inversion: Same-Sex Desires in Italian and British Sexology, c. 1870–1920* (Basingstoke: Palgrave Macmillan, 2012), 187.

[35] Beccalossi, *Female Sexual Inversion*, 189. See also Ivan Crozier, "Nineteenth-Century British Psychiatric Writing about Homosexuality before Havelock Ellis: The Missing Story," *Journal of the History of Medicine and Allied Sciences* 63, no. 1 (2008): 63.

[36] "The Question of Indecent Literature," *Lancet*, November 19, 1898,1344.

[37] "The Question," *Lancet*, 1345. [38] Beccalossi, *Female Sexual Inversion*, 186.

response to *Sexual Inversion*. Sympathetic comments in the medical press suggest, however, that while the book's publishing history served the state as a convenient excuse to prosecute Bedborough and throw the Legitimation League into disarray, it genuinely was an impediment to its reception in medical circles. An editorial in the *Journal of Mental Science* argued that Ellis's reputation as a criminal anthropologist offered a "sufficient guarantee" for his motives in writing the book, but scolded, "Mr. Ellis . . . should have exercised more care with regard to the mode of production and sale of his volume."[39] Another supportive writer, for the *British Medical Journal*, noted that Ellis had, at least, not attempted to advertise it or "expose it for sale other than in a technical sense": signs that his heart was in the right place.[40]

In commenting on *Sexual Inversion*'s circumstances of publication and distribution, writers in the medical press were not simply fretting about its potential to fall into the wrong hands. *Fin de siècle* medical practitioners read a constellation of signs surrounding a publication to authorize it as a legitimate contribution to the field, and *Sexual Inversion* did not meet their criteria. *Sexual Inversion*'s use of literary and historical evidence was unconventional, and could be interpreted as pandering to prurient curiosity. The book's unknown publisher was a more urgent warning sign in a field that had embraced increasingly rigid publishing conventions, however, and Ellis knew it. He had sought to place *Sexual Inversion* with an established general publisher that issued medical works as a kind of compromise, hoping that it would be enough to guarantee that medical practitioners would see the book as a credible intervention in the field. That the *Journal of Mental Science* warned other medical writers to issue accounts of sexual inversion carefully, lest they "become part of the stock-in-trade of the pornographic bookseller," highlights an issue that made *Sexual Inversion*'s unknown publisher especially worrisome to medical readers in the 1890s.[41] The pornography trade was an emerging route for traffic in sexual-scientific material, and it was one that the editors of medical journals like the *Lancet* were all too well aware of.

Semi-Scientific Pornography

In early 1897, on the eve of *Sexual Inversion*'s first, unnoticed English publication and just over a year prior to Bedborough's arrest, staff at the *Lancet* had opened a curious package. It had been posted to the journal's London office from Paris, and contained a small book in two volumes, bound in black leather. Both volumes bore the title *Untrodden Fields of Anthropology* in gold writing. The publisher, a Mr. Charles Carrington, described himself as a publisher of

39 Quoted in Beccalossi, *Female Sexual Inversion*, 189.
40 "Charge of Publishing and Selling Obscene Literature," *BMJ*, November 5, 1898, 1466.
41 Quoted in Beccalossi, *Female Sexual Inversion*, 189.

"medical, folk-lore and scientific works," but the title page did not bear the imprint of any publishing house that the *Lancet* staff had heard of. It was a product of an outfit called the Librairie Des Bibliophiles, based in Montmartre, a bohemian district in Paris known for its raucous cabarets.

The *Lancet* published a scathing review of the book on March 6:

> Mr. Charles Carrington is a person who describes himself as a publisher of medical folk-lore and scientific works. We do not know in which category he would place a book which he has had the insolence to forward us for review, bearing the innocent title of "Untrodden Fields of Anthropology." . . . The book, said to be written by a French army surgeon, is solely a record, and a very badly written record, of garbage from the sewers of human nature. It has no scientific importance whatever. It is of no interest to a student of human nature or natural history. We shall be happy to supply the Paris police with Mr. Carrington's address and to hand over the book to Her Majesty's Postmaster-General, so that he may, if he will, take steps to stay the dissemination of such abominations by the agency of his department.[42]

Carrington was used to being accused of purveying indecent material. Selling it had been his business for nearly two years, and he was already well known to British authorities. Born Paul Ferdinando (1867–1921) to a Jewish tradesman in London's East End, Carrington had run a fraudulent stockbroking firm with two of his brothers, George and Frederick, in the late 1880s and early 1890s. In 1895, after his brothers were indicted in Dublin on nine counts of obtaining money on false pretences, he absconded to Paris, adopted the waspy name Charles Carrington, and set up a publishing business. From Paris, he dominated the British market for luxuriously produced books on sexual subjects, issued in English and French in limited editions. Many of his books were printed in Amsterdam and Brussels and then distributed to British readers through the post or by agents in Carrington's employ.[43]

Carrington modelled his business after those of English publisher-booksellers like Edward Avery, Harry Sidney Nichols, Leonard Smithers, and Charles Hirsch. Inspired by private publishing societies set up by wealthy members of the Cannibal Club earlier in the century, these publishers dealt in expensive, luxuriously produced editions of pornographic, queer, and Decadent literature throughout the 1880s, 1890s, and 1900s.[44] Capitalizing on the hazy line between avant-garde and obscene literature, they simultaneously issued open and clandestine catalogues of works for sale. Sexual-scientific works were among the offerings in both. The same edition of the

42 "A Purveyor of Garbage," *Lancet*, March 6, 1897, 681.

43 Collette Colligan, *A Publisher's Paradise: Expatriate Literary Culture in Paris, 1890–1960* (Amherst: University of Massachusetts Press, 2014), 72–73.

44 See Colligan, *A Publisher's Paradise*, and James G. Nelson, *Publisher to the Decadents: Leonard Smithers in the Careers of Beardsley, Wilde, Dowson* (Philadelphia: Pennsylvania State University Press, 2000), for further information about this publishing culture.

German psychiatrist Richard von Krafft-Ebing's landmark study *Psychopathia Sexualis* (1886) that Rebman sold out of his London bookshop was advertised in one of Smithers's openly published catalogues of rare books alongside a luxury edition of Alexander Pope's *The Rape of the Lock* (1712), for instance, and in a clandestine catalogue beside a collection of "Rare Works on Flagellation."[45] Works like *Psychopathia Sexualis* fit in with these publishers' brand of bookselling, which sought to unify the iconoclasm of the avant-garde, the rarefied appeal of the antiquarian, and the thrill of sexual transgression.

Carrington also had overlapping open and clandestine publishing streams.[46] The books that he circulated underground, through mail-order catalogues and behind the counters of shops in Paris and London, were mostly expensive pornographic novels. They included beautifully bound reprints of eighteenth- and early nineteenth-century English narratives, such as the flagellation fantasy *Venus Schoolmistress* (c. 1808); translations and adaptations of French works, such as *The Double Life of Cuthbert Cockerton* (c. 1898), based on Restif de la Bretonne's *L'Anti-Justine* (1798); piracies of new productions issued by Carrington's competitors; and originals, such as *The Memoirs of Dolly Morton* (1899), a racist flagellation fantasy set in the antebellum United States. Carrington's openly published works were usually less explicit, but they still focused on sexual themes, or were strongly associated with sexual scandal. This list included risqué biographies of aristocrats and celebrities, a number of Oscar Wilde's works after his 1895 trial, translations and imitations of a variety of South Asian and Middle Eastern works on sexuality, and sexual-scientific studies.

The sexual-scientific studies that Carrington sold were quite varied. Half a dozen were volumes in an original book series produced in-house by several writers under the name Jacobus X, the pseudonym of the author of a French travel narrative called *L'Amour aux colonies* (1893) originally issued by the Parisian publisher Isidore Liseaux. This work was the basis for *Untrodden Fields of Anthropology*, the first volume in the series (Figure 7.1). *Untrodden Fields* is an odd book: a cross between an anthropological study and an erotic travelogue. Much of the text is not atypical of late Victorian anthropological writing, which could include lengthy descriptions of "native" bodies and sexual practices. However, Jacobus X's repeated descriptions of sex between indigenous men in the French colonies and leering recollections of his own encounters

45 See Leonard Smithers, *Catalogue of Rare and Curious Books*, April 1895 (London: Leonard Smithers & Co., 1895), 3, C.193.b.56, BL and Charles Carrington, *Bibliotheca Arcana: Being a Rough List of Curious, Rare and Uncommon Books* (Paris: Charles Carrington, 1899), 19 in *Album 7: A Collection of Prospectuses and Catalogues of Erotic and Obscene Books, Pictures and Instruments, 1889–1929*. Unpublished scrapbook. Cup. 364.g. 48, BL.

46 For a full list of Carrington's works and reproductions of his catalogues, see Howard Guacamole [pseud.], *Charles Carrington (1867–1921): Bibliographie eines Verlags* (Norderstedt: Ars Amandi in Kommission, 2005).

Documents on Medical Anthropology

UNTRODDEN FIELDS

OF

ANTHROPOLOGY

OBSERVATIONS ON THE ESOTERIC

Manners and Customs of Semi-Civilized Peoples;

BEING A

RECORD OF THIRTY YEARS' EXPERIENCE IN

ASIA, AFRICA, AMERICA and OCEANIA.

By a French Army-Surgeon.

(*IN TWO VOLUMES*)

Vol. I

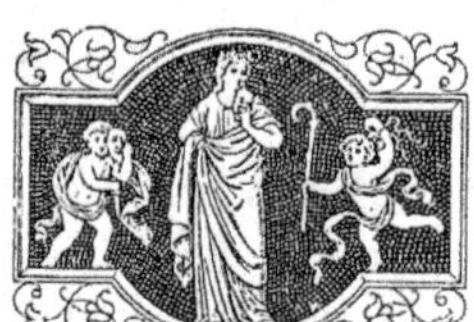

PARIS
Librairie de Médecine, Folklore et Anthropologie
13 Faubourg Montmartre, 13
1898

Figure 7.1 Title page, Jacobus X [pseud.], *Untrodden Fields of Anthropology*, 2nd rev. ed. (Paris: Librairie de Médicine, Folklore, et Anthropologie, 1898). Wellcome Collection, CC BY-NC 4.0.

with indigenous women pushed the envelope even by these standards. Later books in the series were modelled on *Untrodden Fields*'s themes, though not its subject matter. Focused on a variety of supposedly "deviant" sexual practices, these works were cobbled together by drawing on, and in many cases directly translating excerpts from, the work of several Continental sexologists, including Krafft-Ebing and the German psychiatrist Iwan Bloch.[47]

Carrington's broader sexual-scientific catalogue encompassed a spectrum of works, from studies by authors who were widely known and respected in the international scientific community to works whose contributions to scientific debate were questionable in the extreme. He published at least three translations of books by medical authors that the Jacobus X series drew on, including the French physician Charles Samson Féré's *Evolution and Dissolution of the Sexual Instinct* (1904) and the Russian forensic expert Veniamin Mikhaĭlovich Tarnovskiĭ's *The Sexual Instinct and its Morbid Manifestations* (1898). He also sold English and French editions of books written by Krafft-Ebing, Albert von Schrenck-Notzing, Albert Moll, and Magnus Hirschfeld.[48] Yet, his output also included original titles so crude in their descriptions of racialized bodies and sexual violence, and so lacking in anything resembling an argument, that it is difficult to imagine them to be serious scholarship. Carrington's *Flagellation in France: Considered from a Medical and Historical Standpoint* (1898), for instance, is a meandering compilation of anecdotes about beatings in French history, mostly clipped from newspapers, while *Human Gorillas: A Medical, Legal and Historical Study of Rape with Violence* (1901) is a racist mish-mash of reports about sexual assault, bulked up with excerpts from forensic medical studies.[49]

Carrington was clearly interested in exploiting curiosity about racialized bodies and "deviant" – and especially homosexual – sex. The advertisements that he placed in a variety of British newspapers and literary periodicals emphasized this subject matter through thinly coded references. One 1898 newspaper advertisement for *Untrodden Fields*, for instance, tells readers that the work contains "some of the most curious information ever published with relation to sexual matters," and stresses that it makes "special reference" to

47 For more on these titles, see Sarah Bull, "A Purveyor of Garbage? Charles Carrington and the Marketing of Sexual Science in Late-Victorian Britain." *Victorian Review* 38, no. 1 (2012): 69–71.

48 Benjamin Tarnowsky [Veniamin Mikhaĭlovich Tarnovskiĭ], *The Sexual Instinct and Its Morbid Manifestations from the Double Standpoint of Jurisprudence and Psychiatry*, trans. W. C. Costello and Alfred Allinson (Paris: Charles Carrington, 1898); Charles Féré, *Evolution and Dissolution of the Sexual Instinct* (Paris: Charles Carrington, 1904). See Guacamole, *Charles Carrington* for images and transcriptions of sales catalogues that document Carrington's trade in sexual-scientific works that he did not publish.

49 Augustin Cabanès, *Flagellation in France: Considered from a Medical and Historical Standpoint* (Paris: Charles Carrington, 1898); Count Roscaud [pseud?], *Human Gorillas: A Medical, Legal and Historical Study of Rape with Violence* (Paris: Charles Carrington, 1901).

writing by Oscar Wilde, Richard Frances Burton, Cesare Lombroso, Paolo Mantegazza, Krafft-Ebing, and Ellis.[50] These authors were all known to have written about sex between men, or (in Wilde's case) were otherwise associated with it. Carrington promoted the same works in his clandestine sales catalogues, where he framed them in cruder, and sometimes more heterosexual, terms. A description of *Untrodden Fields* in his clandestine catalogue *Forbidden Books* (1902), for instance, declares that a "study of this volume will treat the casual reader as much about the way the women of these countries love and slake their lust as if he had taken a ship and gone out . . . to sample the black and brown lasses."[51]

From the outset, though, Carrington was not solely interested in marketing these works as racy books. He also sought to position himself as a publisher who offered enlightening material on sexual issues for medical practitioners. As the *Lancet*'s response to *Untrodden Fields* suggests, his effort to serve two audiences at once was even less of a success than Ellis's was. Several American medical journals reviewed early books in Carrington's sexual-scientific list, but they found them disappointing. The *Maryland Medical Journal* ventured that *Flagellation in France* was "a curious melange . . . rather amusing and certainly ingenious."[52] The Detroit-based journal *Medicine*, whose editors expressed interest in serious work on flagellation, was harsher, pronouncing *Flagellation in France* "sketchy, discursive, and decidedly 'newspapery'."[53] Carrington's efforts to find a medical audience in Britain were even less fruitful. He claimed to have sent copies of *Untrodden Fields of Anthropology* to six British medical journals in early 1897.[54] The result: one "books received" notice in the *British Medical Journal*, and the review in *The Lancet*.

In the wake of the *Lancet*'s review, Carrington attempted to make *Untrodden Fields* more appealing to scientific practitioners by publishing a second edition designed to convince them of its scholarly merits.[55] He expanded the volumes' physical size, and added a bibliography, an index, an enthusiastic review allegedly written by a physician, and copious footnotes, appendices, and excurses to the original material. Little of the original text was altered, but Carrington changed its tone by cocooning it with the names and words of

50 "Books and Magazines," *Reynolds's Newspaper*, February 27, 1898, 2. For earlier examples, see *Academy*, November 28, 1896, 1282; *Athenaeum*, November 21, 1896, 3604.

51 An Old Bibliophile [Charles Carrington], *Forbidden Books: Notes and Gossip on Tabooed Literature* (Paris: The Author and His Friends [Charles Carrington], 1902), 60.

52 "Flagellation in France," *Maryland Medical Journal* 39 (1898): 541.

53 "Book Reviews: Flagellation in France from a Medical and Historical Standpoint," *Medicine: A Monthly Journal of Medicine and Surgery* 4 (1898): 575.

54 Jacobus X [pseud.], *Untrodden Fields of Anthropology: Observations on the Esoteric Manners and Customs of Semi-Civilized Peoples* [. . .]. (Paris: Librairie de Médecine, Folklore et Anthropologie, 1898), xiii.

55 See Bull, "A Purveyor of Garbage?," 63–67 for a fuller discussion.

influential sexologists, criminologists, anthropologists, and historians, including Krafft-Ebing, Ellis, Symonds, Moll, Ulrichs, Lombroso, and Everard Westermarck. In a new preface, Carrington used these changes to suggest that the book's composition had been more scholarly than it was, glossing over the fact that almost all of the works that his 1898 edition cited were never referred to in *L'Amour aux colonies* or the 1896 *Untrodden Fields*, and that some had not even been published until after both works were issued. This editorial work attests to Carrington's understanding that presentation mattered: scholarly formats and citations spoke to a work's credibility as a scientific intervention. Unfortunately for Carrington, the second edition of *Untrodden Fields* had little hope of success with the mainstream medical community because he was the publisher, and by 1898, Carrington was a pariah in the British medical world.

Carrington had inadvertently made a bad impression on many medical men before he sent his books to medical journals for review. He had started mailing British doctors unsolicited advertising circulars toward the end of 1896, taking the addresses from professional directories.[56] The circulars claimed that his publications were written along "strictly scientific lines," but they also implied that readers might be ashamed of purchasing them. For instance, some of the circulars assured readers that Carrington kept their purchases confidential: "we never publish the names of our subscribers," one said.[57] Such phrases may have been reassuring to Carrington's bread-and-butter customers – collectors of expensive pornography – but they alarmed medical men. A month before it reviewed *Untrodden Fields*, the *Lancet* warned its readers that a "man of filth" calling himself Henri Robert of Paris – one of Carrington's agents, though the *Lancet* suspected that Robert was Carrington himself – had been posting circulars that advertised "pornography . . . of a semi-scientific appearance" to British doctors:

> We know that members of the medical profession are not likely to be attracted by the lubricity of any circular . . . [but] the medical writer might be tempted to purchase the books for other than lewd reasons. Let him not give into temptation. Traffic in these books may not be penal in Paris, but it is penal in England. The man Robert's circulars are posted in England. What is to prevent Robert from communicating to his agents in England the names and addresses of his English clients? On such event blackmail would follow. The recipient of these circulars should send a letter to the Postmaster General and ask his Grace the Duke of Norfolk to earn everyone's gratitude by devising some

[56] PRO HO 45/15139/A59329/2, TNA.

[57] For instance, see *The Genital Laws*, prospectus (Paris: Privately Printed for Students of Psychopathia Sexualis, c. 1900) and *The Genital Laws*, prospectus (Paris: Privately Printed for Students of Anthropology and Private Subscribers, c. 1900) in *Bibliotheca Carringtoniensis*, Part 1 (c. 1896–1906), KIL. "Pornographic Literature," *BMJ*, October 27, 1900, 1269 complains about these specific circulars.

scheme to prevent his Department from being the medium of incentive to vile immorality and even unmentionable crime.[58]

Anxiety about sexual, and especially homosexual, blackmail was rife among medical men in the 1890s. As Angus McLaren has recounted, many believed that the vague language of the Criminal Law Amendment Act, which did not define "gross indecency," made it "an incitement to false accusation."[59] There is no evidence that Carrington had any interest in blackmailing his clients. Nevertheless, his obvious interest in profiting from others' desire to read about sex between men, and his obvious understanding that many readers would not want that desire to become public knowledge, aroused concern in the medical community that his real business was extortion.

Carrington was not the only foreign agent posting circulars advertising sexual-scientific books to British readers. While other publishers and booksellers seem to have escaped suspicions of blackmail, their advertising methods did inspire concern for medicine's reputation. If "obscene quackery" had threatened to undermine the medical profession's claims to authority by unveiling its imbrication in the ethically rocky waters of commercial enterprise, these sellers of sexual-scientific material were thought to undermine medicine's authority through what the *British Medical Journal* called a "masquerade of pornography in the guise of science."[60] This masquerade, medical writers suggested, could involve marketing dubious productions like *Flagellation in France* as medical treatises, using the language of science as cover for selling pornography. However, it could also involve marketing books that had scientific merit in ways that seemed to suggest that they should have their "place in the library of the curious as well as in that of the man of science."[61] Such acts pandered to prurient curiosity about sexual-scientific work and debased it by confounding it with pornography.

The Lancet pressed the Post Office to prevent Carrington from mailing circulars, but stopping him was not easy. The Post Office (Protection) Act of 1884 had given postal authorities license to destroy indecent matter sent through the post. However, they did not have the right to open mail, which made using this power difficult. Postal authorities sometimes opened mail anyway. From 1891, the Home Secretary periodically issued confidential "indecent warrants" which authorized the Postmaster General to seize, open, and document mail going to and from certain, mostly foreign, pornographers.[62]

[58] "A Vile Trade," *Lancet*, February 13, 1897, 468.

[59] Angus McLaren, *Sexual Blackmail: A Modern History* (Cambridge, MA: Harvard University Press, 2002), 18.

[60] Review of *Les eunuques a travers les ages*, by Dr. R. Millant, *BMJ*, April 10, 1909, 905.

[61] Review of *Les eunuques*, *BMJ*, 905.

[62] Colligan, *A Publisher's Paradise*, 36–41; Deana Heath, *Purifying Empire: Obscenity and the Politics of Moral Regulation in Britain, India, and Australia* (Cambridge: Cambridge University Press, 2010), 87–88.

Officials often turned a blind eye to the home-grown trade in expensive pornography. However, they were increasingly preoccupied with cracking down on its entry to the British market from abroad, partly, Jamie Stoops has argued, because this allowed them to frame pornography trafficking as a "foreign problem."[63] The information that the Post Office gathered was used to map pornographers' distribution networks. While their packets were seized and searched, their clients were not tracked. Still, authorities feared scandal if it became known that the government was violating citizens' right to privacy, and so postal surveillance under indecent warrants was a haphazard affair.[64]

Turning postal discoveries into successful prosecutions was also difficult. Police officers arrested Henri Robert in the autumn of 1897, but only by a stroke of luck: Robert had tried to post parcels of pornographic novels by registered mail in Folkstone while he was falling-down drunk.[65] Catching bigger, smarter fish required cooperation with foreign authorities. Unfortunately for British officials, publishers like Carrington based their businesses in France, Belgium, and the Netherlands because obscenity laws applied to a narrower range of material in those countries, and prosecutions for distributing obscene material were generally more difficult to bring.[66] An attempt to prosecute one of Carrington's London-based competitors, Harry Sidney Nichols, on the basis that his new, openly published edition of John Joseph Stockdale's 1821 compilation *Kalogynomia, or The Laws of Female Beauty* was obscene failed in 1900 because Nichols fled to Paris. French authorities refused the British government's request that they arrest Nichols because "the book being apparently in the opinion of the French Police of a medical description, the French Government are, in the absence of some more explicit charge, unable to take any proceedings against Mr. Nichols for the sale of an obscene publication."[67]

In this context, there was little that medical men could do to stop such publishers from doing business, though the *British Medical Journal* and the *Lancet* continued to urge the Postmaster General to stop Carrington's "objectionable circulars" along with those of a "sexual quack" who called himself Dr. Bell.[68] The attempted prosecution of Nichols offered Thomas Bond,

[63] Jamie Stoops, *The Thorny Path: Pornography in Early Twentieth Century Britain* (Montreal: McGill-Queens University Press, 2018), 212. This appears to have been a common strategy. When officials launched a "war on pornography" in Belgium – a major hub of European pornography production – in the 1880s, they focused on preventing its importation from abroad. See Leon Janssens, "Pornography on Rails: Trains and Belgium's "War on Pornography," 1880–1891," *Journal of the History of Sexuality* 32, no. 3 (2023): 269–287.

[64] Colligan, *A Publisher's Paradise*, 30, 40–41. [65] Colligan, *A Publisher's Paradise*, 32.

[66] Colligan, *A Publisher's Paradise*, 20.

[67] Foreign Office to the Marquess of Lansdowne. January 18, 1901. PRO FO 83/2101, TNA.

[68] "The Degradation of the Post-Office," *Lancet*, June 29, 1901, 1843; "Pornographic Literature," *BMJ*, 1269; "The Sexual Quack," *Lancet*, June 16, 1900, 1767.

a surgeon at Westminster Hospital, a rare opportunity to act by serving as an expert witness. Bond pronounced *Kalogynomia* "obscene and ridiculous."[69] Much of the text, he noted, was compiled from works on anatomy and physiology, and rounded out with "voluptuous" discussions of sexual intercourse.[70] Bond found many of the work's statements "incorrect, medically + scientifically," and its plates "disgusting," though he conceded that he would not consider them obscene had they been published in a different book.[71] After he fled the country, of course, Nichols turned the prosecution to his advantage. He now advertised *Kalogynomia* in his clandestine catalogues, where he framed it as a rare collector's item. "This is one of the works . . . which Scotland Yard tried to suppress," Nichols advised readers. "The above described copy is quite perfect, and contains ALL the plates."[72]

Medical men were familiar with the pornography trade's traffic in sexual science in 1897 and 1898. Carrington's books arrived at the offices of medical journals, where their editors looked in askance at their lurid red-and-black title pages. Doctors received his unsolicited circulars at their offices and homes. Some encountered Carrington's advertisements in the periodicals that they perused on Sunday afternoons, and some probably saw sexual-scientific works advertised in his clandestine sales catalogues, crowded together with listings for pornographic novels and photographs. Looking back on Carrington's trade, it is easier to understand why *Sexual Inversion*, with its unknown publisher with unknown motivations, was initially received with such suspicion by British doctors. Ellis and Symonds set themselves a huge challenge in defending same-sex desire as a normal product of human variation during a decade gripped with homophobia. They had increased the challenge by making their argument in a book that did not solely address a medical or a lay audience, but both at once, and by issuing it with a radical publisher. The queer circuits of sexual science's distribution – and the mixed feelings of fear, shame, and desire that they aroused for medical men – magnified these difficulties. In a field that required certainty in the identity of its print culture, *Sexual Inversion* could not be trusted.

Sexual Science and Sexual Ignorance

The circumstances surrounding the Bedborough trial inspire a sense of déjà vu. The state's use of the *Hicklin* definition of obscenity to advance interests that had little to do with concern for readers of *Sexual Inversion* and medics' fears about being damaged by association with an immoral and potentially

69 Metropolitan Police Division, *Examination of Charles Arrow*, 28. PRO CRIM 12/116/ 06/ 04, TNA.

70 *Examination of Charles Arrow*, 22–23.

71 *Examination of Charles Arrow*, 24, 29–30.

72 See no. 34, "Catalogue of Books" in *Album 7*.

extortionate trade are sequels to episodes that we have already visited. The Bedborough trial's portrayal in radical circles and its effect on trade in sexual knowledge also mirror the Knowlton trial and its aftermath in two respects. The right to publish and distribute sex research was immediately framed as a free speech issue in radical communities; and rather than depressing trade in sexual-scientific literature, the controversy around the trial encouraged it. However, the strategies that sexual scientists and their allies developed to distance themselves from damaging associations with disreputable publishers and products, to articulate an identity for sexology, and to justify its existence are worth lingering on, for they differed from strategies examined in the previous chapter in some important ways. Most significantly, they hinged on the promotion of a myth that came to serve as a powerful and remarkably durable rationale for sex research, education, and liberation: the myth of Victorian sexual ignorance.

On Bedborough's arrest, sex radicals hoisted up the banner of free speech. The leftist *Reynolds's Newspaper*, whose editor W. M. Thompson was active in social protest circles, called it a "scandalous" attack on scientific enquiry, while a leading column in the *Adult* cried, "To the Breach, Freemen! . . . An Attack upon the freedom of the press has been made . . . Mr. Bedborough has an unquestionable right to sell such a book."[73] Carrington must not have been able to believe his luck. Free-love advocates were seen as a promising market for sexual material. Throughout 1897, one of Carrington's competitors, Aimé Duringe, had advertised in the *Adult*, placing notices for "books, rare and curious, dealing with subjects not available at English booksellers" by post or in person at his Paris bookshop, which he styled the Cosmos Library.[74] Amid his failing effort to win over medical men, Carrington had started to court the same audience. He sent early volumes in his sexual-scientific catalogue to *Reynolds's Newspaper* for review from 1897, and began to advertise in the *Adult* in February 1898, offering readers discounts.[75] In return, the *Adult* and *Reynolds's Newspaper* published glowing reviews of Carrington's books.

These reviews rapidly came to function as platforms for both periodicals to decry what their editors saw as British sexual conservatism, and, after May 1898, Bedborough's arrest for selling *Sexual Inversion*. A review of Carrington's edition of Tarnovskiĭ's *Sexual Instinct*, published in *Reynolds's Newspaper* in October 1898, for instance, told readers:

> The subject with which this book deals is one of increasing interest. The physicians of other countries have devoted much more study of it than those of our own, yet the

[73] "Booksellers and Erotic Literature: Astounding Revelations," *Reynolds's Newspaper*, June 12, 1898, 3; "To the Breach," *Adult*, July 1898, 159.

[74] See "Cosmos Library," *Adult*, September 1897, 32. For information about Duringe, see Colette Colligan, "Digital Discovery and Fake Imprints: Unmasking Turn-of-the-Century Pornographers in Paris," *Book History* 22, no. 1 (2019): 249–279.

[75] See advertisements in *The Adult*, February 1898, 2; May 1898, 2; October, 1898.

> morbid manifestations of the passions, both from the view of psychiatry and of jurisprudence are becoming of ever-growing importance. The conservative tendencies of our own people are curiously illustrated by the circumstance that a work dealing with similar topics by the distinguished author, Dr. Havelock Ellis, is now the subject of prosecution. We shall learn in a fortnight's time whether or not England is the only country which regards as a crime the investigation of the inclinations of that creature which, we are told, God made in His own image.[76]

Even Carrington's more dubious productions were praised in these venues for shedding light on "suppressed" topics. A paragraph in the *Adult* on his gossipy chronicle of sexual scandals *Curious By-Paths of History* (1898) called it "well worth reading, if only because of the great pains invariably taken to suppress these things."[77] Carrington's second edition of *Untrodden Fields* was celebrated for affording "a long-sought opportunity of noticing practices and customs which interest all mankind, and which 'Society' would not hear mentioned."[78]

Obscenity trials – and reviews like these – sold books. Carrington immediately capitalized on the situation. First, he donated money to the Free Press Defence Committee, a group set up to fund Bedborough's defence at trial.[79] Then he began to re-use excerpts from the reviews in advertisements, even as he set about expanding his sexual-scientific catalogue at a rapid clip. He reprinted part of *Reynolds's* review of Tarnovskiĭ's *Sexual Instinct*, for example, in a circular appended to the back of pages of his 1899 volume in the Jacobus X series, *The Ethnology of the Six Sense*, using it to align both works with *Sexual Inversion* and frame himself as a "defender of truth."[80] Carrington thus neatly associated new productions, including blatant piracies and dubious compilations, with the works of authors who had gained respect in the international scientific community. He represented himself and his books as defenders of free speech in sexual matters, even as he banked on their appeal as containers of "forbidden" knowledge.

Weissenfeld also expanded his trade in sexual-scientific literature.[81] Over the next four years, he sold translations of Continental sexology issued by Rebman, Walter Scott, and Carrington in London and the surrounding area; published his own translations of books by Féré and Joanny Roux; and issued

[76] "Books Received: *The Sexual Instinct*," *Reynolds's Newspaper*, October 16, 1898, 2.

[77] "Books Received: *Curious By-Paths of History*," *Adult*, April 1898, 88–89.

[78] "Books Received: *Untrodden Fields of Anthropology*," *Adult*, September 1898, 250–252.

[79] "The Free Press Defence Committee: The Bedborough Case Balance Sheet" ([London?]: The Executive of the Free Press Defence Committee, 1899), 4.

[80] "List of Mr. Carrington's New and Forthcoming Works in English and French," 425, appended to Jacobus X [pseud.], *The Ethnology of the Six Sense* (Paris: Charles Carrington, 1899), CUP.364.c.92, BL.

[81] For a fuller account of Weissenfeld's publishing activities, see Ross Brooks, "Bad Sexology: The Scientific Publications of the University Press (Watford and London), 1897–1901," *Social History of Medicine* 36, no. 4 (2023): 615-641.

a new edition of *Sexual Inversion* allegedly printed in Leipzig. He also issued several home-grown productions, such as Walter Gallichan's *Chapters on Human Love* (1898), that aimed to popularize ideas in Continental sexology. Like Carrington's, Weissenfeld's marketing for this material heavily emphasized its "suppressed" status. The first page of his 1901 *Catalogue of Scientific Works on the Psychology and Pathology of Sex* features the headline "The Corruption of the Morals of Her Majesty's Subjects." Below this headline, Weissenfeld published a dramatic account of a police raid on his home in Watford, where, he reported, copies of Gallichan's *Chapters* and volumes in Ellis's *Psychology of Sex* series were seized and carted away. "The Bench ... ordered THE DESTRUCTION BY FIRE of indicted books," the account finishes. Weissenfeld framed his books as martyrs for free speech, sanctified in fires lit by "prudes on the prowl."[82]

Rebman issued increasing numbers of sexual-scientific publications too, though the Bedborough trial does seem to have concerned him. The preface to his tenth edition of Krafft-Ebing's *Psychopathia Sexualis*, published a year after the Bedborough trial, is appended with a notice that advises readers that the "sale of this book is rigidly restricted to members of the medical and legal professions."[83] There is evidence that some booksellers restricted sales of *Psychopathia Sexualis* and other sexual-scientific works for decades after the Bedborough trial. However, as Phillip Kuhn has argued, it is doubtful that they were restricted as much as this disclaimer suggests: reportedly, Rebman's 1899 edition of *Psychopathia Sexualis* sold in large numbers.[84]

Did Rebman advertise restrictions on the work because he worried that he might be prosecuted for selling it? Or did he want to perform respectability for his medical customers in the wake of the Bedborough trial? If the former, his fears were eventually realized: in 1909, following a complaint lodged at the Home Office, the police seized copies of Rebman's 1908 English edition of Iwan Bloch's *Das Sexualleben unserer Zeit in seinen Beziehungen zur modernen Kultur* (1906), *The Sexual Life of our Time in its Relations to Modern Civilization*, which was framed as a comprehensive encyclopedia of the sexual sciences. In the end, the magistrate ordered the books impounded rather than destroyed as he agreed that Bloch's work was scientific, and Rebman resumed selling them three months later. Kuhn speculates that Rebman and the Home Office cut a deal: if Bloch's book carried a disclaimer, Rebman could sell it. "It

82 *A Catalogue of Scientific Works on the Psychology and Pathology of Sex* (London: University Press, c. 1901), 258776 f.4, Bodleian Library.

83 Richard von Krafft-Ebing, *Psychopathia Sexualis, with Especial Reference to Contrary Sexual Instinct: A Medico-Legal Study*, trans. Charles Gilbert Chaddock [1892] (London: F. J. Rebman, 1899), unpaginated publisher's preface.

84 Kuhn, "Sexual Life," 48.

must be clearly understood that this is a work belonging to the category of 'adult literature'," the preface of a new edition states.[85]

Kuhn argues that Rebman found himself in this situation because sex research had gained more acceptance by 1909.[86] Medical journals reviewed sexual-scientific studies more regularly and generously. Prior to the police raid, Rebman had dropped disclaimers from his translations of Continental studies, and was advertising them in mainstream periodicals. His translation of Bloch's book had been favourably reviewed in a variety of British newspapers in 1908.[87] The fact that a complaint was lodged against the book was less a sign that efforts to make sexology respectable had failed than it was a sign of their mounting success: sex research now enjoyed the kind of visibility that made a complaint to the Home Office possible in the first place. Some of this acceptance was probably linked to the outcry against the Bedborough trial, in which foreign scientists joined British social protestors in arguing that the trial was an attack on free speech and scientific progress. However, as Fisher and Funke have shown, sexologists and their allies were also working to cultivate acceptance through a more complex version of that argument, one that relied on two claims to authorize sexology as a scientific field and distance it from associations that threatened it. One of these claims was that sexual expression and discussion were "natural" and "healthy." The other was that both had been suppressed, and that their suppression had destroyed people's natural relationship with sex.[88]

Aspects of this argument can be traced all the way back to Richard Carlile, who opined that sex was "natural, wholesome, and clean" and that religious opposition to non-marital sex was a "perverted" form of vice, but it evolved alongside free-speech arguments for sexual causes from the 1880s and was further elaborated by sex reformers and sexual scientists after 1898.[89] Havelock Ellis's 1922 essay "The Revaluation of Obscenity" is emblematic of the argument in its fully fledged form. In the essay, Ellis pleads with readers to cast off outmoded ideas about the dangers of frank sexual discussion and abolish laws that would impede it for their own good. Although obscenity was defined in British law as that which had the tendency to deprave and corrupt,

85 Kuhn, "Sexual Life," 50–54. Considering their earlier attitude toward defences of sexual content in medical books, it is interesting that medical reviewers seem to have approved of disclaimers in this context. See "Sexual Psychology," *BMJ*, April 10, 1909, 904.

86 Kuhn, "Sexual Life," 54. 87 Kuhn, "Sexual Life," 49–50.

88 Fisher and Funke, "Are We to Treat," 85–91.

89 Quoted in M. L. Bush, *What Is Love? Richard Carlile's Philosophy of Sex* (London: Verso, 1998), 19; Fisher and Funke, "Are We to Treat," 90. Writers of modernist literature, whose circles overlapped with Ellis's, made a version of the same argument to justify sexual details in literary works. For instance, see D. H. Lawrence, *Pornography and Obscenity* (London: Faber and Faber, 1929); Virginia Woolf, "The Censorship of Books," *Nineteenth Century and After* 105 (1929): 446–447; E. M. Forster, "The Censorship of Books," *Nineteenth Century and After* 105 (1929): 444–445.

Ellis argues that most works labelled obscene merely expressed "the naturalistic aspect of sexual processes."[90] Framing obscenity as a permanent element in human life across all cultures and classes, Ellis maintains that it presented no danger to its viewers. Indeed, for Ellis, obscenity was a beautifully "open and wholesome" mode of expression.[91]

Spinning a kind of narrative that Michel Foucault would parody half a century later in his foundational *History of Sexuality*, Ellis then argues that while obscenity circulated freely in England during the early modern period – the "Golden Age of British history" – and remained a feature of "primitive" societies, "Victorianism" stole it from his own society by depriving sexual representations of "all naturalistic character" and bathing them in "a vague and frequently quite impenetrable mist."[92] Victorian censorship, Ellis suggests in this essay, and other sexologists argued elsewhere, fostered fear and ignorance of sex. Yet, it was sexual ignorance that presented the real danger to society: sexual ignorance led people away from their natural relationship with sexuality, leading to "years of heartache and blind questioning," and even "abnormal" sexual behaviour.[93]

Even as sexologists and their allies defended sex and its "obscene" expression in art, literature, and science as "natural," they decried the existence, and even advocated the suppression, of pornography – a media form that they rarely attempted to define but chronically cast as inaccurate, immoral, and, most of all, "unnatural."[94] This side of the argument elaborated on hostile stances that many sex radicals, from Carlile on, had taken toward sexual entertainment, and "The Revaluation of Obscenity," again, offers a pretty good illustration of it. In the essay, Ellis goes to pains to distinguish "naturalistic" obscenity from pornography through an extended anecdote about a book that he purchased on holiday in Seville, which he claims to have found "pathetically crude and unpleasant," a "vulgar, disgusting, and stupid" piece of work.[95] According to Ellis, it was the suppression of naturalistic forms of sexual expression that made such works "attractive and profitable": in the absence of censorship, interest in pornography would disappear.[96] As H. G. Cocks has shown, some sex reformers went further than Ellis, advocating the destruction of pornography on the grounds that it was "unhealthy."[97]

90 Havelock Ellis, "The Revaluation of Obscenity," in *On Life and Sex*, ed. Havelock Ellis (London: W.M. Heinemann, 1948), 207.

91 Ellis, "Revaluation of Obscenity," 212.

92 Michel Foucault, *The History of Sexuality. Volume 1: An Introduction*, trans. Robert Hurley (1978; repr., New York: Random House, 1990), 3–5; Ellis, "Revaluation of Obscenity," 206, 209, 216.

93 Fisher and Funke, "Are We to Treat," 90–91.

94 Cocks, "Saucy Stories," 472–473.

95 Ellis, "Revaluation of Obscenity," 224.

96 Ellis, "Revaluation of Obscenity," 221–223.

97 Cocks, "Saucy Stories," 474.

Decrying the censorship of "naturalistic" sexual discussion on the grounds that it led to sexual ignorance and condemning pornography as an "unnatural" perversion of wholesome sexual expression enabled sexologists and their allies to accomplish two things. First, as Fisher and Funke emphasize, it made the case for their own work. According to this narrative, Victorian censorship had damaged personal well-being and public morality by making people ignorant of sex. Sex researchers could heroically repair the damage by bringing the truth of sex "into the pure air" of the dawning twentieth century.[98] At the same time, by identifying pornography as a grotesque product of their grandparents' era, sexologists bounded sexual knowledge, distancing their literature from a media form that often met with disgust at a time when sexual science and sexual entertainment continued to overlap in the book trade. Through the first half of the twentieth century, booksellers continued to sell sexual-scientific literature by Ellis, Bloch, and others alongside pornographic, pulp, and fetish material, and publishers increasingly incorporated sexual-scientific language into this material to justify its existence and try to circumvent censorship themselves.[99] The argument outlined here repudiated this troublesome boundary-blurring.

It was a neat argument. However, it was not without its contradictions. One contradiction, which Fisher and Funke explore in more detail, was that it was founded on the idea "that natural sexual impulses needed guiding, since the sexual instinct was a volatile and changeable force that could easily be influenced and even corrupted by external influences."[100] This idea justified sex research and the circulation of its findings beyond scientific communities. However, it also led sexologists to become censors themselves. Sexual knowledge, they agreed, was a powerful thing. It needed to reach the right readers in the right ways, lest their natural instincts be led astray. Even as some sexologists complained that their works had limited circulation in public libraries and called for reforms to the law so that they might write and publish without fear of restriction, they not only supported restrictions on trade in sexual entertainment but also restricted access to sexual-scientific knowledge. In addition to censoring their own writing (Ellis, for example, admitted to omitting "any crude + repellent details which did not seem . . . necessary to the comprehension of the matter at hand" in his publications), sexual-scientific authors embraced the kinds of disclaimers that Rebman had appended to Krafft-Ebing's *Scientia Sexualis*, underscoring that their publications were intended for professional or adult readers only.[101] Organizers restricted admission to events like the 1929 World Congress of the International Society for Sex Research, where delegates delivered

98 Havelock Ellis to Bronislaw Malinowski, December 26, 1923, MALINOWSKI 29/4, LSE.

99 Cocks, "Saucy Stories," 475–481.

100 Fisher and Funke, "Are We to Treat," 81.

101 Havelock Ellis to Bronislaw Malinowski, January 10, 1924, MALINOWSKI 29/4, LSE; Fisher and Funke, "Are We to Treat," 95.

impassioned speeches against the scourge of censorship, to "serious students of this field of science."[102]

This argument also elided sexology's debts to pornography. The most dangerous aspects of sexology for its image as a scientific field lay with its reliance on social networks and ways of knowing that could raise questions about its objectivity, its motivations, its identity as science. Pornographers' relationship with sexual science was more complicated than the editors of the *Lancet* assumed. As I suggested earlier, the pornography trade played a role in sexology's development by circulating its literature. By bringing sexual-scientific books across borders, pornographers enabled exchanges between sex researchers, and even introduced new works into the sexological canon. Havelock Ellis, Iwan Bloch, Albert Moll, Ferdinand Karsch-Haack, and Georg Merzbach all cited editions of studies published by Carrington, including volumes in his Jacobus X series, which they took far more seriously than the *Lancet*'s editors.[103] More problematically for sexology's image, however, early sexologists also engaged with pulp and pornographic literary works to various degrees as they sought out new sources of insight into the workings of sexual nature. This engagement brought sexual-scientific and pornographic print cultures closer together, and in some cases collapsed distinctions between them altogether. While their vague use of the terms meant that they were open to interpretation, the distinctions between "obscenity" and "pornography" that figures like Ellis made in their public writing were rather misleading.

Erotic literature's influence on early sexology seems to be related to its practitioners' interest in adapting methods used in earlier antiquarian and anthropological studies of ancient and foreign sexuality, and is clearest in Continental sexology.[104] Scholarship on erotic literature and sex research overlapped in the practices of figures like Paul Englisch, who wrote

[102] Quoted in Fisher and Funke, "Are We to Treat," 95.

[103] Ferdinand Karsch-Haack, *Das gleichgeschlechtliche Leben der Naturvölker* (München: E. Reinhardt, 1911), 551, 632, 682; Georg Merzbach, *Die krankhaften Erscheinungen des Geschlechtssinnes* (Wien: Hölder, 1909), 461. Iwan Bloch, *Das Sexualleben unserer Zeit in seinen Beziehungen zur modernen Kultur* (Berlin: L. Marcus, 1919), 644; Albert Moll, *Das Sexualleben des Kindes* (Leipzig: Vogel, 1908), 135; Havelock Ellis, *Studies in the Psychology of Sex: The Sexual Impulse* (Philadelphia, PA: F.A. Davis, 1904), 38, 83–84. These works may have been purchased through third-party dealers, as suggested in Havelock Ellis to Edward Carpenter, November 12, 1916, ADD MS 70536, BL.

[104] There are striking overlaps between methods and perspectives that sexual scientists brought to working with pornographic literature and bibliography (a field with roots in antiquarianism) and the methods and perspectives that they brought to working with erotic artefacts, building on earlier work by antiquarians and, later, anthropologists. See Jana Funke, Kate Fisher, Jen Grove, and Rebecca Langlands, "Illustrating Phallic Worship: Uses of Material Objects and the Production of Sexual Knowledge in Eighteenth-Century Antiquarianism and Early Twentieth-Century Sexual Science," *Word & Image* 33, no. 3 (2017): 324–337 and Helen Wickstead, "Sex in the Secret Museum: Photographs from the British Museum's Witt Scrapbooks," *Photography and Culture* 11, no. 3 (2018): 351–366.

a substantial history of erotic literature in the 1930s, and Iwan Bloch, the discoverer of the Marquis de Sade's lost novel *Les 120 journées de Sodome* (*The 120 Days of Sodom*).[105] A number of sexologists also drew directly on pulp and pornographic representations of sexual behaviour and desire to formulate theories about sexual perversions. Krafft-Ebing famously drew on the writings of Sade and Leopold von Sacher-Masoch, author of the explicit novel *Venus im Pelz* (*Venus in Furs*) (1870), to frame the pathologies of sadism and masochism, for instance, while the French psychologist Alfred Binet cited Jules Amédée Barbey d'Aurevilly's erotically charged novels *Les diaboliques* (*The She-Devils*) (1874) and *Une vieille maîtresse* (*An Old Mistress*) (1851) in his study *Le fétichisme dans l'amour* (*Fetishism in Love*) (1897).[106]

As Birgit Lang has emphasized, these researchers' understandings of how literary representations of desire functioned as evidence of sexual phenomena differed, and changed over time.[107] Krafft-Ebing initially recognized his patients' identification with literary characters and scenes, but only gradually came to believe that they reflected real-life desires.[108] Binet had no trouble seeing literature as a source of insight into human sexuality, but felt the need to establish the accuracy of its representations, and would question authors about the basis of their descriptions.[109] Bloch took the concept of the literary author as observer of sexual nature further still, arguing that sexually explicit literature could be a form of sexual science in its own right. His prime example was Sade's work: in Bloch's view, Sade's attempt to catalogue sexual perversions in *Les 120 journées de Sodome* made him a pioneering "Sexualphilosoph" (sexual philosopher).[110]

During a period in which bibliographers were framing bibliography as a science – one that, like botany or anthropology, relied on specialized knowledge and involved systematic observation and classification – bibliographies could also be thought of as sexual-scientific studies.[111] Bloch's belief that bibliographies of erotic books like those of the British collector Henry Spencer Ashbee recorded observations of sexual culture led him to transform a work of bibliography that was a fixture of the pornography trade into a work of sexual science, subsuming it into

[105] Sarah L. Leonard, "Pornography and Obscenity," in *Palgrave Advances in the Modern History of Sexuality*, ed. H. G. Cocks and Matt Houlbrook (Basingstoke: Palgrave Macmillan, 2006), 184; Neil Schaeffer, *The Marquis de Sade: A Life* (Cambridge, MA: Harvard University Press, 1999), 383.

[106] Anna Katherina Schaffner, "Fiction as Evidence: On the Uses of Literature in Nineteenth-Century Sexological Discourse," *Comparative Literature Studies* 48, no. 2 (2011): 165.

[107] Schaffner, "'Fiction as Evidence,'" 169–182; Birgit Lang, "The Shifting Case of Masochism: Leopold von Sacher-Masoch's *Venus im Pelz* (1870)," in *A History of the Case Study: Sexology, Psychoanalysis, Literature*, ed. Birgit Lang, Joy Damousi, and Alison Lewis (Manchester: Manchester University Press, 2017), 23–26.

[108] Lang, "Shifting Case," 23–26. [109] Schaffner, "Fiction as Evidence," 169–175, 190.

[110] Schaffner, "Fiction as Evidence," 190.

[111] Thomas G. Tanselle, "Bibliography and Science," *Studies in Bibliography* 27 (1974): 55–89.

the discipline. His three-volume study *Das Geschlechtsleben in England* (*Sexual Life in England*) (1901–3), published under the pseudonym Eugène Dühren, drew heavily on Ashbee's three bibliographies, *Index Librorum Prohibitorum* (1877), *Centuria Librorum Absconditorum* (1879), and *Catena Librorum Tacendorum* (1885), which contain lengthy excerpts from Ashbee's gossipy, opinion-filled commentary on a wide range of pornographic productions. Ashbee's name never appears in *Das Geschlechtsleben in England.* Bloch promised that he would only cite Ashbee using the pseudonym that he used to publish the bibliographies, Pisanus Fraxi.[112] However, Ashbee's pseudonym, his readings of erotic literature, and his views about what it reveals about human sexuality dominate the study.

In addition to citing Ashbee as an authority on subjects ranging from the idea that "passive flagellation plays a great part as a simple preliminary to intercourse" in England to the notion that the pornographic novel *Letters from Laura and Eveline* (1883) provides a valuable illustration of sex between "hermaphrodites," Bloch paraphrases from the bibliographies at length. Even the theoretical basis for Bloch's study – that impressions of a foreign sexual culture "may best be tested for correctness by examining its most blatant expression in erotic literature" – seems to be modelled on Ashbee's justification for compiling his bibliographies:[113]

> Erotic Novels... "hold the mirror up to nature" more certainly than do those of any other description ... [T]heir authors have, in most instances, been eyewitnesses of the scenes they have described ... themselves enacted, in part, what they have portrayed. Immoral and amatory fiction ... must unfortunately be acknowledged to contain ... a reflection of the manners and vices of the times – of vices to be avoided, guarded against, reformed, but which unquestionably exist, and of which an exact estimate is needful to enable us to cope with them.[114]

As Heike Bauer has shown, sexologists frequently translated and adapted sexual-scientific studies for new audiences and new cultural contexts.[115] In this light, *Das Geschlechtsleben in England* can be thought of as a translation,

[112] Ian Gibson, *The Erotomaniac: The Secret Life of Henry Spencer Ashbee* (Boston, MA: Da Capo, 2001), 141. For another letter between Ashbee and Bloch, see Iwan Bloch to Henry Spencer Ashbee, July 20, 1900, Bloch Collection, Magnus-Hirschfeld-Gesellschaft.

[113] Iwan Bloch, *Sexual Life in England, Past and Present*, trans. W. H. Forstern (London: Francis Aldor, 1938), 499. The untranslated passage reads: "Dieses allgemeine Urteil über die Bedeutung des Erotischen in der Poesie und Prosa der Völker lässt sich auf seine Richtigkeit am besten prüfen, wenn man den krassesten Ausdruck des Erotischen, wie er in der sogenannten „erotischen" Litteratur im engeren Sinne sichtbar wird." Eugène Dühren, *Das Geschlechtsleben in England, mit besonderer Beziehung auf London*, vol. 4 (Berlin: M. Lilienthal, 1903), 320.

[114] Pisanus Fraxi [Henry Spencer Ashbee], *Catena Librorum Prohibitorum: Bio-Biblio-Iconographical and Critical Notes on Curious, Uncommon, and Erotic Books* (London: Privately Printed, 1885), xxxv–li.

[115] Heike Bauer, *English Literary Sexology: Translations of Inversion, 1860–1930* (Basingstoke: Palgrave Macmillan, 2009), 15–16.

one that not only renders parts of Ashbee's English bibliographies into German but also reinscribes erotic bibliography as sexual science.

It is more difficult to trace pornography's influence on British sex research. Overt engagements with pornography as source material were absent here; yet, some sexologists do seem to have been interested in its potential as source material. Ellis – the self-professed hater of pornographic novels – collected erotic artwork, and reportedly "cheap sado-masochistic semi-pornography of the kind published in Paris by the [erotic book publisher] 'Select Bibliothèque'."[116] Like Bloch and Englisch, Ellis was also deeply familiar with bibliographies of erotic literature, including Ashbee's works (which he viewed at the British Museum Library); Guillaume Apollinaire, Fernand Fleuret, and Louis Perceau's *L'Enfer de la Bibliothèque nationale* (1913); and Hugo Hayn and Alfred Gotendorf's eight-volume *Bibliotheca Germanorum Erotica et Curiosa* (1912–14).[117] His familiarity with these bibliographies was well known to his colleagues: those interested in translating or reprinting them, or in writing their own, approached him for assistance.[118]

Yet, Ellis was loath to make his interest in erotic material public. He refused an invitation from the anthropologist Bronislaw Malinowski to write the introduction to the bibliographer Alfred Rose's bibliography of erotic books *Registrum Librorum Eroticorum* (1936), even though Malinowski was convinced that the work had great "importance for the students of the psychology of sex" and felt he would agree.[119] And he was incredibly defensive about his collection of erotic artwork, even in private correspondence. In 1936, Ellis wrote to the binder Mills Whitman, asking Whitman to prepare some books from his collection for sale. At the outset, he warned Whitman that he might find one of them "rather alarming! I have for years possessed, in ten parts, a famous work which is no doubt the best collection of erotic works of art there is – copies of paintings, drawings, etc. by famous artists." Then he added, "a serious work of course, not 'pornographic' or I would not possess it. But from the police & magisterial point of view it is definitely 'obscene'."[120]

Ellis's decision to underline the word "serious" in this private letter, straining to distance himself on the page from that which might call his credibility into question, is an apt metonym for the trajectory of the history that this chapter,

116 Gershon Legman, "The Lure of the Forbidden," in *Libraries, Erotica, and Pornography*, ed. Martha Cornog (Phoenix, AZ: Oryx Press, 1991), 55.

117 Patrick Kearney, *The Private Case: An Annotated Bibliography of the Private Case Erotica Collection in the British (Museum) Library* (London: J. Landesman, 1989), 356–357.

118 Havelock Ellis, Letter to Montague Summers, December 28, 1926, typescript insert in Kearney, *The Private Case*, 356 in RAR 808.803, BL.

119 Bronislaw Malinowski to Havelock Ellis, May 8, 1934, MS, Archives and Manuscripts, ADD MS 70539, BL.

120 Havelock Ellis to Mills Whitman, August 8, [19]36, WMS 4, MS 8106/55, WL.

and this book, has traced. The nineteenth century witnessed the consolidation of new businesses, movements, and institutions that claimed authority over sexual knowledge. Their agents were united in their representation of sexual knowledge as something that they had, and that other people lacked. Where they departed was in their beliefs about how that knowledge should be used, not least by those who put it into circulation. Above all, regular medical practitioners, sex reformers, and sexual scientists desired to be taken seriously during an era in which rationality and restraint were prized. They wanted to be – and to be seen as – agents who were working for the common good, above the profit-making and pleasure-seeking that their sometime competitors, sometime collaborators openly embraced. Through the precarious narratives that they created to frame sexual knowledge, and claim it for themselves, sexual knowledge's production and distribution were situated as enterprises of vital social importance, *serious* enterprises untainted by the pleasures of desire and the messy, morally compromised affinities of the market.

Conclusion

Victorian Ignorance

This book has focused on the sellers of sexual knowledge. By examining their activities, hopes, and anxieties, I have aimed to bring into focus challenges that agents across the political spectrum encountered as they sought to sell sexual knowledge in print. *Selling Sexual Knowledge* has shown that print was, and was understood to be, crucial to circulating knowledge, advancing causes, consolidating collective identities, and establishing moral and epistemic authority. It has also illustrated how difficult would-be authorities in sexual matters could find exploiting these affordances of print in a context in which it could always be co-opted, recast, and misunderstood. And it has charted how they sought to remedy problems they encountered by managing print and interpretation. By way of conclusion, I want to turn to a figure that has haunted this book but rarely been the focus of its attention: the reader. More accurately, I want to more closely consider the meaning of the history this book has traced for readers of two kinds. One is the Victorian reader: the kind of non-expert reader who would have seen, bought, read, lent, borrowed, hidden, thrown out, or ignored works mentioned in *Selling Sexual Knowledge*, from *The Secrets of Nature Revealed* to *Sexual Inversion*. The other is the kind of reader that this book is intended for: the scholarly reader trying to make sense of the past by sifting through its remains.

It was my interest in what and how ordinary Victorians read to learn about sex that led me to the research that informs this book. That such readers' stories ended up appearing in it infrequently is partly a result of the challenges of finding them. Reading is a process that is often internal and always ephemeral. Evidence of reading experiences – like evidence of sexual acts – is hard to locate, and difficult to interpret.[1] This is true even of accounts in letters, diaries, and autobiographies, which frequently record acts of reading decades after the fact, and do not document reading experiences evenly. There are far fewer accounts of reading about sex from the Victorian period than there are accounts

[1] See, respectively, Robert Darnton, "First Steps toward a History of Reading," *Australian Journal of French Studies* 51, no. 2/3 (2014): 152–177 and Valerie Traub, *Thinking Sex with the Early Moderns* (Philadelphia: University of Pennsylvania Press, 2015).

of reading Shakespeare.[2] Indeed, scholars had discovered so few by the early 2000s that Jonathan Rose, an indefatigable historian of reading, concluded that the circulation of sexual information in cheap print must have been very constricted.[3] Early twentieth-century accounts from readers looking back on the Victorian period are more plentiful, but most do little to trouble this view: they invariably focus on their authors' confusion about sex, recalling the Victorian era as an era of extreme sexual ignorance.[4]

These elements of the historical record would seem to contradict the picture that *Selling Sexual Knowledge* has painted of the Victorian print world: a world in which the constant, unruly circulation of information about sex and reproduction was a source of great anxiety for groups working hard to establish themselves as authorities in these matters. Here, I want to consider that picture in relation to readers' claims about sexual ignorance, claims that also flowed from the pens of sexologists in the last chapter of the book. To do so, I will draw on the work of Kate Fisher, whose notion of an "epistemology of sexual ignorance" is enormously helpful for understanding of how a period that witnessed massive expansions in the production and circulation of works on sexual matters could have been remembered for so long and by so many for its dearth of sexual understanding.[5] This will enable me to offer a deeper reflection about what the changing print culture that *Selling Sexual Knowledge* has examined meant for Victorian readers. It will also offer me an opportunity to say a few words about the larger significance of the book's argument for scholarly readers.

Fisher argues that claims about sexual ignorance are a modern phenomenon that have less to do with what or how much people know about sex than they have to do with how sexual knowledge is constructed. To "conceptualize knowledge of sex and reproduction as requiring a journey out of ignorance derives from a distinctly modern understanding" of sexual knowledge, Fisher writes, an understanding that only makes sense "once an emphasis on core facts has replaced a premodern view of knowledge as a pluralistic mix of natural wisdom, bodily awareness, scholarly learning, lore and experience."[6] When "sexual knowledge" came to mean "biological facts," sexual ignorance became

2 For a repository of traces of reading experience, see UK RED: Reading Experience Database, Open University. Accessed August 26, 2023, www.open.ac.uk/Arts/reading/UK/.

3 Jonathan Rose, *The Intellectual Life of the British Working Classes*, 2nd ed. (New Haven, CT: Yale University Press, 2010), 207.

4 Rose, *Intellectual Life*, 209–211. See also Kate Flint, *The Woman Reader, 1837–1914* (Oxford: Clarendon, 1995), 214–218 and Lisa Z. Sigel, *Making Modern Love: Sexual Narratives and Identities in Interwar Britain* (Philadelphia, PA: Temple University Press, 2012), 45.

5 Kate Fisher, "Modern Ignorance" in *Reproduction: Antiquity to the Present*, ed. Nick Hopwood, Rebecca Fleming, and Lauren Kassell (Cambridge: Cambridge University Press, 2018), 471–472.

6 Fisher, "Modern Ignorance," 471–472.

a natural state. From the late eighteenth century, to become knowledgeable about sex meant acquiring empirical information. One needed to scrutinize a model or a specimen in a museum; consult with an expert; or read a book written by an expert to *know* about sex, even – as anatomical museum owners' entreaty to visitors, "Know Thyself!" suggests – to understand one's own body and desire.

Opportunities for learning about sex in this way were everywhere during the Victorian period: works that addressed reproduction and sexual health were cheap, plentiful, and visible. And yet, it is not difficult to imagine that the kind of print culture described in this book would only have made many people feel more ignorant.[7] We should consider that medical works typically demanded prior knowledge that people did not always possess. Significantly, most accounts of reading about sex during the Victorian period are accounts of *first* experiences, the experiences of children or teenagers who had not experimented much sexually.[8] As we have seen, however, the vast majority of medical titles in circulation assumed sexual experience. They aimed to enlighten grown-up, sexually active readers about the physiology of reproduction, the symptoms of venereal disease, means by which pregnancy might be prevented, or the nature of desire. They did not usually explain what heterosexual, let alone homosexual, sexual acts were, how they were performed, or exactly how they related to pregnancy or venereal disease. It was only in the last decades of the century that those who claimed authority in sexual matters began to consider such knowledge "scientific" and necessary to offer to the public in print. In this context, it is little wonder that Victorian accounts of youthful reading speak so often of confusion.

Many medical works also used terms that were not universally understood. Alan Clark, the son of Bolton textile workers, found language and diagrams in the medical textbooks that he perused at the public library "incomprehensible."[9] I have argued that the increasing specialization of the language in such works made experiences like Clark's more and more likely. However, it is not clear that many works aimed at popular audiences would have been much more understandable to working-class readers, particularly in the early decades of the Victorian period, when they were routinely made by cutting and pasting parts of more specialized publications. Even medical terms in Holywell Street catalogues could confuse, as marginalia translating "labia" to "cunt" suggests.[10] And although middle-class men

7 Fisher surveys some of these effects in broader terms than I do here, covering a longer period, in "Modern Ignorance," 480–483.

8 Rose, *Intellectual Life*, 207–211; Flint, *The Woman Reader*, 214–218.

9 Rose, *Intellectual Life*, 210.

10 *A Select Catalogue of Books, Facetious and Amorous* ([London]: s.n., n.d.), DA 676, box 6, item 51, MSCE. This may explain the popularity of *Aristotle's Masterpiece*, a work that addressed procreation in older and probably more accessible terms.

like George Bedborough easily deciphered terms increasingly used in advertising, such as "curious," "from life," and "skin diseases," as Fisher points out, such euphemisms could bewilder the uninitiated.[11] Medical works on sexual matters were cheap and plentiful, and information about how to acquire them was everywhere. Yet, purchasing them and understanding what they contained both required specific kinds of literacy.

The ways these works were framed is equally, if not more, significant. Like making sexual-scientific authority, the narrower activity of selling information about sex and reproduction necessarily involved producing ignorance. Sellers of sexual knowledge interpolated readers with very different levels of interpretive agency. However, as I emphasized at the end of the last chapter, they all portrayed sexual knowledge as something that they had and that others lacked. This framing played a major role in the promotion of popular medical works during the first decades of the Victorian period. Pornographers framed such works as containers of "secret" knowledge, even in cases when they had circulated for centuries. Consulting surgeons framed their manuals as containers of elite knowledge that was only now being made accessible to the common man or woman. That these works were distributed by post in sealed envelopes – sometimes, advertisements suggest, to people ordering them under assumed names – also seems significant. Such modes of marketing and distribution, as Fisher argues, could make sexual knowledge feel rare, forbidden, and suppressed even when it was none of these things.[12]

In the hands of late nineteenth-century sex reformers and sexologists, this framework was adapted in ways that offered sellers of sexual knowledge a still more powerful justification for their ambitions.[13] Medical publications had long been portrayed as containers of knowledge that could enable people to manage their bodies, desires, and relationships in better ways. Now, they were portrayed as containers of knowledge that had the power to dispel a deep-seated cultural ignorance of sex that destabilized relationships, fostered confusion, guilt, and shame, and even produced "abnormal" sexual behaviour. This representation of sexual ignorance as a kind of social disease and of sexual-scientific knowledge as its cure was a fixture of sex reform and advice literature through the first half of the twentieth century. By the end of the 1940s, as Matthew Lavine has observed, authors' perennial diagnoses of sexual ignorance and perennial claims that they were "the first to shatter the taboo" by dispelling it had become such tired tropes that they practically parodied themselves.[14] Exhausted, they faded amid the rise

11 Fisher, "Modern Ignorance," 481. 12 Fisher, "Modern Ignorance," 481.

13 Simon Szreter and Kate Fisher, *Sex before the Sexual Revolution: Intimate Life in England, 1918–1963* (Cambridge: Cambridge University Press, 2010), 66; Fisher, "Modern Ignorance," 475.

14 Matthew Lavine, "'Advanced Marriage Technique': Sex as a Perfectible Skill in Mid-Twentieth-Century American Marriage Manuals," *Journal of Family History* 46, no. 4 (2021): 476.

of the so-called sexual revolution. Modern Britain was cast as a sexualized society, one in which – for better or, in the eyes of many, worse – everyone knew about sex. In this context, personal claims of sexual ignorance began to fade too.

What lingered on was the history of sexual knowledge that was established alongside the tropes that Lavine describes. That history, as Havelock Ellis's "The Revaluation of Obscenity" suggests, identified the Victorian period as the nadir of sexual understanding in the West, an era marked by an anxiety about sex that was so potent and so pervasive that sexual discussion was almost entirely repressed and, where it could not be repressed, was suppressed. Major elements of this narrative have been debunked time and again. As Lesley Hall has noticed, hardly a year goes by before another popular history appears to tell us that the Victorians knew about sex, and that they had a lot of it, in a lot of different ways.[15] For most of the time I spent working on this book, I had no desire to join the chorus. Arguments against the idea of Victorians' ignorance of sex have become almost as shopworn as previous arguments for it. Over time, however, I came to believe that aspects of the narrative that Ellis helped construct remain influential, even in sophisticated scholarship on Victorian sexuality. Michel Foucault's argument that viewing a period in the relatively recent past as an era of sexual repression is appealing because it enables us to see ourselves as liberated offers one explanation for its stubborn stranglehold on popular culture.[16] However, I would argue that what remains of its influence on scholarship has more to do with the hall of illusions that nineteenth- and early twentieth-century contests for sexual authority produced.

One of the most significant challenges that historians of sexuality have faced – a challenge famously identified by Foucault in the 1970s – is figuring out how to interpret historical claims about sexual knowledge and its circulation. Interpreting claims about sexual ignorance, as Fisher argues, requires a fine-grained understanding of the frameworks in which sexual knowledge was situated. Without a detailed grasp of how sexual knowledge was conceptualized and how it was mediated, all we can do is take historical claims about sexual ignorance at face value. And taking these claims at face value is easy to do when the cultural narratives that we have received from (late) Victorians tell us that we should. *Selling Sexual Knowledge* has argued something similar of Victorian claims about obscenity and censorship. Scholars developed sophisticated understandings of how obscenity was constructed decades ago, showing that Victorian models of obscenity relied on paternalistic ideas about reading that framed certain groups as especially vulnerable to media influences.

[15] Lesley Hall, "The Victorians: Our Others, Our Selves?" in *Sex, Knowledge, and Receptions of the Past*, ed. Kate Fisher and Rebecca Langlands (Oxford: Oxford University Press, 2015), 161.

[16] Michel Foucault, *The History of Sexuality. Volume 1: An Introduction*, trans. Robert Hurley (1978; repr., New York: Random House, 1990).

However, like claims about sexual ignorance, Victorian claims about obscenity are too often accepted at face value as uncomplicated expressions of belief, and claims about what was censored on the grounds of obscenity too often accepted as fact. And it is easy to accept these claims, because they affirm another idea that we inherited from late Victorian sellers of sexual knowledge: that the Victorians were uniquely anxious about sex, and that this anxiety translated into concerted (if not always consistent or successful) attempts to regulate the circulation of knowledge about it.

This book has made my case for the idea that understanding Victorian claims about medical obscenity and censorship requires understanding sexual knowledge's situation in print. My work often led me away from topics typically associated with work in the history of sexuality. When I shared early, messy drafts of this book, some colleagues expressed frustration that I seemed more interested in medical practitioners' debates about what an advertisement was than I was in how works at issue in obscenity trials represented sex. Yet, as I hope I have demonstrated, understanding how medical print culture operated in practical terms furnishes a richer context for interpreting Victorian claims about obscenity. It enables us to understand that the circulation of sexual knowledge did become the subject of highly politicized debates as it was consolidated as a field of medical expertise, debates that often focused on young, male, and working-class readers and their supposed vulnerability to the influences of print. Yet, because they offered ways of managing how books, people, movements, and institutions were understood, claims about obscenity and censorship were deeply entangled with contests over what constituted expert knowledge, who could make it known, and for what purposes. Alongside sexual ignorance, medical obscenity and medical censorship were to a great extent produced by would-be authorities to sell sex as a field of expertise and direct its applications.

Appendix A: Holywell Street Publishers' Catalogues

This appendix provides a list of catalogues associated with the early-Victorian trade in sexual entertainment that inform Chapter 1 and parts of Chapter 4.

Brook, H. G. *Catalogue of Fast and Funny Literature*. London: H.G. Brook, n.d. DA 676, box 1, item 52, MSCE.

A Catalogue of Books, Principally Facetious and Humorous. London: Hicks and Smith, n.d. DA 676, box 1, item 50, MSCE.

[Dugdale, William]. "A Catalogue of Books, Principally Facetious and Humorous." In *The Exquisite: A Journal of Fun, Frolic, and Facetiae*. London: H. Smith, n.d. DA 676, box 3, item 31, MSCE.

[Dugdale, William]. "Catalogue of Books Published by H. Smith." In *Hints to Men about Town, or Waterfordania: Containing a List and Description of the Most Known, Swell, Flash-up, and Downright Introducing Houses and Celebrated Seraglios* [. . .]. London: Henry Smith, c. 1841. DA 679.H666, MSCE.

[Dugdale, William]. "Catalogue of Books Published by H. Smith, 37, Holywell Street, Strand." In Henry Horne [pseud.]. *Marriage, Historically, Philosophically, Legally, Physiologically, and Pathologically Examined*. London: H. Smith, c. 1842. 162.3 H81 m, KIL.

[Dugdale, William]. "Catalogue of a New Assortment of Scarce and Amorous Literature." and "Works Sold by H. Smith." In Alexander [*sic*] Dumas, *The Lady of the Camelias* [*sic*]. London: H. Smith, c. 1855. C.194.a.447(1), BL.

[Dugdale, William]. "Works Published by H. Smith." In *The Philosophy of Kissing Anatomically and Physiologically Explained*. London: Henry Smith, c. 1840. 41132/P, WL.

[Duncombe, Edward?]. *Catalogue of Select Works, Funny, Flash, and Facetious, of the Best Description, Richly Embellished with Plates*. [London?]: s.n., c. 1840. DA 676, box 1, item 53, MSCE.

[Duncombe, Edward?]. *Catalogue of Select Works, Funny, Flash, and Facetious, of the Best Description, Richly Embellished with Plates*. [London?]: s.n., c. 1840. DA 676, box 1, item 54, MSCE.

[Duncombe, Edward]. *Marriage Physiologically Discussed*. London: John Wilson, n.d. DA 676, box 5, item 22, MSCE.

Dyer, Edward. *A Catalogue of Facetious and Humorous Books*. London: Edward Dyer, n.d. DA 676, box 1, item 51, MSCE.

Dyer, Edward. "A Catalogue of Books, Principally Facetious and Humorous." In *The Exquisite: A Journal of Fun, Frolic, and Facetiae*. London: Edward Dyer, n.d. DA 676, box 3, item 30, MSCE.

Jackson & Co. "The Following Works to Be Had at Jackson and Co." In *The Daughters of Thespis; or, a Peep Behind the Curtain! Comprising Biographical Sketches, Brilliant Repartees, Witty Sallies, Extraordinary Adventures, and Amusing Anecdotes* [. . .]. London: Jackson and Co., 1841. PN 2597 D328 HRC-TA, HRC.

Metford, M. [John Duncombe]. "Books Published and Sold by M. Metford." In *A Peep into the Holy Land, or, Sinks of London Laid Open*! London: John Duncombe, n.d. DA 688.P37, MSCE.

A Select Catalogue of Books; Facetious and Amorous. [London]: s.n., n.d. DA 676, box 6, item 51, MSCE.

A Select Catalogue of Books; Facetious and Amorous. [London]: s.n., n.d. DA 676, box 6, item 52, MSCE.

A Select Catalogue of Books, Facetious and Amorous. [London]: s.n., n.d. DA 676, box 6, item 53, MSCE.

Ward, W. [Thomas Paine Carlile?]. *Ward's New Catalogue of Parisian Novelties*. Strand: W. Ward, c. 1850. DA 676, box 8, item 22, MSCE.

Ward, Wm. [Thomas Paine Carlile?]. *The Man of Pleasure's Illustrated Pocket-Book for 1850*. London: Wm. Ward's Bachelor's Repository of Arts, 1850. DA 679.M285, MSCE.

Appendix B: Translations of Consulting Surgeons' Manuals

This appendix provides bibliographic information for translations of four manuals associated with consulting surgeons discussed in Chapter 2, in all of the languages that the manuals were translated into to my knowledge. Readers should be aware that this appendix is not a comprehensive list of translated editions, however: as with the English versions, translations of these manuals were issued in many editions, over many years, by many different publishers in different countries. Most of the translations listed in this appendix have been digitized by the institutions that own them or by external organizations, such as Google Books. Where possible, I have provided location information for original print copies.

Translations of J. L. Curtis, *Manhood: The Causes of Its Premature Decline.*

Curtis, J. L. *De la virilidad, de las causas de su decadencia prematura é instrucciones para restablecerse perfectamente* [...]. Barcelona: Imprenta de Oliveres Hermanos, 1847. S.65, New York Academy of Medicine Library.

Curtis, J. L. *Manddom: Aarsagerne til dens for tidlige Aftagelse og Anviisning til den fuldstændige Gjenerholdelse* [...]. Kjøbenhavn: Ludvig Jordans Forlag, 1850. 1–123 6118, Det Kongelige Bibliotek.

Curtis, J. L. et Compagnie, *De la virilité, des causes de son déclin prématuré et instructions pour en obtenir le parfait rétablissement* [...]. Paris: Charpentier, 1851. Path. 1482 o, Bayerische Staatsbibliothek.

Curtis, J. L. *Mannheit: die Ursachen ihrer vorzeitigen Abnahme und Belehrungen über ihre vollständige Wiederherstellung* [...]. Leipzig: Orthaus, 1851. Spez. Path.7186, Bibliotheca Albertina, Universitätsbibliothek Leipzig.

Curtis, Joseph. L. *Mężkość: przyczyny przedwczesnego jej upadku i wskazówki dotyczące środków spiesznego powrotu do zdrowia: dziełko poświęcone osobom cierpiącym w skutek nierządu* [...], translated by Seweryn

Zdzitowiecki. Warszawa: Karola Bernstejna, 1861. Magazyn Książek, 1.465.430 A, Biblioteka Narodowa.

Curtis, Joseph. L. *Manbaarheid, de oorzaken van haar ontijdig verval en wenken om dat volmaakt te genezen* [. . .]. Rotterdam: Stoeller [Rothmeijer], 1872. UBM: 645 J 31, Bibliotheek Universiteit van Amsterdam.

Translations of Samuel La'Mert, *Self-Preservation*

La'Mert, Samuel. *La préservation personnelle: traité médical sur les maladies des organes de la generation résultant des habitudes cachées, des excès de la jeunesse ou de la contagion* [. . .]. Paris: Ledoyen et Laroque, 1847. WJA L228s 1847, NLM.

La'Mert, Samuel. *Het zelfbehoud: geneeskundige verhandeling over de ziekten der geslachtsdelen, als gevolgen van Geheime gewoonten, uitspattingen der jeugd of besmetting* [. . .], translated by P. J. Koorn. Amsterdam: F. Canongette, 1849. UBM: 645 E 21, Bibliotheek Universiteit van Amsterdam.

La-Mert, Samuel. *La preservación personal: o tratado médico popular sobre las enfermedades de la juventud y de la edad viril, la impotencia prematura* [. . .]. Madrid: Librería de la Viuda e Hijos de Mayol, 1849. Europeana.

La'Mert, Samuel. *A preservação pessoal: tratado medical sobre as doenças dos orgãos da geração; resultantes dos habitos clandestinos dos excossos da mocidade ou do contagio com observações practicas sobre a impotencia prematura*. Rio de Janeiro: Prius & Co, c. 1850. WJA L228p 1840, NLM.

La'Mert, Samuel. *Der persönliche Schutz. Medizinische Abhandlung über die Krankheiten der Geschlechtstheile, welche aus den geheimen Lastern, den Ausschweifungen der Jugend und der Ansteckung hervorgehen* [. . .]. Antwerpen: Kornicker, 1850. WJA L228s 1850, NLM.

La'Mert, Samuel, *Della preservazione individuale; trattato igienico popolare sopra le malatie degli organi sessuali procedenti da occulte abitudini, da giovanili intemperanze o da contagio, con osservazioni pratiche sopra l'impotenza prematura*. Milano: Oliva, 1855. WJA L228s 1855, NLM.

La'Mert, Samuel. *Fat Mod!: Lægeanviisning til hurtig og sikker Helbredelse for alle dem, som lide af Svækkelse, en Følge af hemmelige Ungdomssynder, Udsvævelser med Fruentimmer, Syphilis m. m.* [. . .]. Kjøbenhavn: Oversætterens Forlag: i Commission hos V. Pio, 1866. 130019425496, Det Kongelige Bibliotek.

Lamerta, Doktora. *Kartiny poslīēdstviĭ razvrata, ili, Razrushitel'noe vlīīānie prirody na līūdeĭ, predaīūshchikhsīā līū bostrastīīū: nastol'naīā kniga dlīā vracheĭ i vospitateleĭ*. Moskva: V Tip. L. Stepanovoĭ pri Imperatorskikh Moskovskikh Teatrakh, 1859. WJA L228sR 1859, NLM.

Translations of Samuel La'Mert, *The Science of Life*

La'Mert, Samuel. *De kennis des levens of hoe men moet leven en waarvoor men moet leven* [...]. Amsterdam: s.n., 1849. UBM: 659 G 30, Bibliotheek Universiteit van Amsterdam.

La'Mert, Samuel. *La science de la vie; ou, Comment il faut vivre et pourquoi il faut vivre, suivie d'observations pratiques sur la santé, la diète et la longévité, et d'un extrait des Théories populaires de Liebig sur la vie, la santé et les maladies* [...]. Bruxelles: J. de Wallens et cie, 1849. Magazyn Książek, 288.895, Biblioteka Narodowa.

La'Mert, Samuel. *Lebenskunst: Inbegriff praktischer Anweisungen zur Verlängerung des menschlichen Lebens; eine vollständige Lösung der großen Frage* [...], edited by L. Raudnitz. Leipzig: Spamer, 1850. 22.311.25, Universitätsbibliothek Gießen.

La'Mert, Samuela. *Nauka życia czyli jak i dlaczego żyć trzeba: dzieło zawierające praktyczne uwagi o zdrowiu oraz wyjątki z teorii popularnych Liebiga o życiu, zdrowiu i chorobach* [...]. Warszawa: G.L. Glücksberg, 1850. Magazyn Książek; 49.562, Biblioteka Narodowa.

Translations of R. and L. Perry & Co, *The Silent Friend*

R. et L. Perry et Ce. *L'ami discret, ouvrage pratique sur l'anatomie et la physiologie des organes générateurs et leurs maladies, avec des observations sur l'onanisme*. Paris: Hermann, 1854. 617.463, BNF.

R. e L. Perry e Ca. *L'amico discreto; trattato pratico, sopra l'anatomia e la fisiologia degli organi genratori e le loro malattie*. Torino: Schieppati, c. 1855. WJA P464s 1855, NLM.

Bibliography

1 Primary Sources

(i) Archives and Libraries

Archive of British Printing and Publishing (University of Reading)
Archives of the Royal College of Surgeons of England
Bayerische Staatsbibliothek
Beinecke Library (Yale University)
Bibliotheca Albertina (Universitätsbibliothek Leipzig)
Bibliotheek Universiteit van Amsterdam
Bibliothèque Nationale de France
Biblioteka Narodowa
British Library
Cambridge University Library
Columbia University Rare Book and Manuscript Library
Det Kongelige Bibliotek
Frances A. Countway Library of Medicine (Harvard University)
Harry Ransom Center (University of Texas, Austin)
Hoare's Bank Museum
Kinsey Institute Library and Special Collections (Indiana University)
London Metropolitan Archives
London School of Economics
Magnus-Hirschfeld-Gesellschaft
McGill University Libraries
Michael Sadleir Collection of Ephemera, 1748–1887 (Lilly Library, Indiana University)
Morris Library (Southern Illinois University)
National Archives, UK
National Library of Medicine, USA
New York Academy of Medicine Library
State Library of New South Wales
State Library of Victoria
Sydney Jones Library (University of Liverpool)
Universitätsbibliothek Gießen

University of Reading
University of Toronto Libraries
Wellcome Library

(ii) Online Resources

19th Century UK Periodicals
British Library Newspapers, 1800–1900
British Newspaper Archive
Canadiana
Curran Index to Nineteenth-Century Periodicals
England & Wales, Civil Registration Death Index, 1837–1915
Europeana
Google Books
Hansard
HathiTrust Digital Library
London Low Life
Old Bailey Proceedings Online
Proquest Historical Newspapers
Readex: World Newspaper Archive
Reading Experience Database, 1450–1945
RetroNews: Le site de presse de la BnF
Trove
University of Leeds Digital Library

(iii) Legislation

Anatomy Act, 1832, 2 & 3 Will. 4. c. 75
Criminal Law Amendment Act, 1885, 48 & 49 Vict. c. 69
Indecent Advertisements Act, 1889, 52 & 53 Vict. c. 33
Medical Act, 1858, 21 & 22 Vict. c. 90
Metropolitan Police Act, 1839, 2 & 3 Vict. c. 47
Obscene Publications Act, 1857, 20 & 21 Vict. c. 83
Post Office (Protection) Act, 1884, 47 & 48 Vict. c. 76
Repeal of Certain Stamp Duties Act, 1853, 16 & 17 Vict. c. 63
Vagrancy Act, 1824 (5 Geo. 4 c. 83)
Vagrancy Act, 1838, 1 & 2 Vict. c. 17

(iv) Newspapers and Periodicals

Aberdeen Journal
Academy
Adult (UL)
American Medical Monthly

Annals of Philosophy
Anthropological Review
Association Medical Journal (later: *British Medical Journal*)
Athenaeum
Bee-Hive
Bell's Life in London and Sporting Chronicle
Bell's Penny Dispatch and Sunday Chronicle
Berkshire Chronicle
Berrow's Worcester Journal
Beverley and East Riding Recorder
Birmingham Daily Gazette
Bookseller
Boston Medical and Surgical Journal
Bristol Mercury
Bristol Times and Mirror
British and Foreign Medical Review
Caledonian Mercury
Chambers's Edinburgh Journal
Cheshire Observer and General Advertiser
Clinic
Comercio (Lima)
Courier (Tasmania)
Daily News (London)
Daily Post (Liverpool)
Derby Mercury
Derbyshire Times and Chesterfield Herald
Deutsche Zeitung Frankfurt
Diario de avisos, y semanario de las provincias (Caracas)
Diario de la Marina (Havana)
Dublin Medical Press
Dublin Quarterly Journal of Medical Science
Edinburgh Christian Magazine
Edinburgh Evening News
Edinburgh Medical and Surgical Journal
Edinburgh Medical Journal
Elgin Courant, and Morayshire Advertiser
Englishwoman's Domestic Magazine
Era
Examiner
Exquisite (BL)
Farmer's Magazine
Fly
Freeman's Journal and Daily Commercial Advertiser
Friend of India
Gems for Gentlemen (BL)
Gentleman's Magazine
Glasgow Sentinel

Hampshire Chronicle
Haszard's Gazette (Charlottetown)
Health
Herapath's Railway Journal
Hereford Journal
Hull Daily Mail
Hull Packet and East Riding Times
Illustrated London News
Illustrated Police News
Illustrated Sporting News and Theatrical and Musical Review
Investor's Chronicle and Money Market Review
John Bull and Britannia
Jornal do Commercio (Rio de Janeiro)
Journal of Mental Science
Judy
Ladies' Monthly Museum
Lancet
Lancet General Advertiser
Law Times
Leeds Mercury
Leeds Times
Literary and Biographical Magazine and British Review
Literary World (New York)
Liverpool Mercury
Lloyd's Weekly Newspaper
London Evening Standard
London Investigator
London Medical and Surgical Journal (later: *Provincial Medical Journal and Retrospect of the Medical Sciences*; merged with *Association Medical Journal*)
London Review
Malthusian (UL)
Malthusian Herald (BL)
Manchester Courier
Manchester Evening News
Manchester Weekly Times
Maryland Medical Journal
Medical Circular and General Medical Advertiser
Medical Examiner (Philadelphia)
Medical Press and Circular
Medical Press and Circular Advertiser
Medical Times and Gazette
Medical Times and Gazette Advertiser
Medicine (Detroit)
Medico-chirurgical Review
Mercurio de Valparaiso
Morning Advertiser

Morning Chronicle
Morning Herald
Morning Post
Morpeth Herald
Movement and Anti-Persecution Gazette
Myra's Journal of Dress and Fashion
North Wales Chronicle
Northampton Mercury
North-China Herald and Supreme Court & Consular Gazette
Northern Star and Leeds General Advertiser
Nuneaton Chronicle
Onze Tolk (Nijmegen)
Oracle of Reason
Pall Mall Gazette
Pasatiempo (Bogota)
Patrie (Paris)
Paul Pry (BL)
Peeping Tom
Penny Magazine
People's Paper
Pick-Me-Up
Poor Man's Guardian
Portland Guardian and Normanby General Advertiser (Victoria)
Preston Guardian
Punch
Railway Chronicle
Rambler's Magazine
Reasoner
Republican
Reynolds's Newspaper
Reynolds's Weekly News
Saint James's Chronicle
Satirist; or, the Censor of the Times
Saturday Review
Secular Chronicle
Sheffield Daily Telegraph
Sheffield Independent
Shrewsbury Chronicle
Simmond's Colonial Magazine and Foreign Miscellany
Solicitor's Journal & Reporter
South Australian Register
South Wales Echo
Sporting Times
Standard
Star and Conception Bay Semi-Weekly Advertiser (Newfoundland)
Students' Journal and Hospital Gazette
Tamworth Herald

Times
Times of India
Western Mail
Western Times
Westminster Review
World of Fashion and Continental Feuilletons
Wrexham Advertiser and North Wales News

(v) Other Published Primary Material

"Abortion." In *Encyclopædia Britannica: or, A Dictionary of Arts, Sciences, and Miscellaneous Literature*, 37. 5th ed. Edinburgh: Printed at the Encyclopaedical Press, 1817.

Acton, William. *The Functions and Disorders of the Reproductive Organs*. London: John Churchill, 1857a.

Prostitution, Considered in Its Social, Moral, and Sanitary Aspects. London: John Churchill, 1857b.

Allbutt, Henry Arthur. *Evils Produced by Over-Childbearing and Excessive Lactation*. [London]: [Malthusian League], [1878].

The Wife's Handbook. 7th ed. London: R. Forder, 1888.

Allinson, Thomas Richard. *A Book for Married Women*. London: F. Pitman, 1894.

Anderson, Gideon. *Thoughts on Animalcules; or, A Glimpse of the World Revealed by the Microscope*. London: John Murray, 1846.

Aristotle [pseud.]. *The Works of Aristotle: In Four Parts. Containing I. His Complete Master Piece;* [...] *To Which Is Added, the Family Physician* [...]. London: Published for the Booksellers, 1790.

Aristotle's Master-Piece; or, Every Woman's Book! Displaying All the Secrets of Nature, as Exhibited in the Creation of Man! London: Printed for James Duncombe, c. 1830.

Revised Edition of the Works of Aristotle, the Famous Philosopher, Containing His Complete Masterpiece and Family Physician, his Experienced Midwife, his Book of Problems, and Remarks on Physiognomy. London: J. Smith, [1857].

Armstrong, John. *The Young Woman's Guide to Virtue, Economy, and Happiness*. Newcastle: Mackenzie and Dent, 1826.

Atkinson, William. *Popery Unmasked and Her Supporters Exposed*. Leeds: T. Inchbold, 1829.

Bacot, John. *A Treatise on Syphilis*. London: Longman, Rees, Orme, Brown and Green, 1829.

Beach, Wooster. *The American Practice of Medicine*. 2nd ed. New York: Kelley & La'Tourette, 1836.

Becklard, Eugène, and M. Sherman Wharton. *The Physiologist, or, Sexual Physiology Revealed: Being Mysteries and Revelations in Matters of Great Importance to the Married and Unmarried of Both Sexes* [...]. (s.l.: s.n., 1846).

Bell, T. [pseud.]. *Kalogynomia, or The Laws of Female Beauty: Being the Elementary Principles of that Science*. London: J.J. Stockdale, 1821.

Besant, Annie. *Autobiographical Sketches*, edited by Carol Hanbery MacKay. Peterborough: Broadview, 2009.

The Law of Population: Its Consequences, and Its Bearing upon Human Conduct and Morals. London: Freethought Publishing Company, [1878].

The Law of Population: Its Consequences, and Its Bearing upon Human Conduct and Morals. London: Freethought Publishing Company, 1887.

Black, Donald Campbell. *On the Functional Diseases of the Renal, Urinary, and Reproductive Organs, with a General Review of Urinary Pathology*. London: J & A Churchill, 1872.

On the Functional Diseases of the Renal, Urinary, and Reproductive Organs, with a General Review of Urinary Pathology. 2nd rev. ed. London: J & A Churchill, 1875.

Bloch, Iwan. *Das Sexualleben unserer Zeit in seinen Beziehungen zur modernen Kultur*. Berlin: L. Marcus, 1919.

Sexual Life in England, Past and Present, translated by W. H. Forstern. London: Francis Aldor, 1938.

The Bombay Almanack and Book of Direction for 1858. Bombay: Bombay Gazette Press, 1858.

Bradlaugh, C., and W. Simpson. *Disestablishment and Disendowment of the English Church*. London: Charles Watts, 1876.

Brodum, William. *A Guide to Old Age, or Cure for the Indiscretions of Youth*. 2 Vols. London: J.W. Meyers, 1797.

Burn, J. D. *The Language of the Walls: And a Voice from the Shop Windows; or, The Mirror of Commercial Roguery. By One Who Thinks Aloud*. Manchester: Abel Heywood, 1855.

Burke, William. *The Popular Compendium of Anatomy: or, A Concise and Clear Description of the Human Body; with the Physiology, or Natural History of the Various Actions and Functions of Its Different Organs and Parts*. London: Printed for S. Highley, 1804.

Cabanés, Augustin. *Flagellation in France: Considered from a Medical and Historical Standpoint*. Paris: Charles Carrington, 1898.

Carlile, Richard. *Every Woman's Book; or, What is Love? Containing Most Important Instructions for the Prudent Regulation of the Principle of Love, and the Number of a Family*. London: R. Carlile, 1826.

Every Woman's Book; or, What is Love? Containing Most Important Instructions for the Prudent Regulation of the Principle of Love, and the Number of a Family. London: A. Carlile, 1838.

A Catalogue of Scientific Works on the Psychology and Pathology of Sex. London: University Press, [1901].

Caton, T. M. *A Practical Treatise on the Prevention and Cure of the Venereal Disease*. London: Samuel Highley, 1809.

Chapman, John. *Cheap Books and How to Get Them*. London: John Chapman, 1852.

Christie, W. D. *John Stuart Mill and Mr. Abraham Hayward, Q.C.* London: Henry S. King & Co, 1873.

Christianity in Relation to Freethought, Skepticism, and Faith: Three Discourses by the Bishop of Peterborough with Special Replies by Mr. Charles Bradlaugh. London: Austin & Co, 1873.

Churchill, John. *The Medical Intelligencer*. London: John Churchill, 1853–1857.
Clarke, James Fernandez. *Autobiographical Recollections of the Medical Profession*. London: J & A Churchill, 1874.
Cobbett, William. *Cobbett against Himself*. London: T. Gilet for John Joseph Stockdale, 1807.
Cooper, Alfred. *Syphilis*. 2nd ed, edited by Edward Cotterell. London: J & A Churchill, 1895.
Cooper, Astley. *Lectures on the Principles and Practice of Surgery*. 2nd ed. London: F. C. Westly, 1830.
Courtenay, Francis Burdett. *Practical Essays on the Debilities of the Generative System*. London: T. Hill, 1839.
Revelations of Quacks and Quackery: A Series of Letters by "Detector" reprinted from "The Medical Circular." 3rd ed. London: Baillière, Tindall & Cox, 1865.
Cowan, Charles. *The Danger, Irrationality, and Evils of Medical Quackery*. London: Sherwood, 1839.
Curtis, J. L. *Manhood: The Causes of Its Premature Decline, with Directions for Its Perfect Restoration* [...]. London: Published by the Authors, 1840.
De la virilité, des causes de son déclin prématuré et instructions pour en obtenir le parfait rétablissement [...]. Paris: Charpentier, 1851.
Manhood: The Causes of Its Premature Decline, with Directions for Its Perfect Restoration [...]. London: Published by the Author, 1852.
De la virilidad: de las causas de su decadencia prematura é instrucciones para obtener su completo restablecimiento [...]. Madrid: C. Bailly-Bailliere, 1853.
Curwen, Henry. *A History of Booksellers, the Old and the New*. London: Chatto and Windus, 1874.
Dallas, Robert Charles. *Elements of Self-Knowledge; Intended to Lead Youth into an Early Acquaintance with the Nature of Man, by an Anatomical Sketch of the Human Frame, a Concise View of the Mental Faculties, and an Enquiry into the Genuine Nature of the Passions*. London: B. Crosby, 1805.
Dawson, Richard. *An Essay on Marriage; Being a Microscopic Investigation into Its Physiological and Physical Relations* [...]. London: Hugh Hughes, 1848.
Deslandes, Léopold [pseud.]. *Manhood: The Causes of Its Premature Decline: with Directions for Its Perfect Restoration*. Boston: Otis, Broaders, 1842.
Discussion on Secularism: Report of a Public Discussion between the Rev. Brewin Grant, B.A., and George Jacob Holyoake, Esq [...]. Glasgow: Robert Stark, 1854.
Douglas, G. A. *The Nature and Causes of Impotence in Men, and Barrenness in Woman, Explained*. 3rd ed. London: Printed for J. Brett, 1758.
Douse, W. J. *A True Remedy for Poverty!* Nottingham: W. J. Douse, [1895].
Drysdale, Charles R. *The Principles of Population*. [London]: [Malthusian League], [1878].
The Struggle for Enjoyable Existence. [London]: [Malthusian League], 1878.
[Drysdale, George]. *Physical, Sexual, and Natural Religion*. London: Edward Truelove, 1855.
Durand, Jean Baptiste Léonard. *A Voyage to Senegal: or, Historical, Philosophical, and Political Memoirs, Relative to the Discoveries, Establishments, and Commerce of Europeans in the Atlantic Ocean* [...]. London: Richard Phillips, 1806.

Dühren, Eugène [Iwan Bloch]. *Das Geschlechtsleben in England, mit besonderer Beziehung auf London*. Vol. 4. Berlin: M. Lilienthal, 1903.

Dwight, Timothy. *Theology: Explained and Defended, in a Series of Sermons*. Vol. 3. New Haven, CT: S. Converse, 1825.

Eliot, George. *The Journals of George Eliot*, edited by Margaret Harris. Cambridge: Cambridge University Press, 1998.

Ellis, Havelock. *A Note on the Bedborough Trial*. London: University Press, 1898.

Studies in the Psychology of Sex: The Sexual Impulse. Philadelphia, PA: F.A. Davis, 1904.

My Life: The Autobiography of Havelock Ellis. Boston, MA: Houghton Mifflin, 1939.

"The Revaluation of Obscenity." In *On Life and Sex*, edited by Havelock Ellis, 206–230. London: W.M. Heinemann, 1948.

Encyclopaedia Perthensis; or, Universal Dictionary of the Arts, Sciences, Literature, &c, Edinburgh: John Brown, Anchor Close, 1816.

Féré, Charles Samson. *Evolution and Dissolution of the Sexual Instinct*. Paris: Charles Carrington, 1904.

"A Few Words to News-Readers." London: W. Eglington, 1850.

First Report of the Postmaster General on the Post Office: Presented to Both Houses of Parliament by command of Her Majesty. London: George E. Eyre and William Spottiswoode, 1855.

Forster, E. M. "The Censorship of Books." *The Nineteenth Century and After* 105 (1929): 444–445.

Fraxi, Pisanus [Henry Spencer Ashbee], *Catena Librorum Prohibitorum: Bio-Biblio-Icono-graphical and Critical Notes on Curious, Uncommon, and Erotic Books*. London: Privately Printed, 1885.

"The Free Press Defence Committee: The Bedborough Case Balance Sheet." [London?]: The Executive of the Free Press Defence Committee, 1899.

Frost, Thomas. *Reminiscences of a Country Journalist*. London: Ward and Downey, 1886.

Fyfe, Andrew. *A Compendium of the Anatomy of the Human Body: Intended Principally for the Use of Students*. Vol. 2. Edinburgh: Pillan and Sons, 1810.

Glenn, Robert George. *A Manual of Laws Affecting Medical Men*. London: J & A Churchill, 1871.

Good, John Mason. *The Study of Medicine*. 3rd rev. ed., vol. 4. London: Thomas and George Underwood, 1829.

Goss, Horace. *Woman: Her Physiology and Functions*. London: Published by the Authors, 1853.

Graham, James. *A Lecture on the Generation, Increase, and Improvement of the Human Species*. [London]: Typis excusum Jac. Graemaei, c. 1783.

Graham, T. [G.A. Douglas]. *Conjugal Love; or, The Mysteries of Hymen Unveiled*. London: H. Smith [William Dugdale], n.d.

Granville, A. B. *Graphic Illustrations of Abortion and the Diseases of Menstruation*. London: John Churchill, 1834.

Gulliver, George. *Elements of the Minute Anatomy of Man and the Mammalia*. London: Baillière, 1842.

H., M. G. *Poverty: Its Cause and Cure*. London: Edward Truelove, 1860.

Hall, A. G. *Womanhood: Causes of Its Premature Decline, Respectfully Illustrated: Being a Review of the Changes and Derangements of the Female Constitution* [. . .]. Rochester, [NY]: E. Shepard, 1845.

Hamilton, Lady Augusta. *Marriage Rites, Customs, and Ceremonies of the Nations of the Universe*. London: J. Smith, 1822.

Heron, Robert. *A Collection of Late Voyages and Travels, Chiefly Translated and Arranged from the French and other Foreign Publications of Neibuhr, Mariti, Beauchamp, &c* [. . .]. [London?]: Watson and Co., 1797.

Hints to Men about Town, or, Waterfordiania: Containing a List and Description of the Most Known, Swell, Flash-up, and Downright Introducing Houses and Celebrated Seraglios [. . .]. London: Henry Smith [William Dugdale], c. 1841.

Horne, Henry [pseud.]. *Marriage, Historically, Philosophically, Legally, Physiologically, and Pathologically Examined*. London: H. Smith [William Dugdale], c. 1842.

Imray, Keith. *A Popular Cyclopedia of Modern Domestic Medicine*. American ed. New York: Gates, Stedman and Company, 1850.

Intercidona [pseud.]. *The Connubial Guide, or, Married People's Best Friend*. London: John Wilson [Edward Duncombe], c. 1843.

Jacques, I. A., & Co. *The Secret Preceptor; or, the Grandeur & Vigour of Man, Physically, Mentally, and Morally Vindicated, Illustrated & Displayed* [. . .]. London: Published by the Authors, [1852].

Jordan, J. & Co. *Human Frailty: A Popular Work on the Awful Results Produced by the Dangerous Effects of an Inordinate Indulgence of the Passions* [. . .]. London: Published by the Authors, 1842.

Jraham [*sic*], James [James Graham]. *On Impotence and Sterility, or, Private Advice To Those Married Ladies Who Have Been Unable, but Are Eagerly Desirous to Have Children*. London: H. Smith [William Dugdale], n.d.

Kahn, Joseph. *Catalogue of Dr. Kahn's Anatomical Museum*. London: J. Golbourn, 1851.

Atlas of the Formation of the Human Body: In the Earliest Stages of Its Development [. . .]. London: John Churchill, 1852.

Catalogue of Dr. Kahn's Anatomical and Pathological Museum. London: J. Golbourn, [1853].

Men with Tails: Remarks on the Niam-Niams of Central Africa; Comprising an Introduction, by Dr. Kahn; and an Essay on the Anatomical View of the Question by Dr. Sexton [. . .]. London: W. J. Colbourn, 1855.

Handbook of Dr. Kahn's Museum. [London]: W. Snell, 1863.

Kahn, L.J. [Louis]. *Nervous Exhaustion: Its Cause and Cure. Comprising a Series of Eight Lectures on Debility and Disease, as Delivered Nightly at Dr. Kahn's Museum of Anatomy* [. . .]. New York: s.n., 1870.

Karsch-Haack, Ferdinand. *Das gleichgeschlechtliche Leben der Naturvölker*. München: E. Reinhardt, 1911.

Knowlton, Charles. *Fruits of Philosophy, or, The Private Companion of Young Married People*. London: Dugdale, Russell Court, Drury Lane, 1838.

Fruits of Philosophy, or, The Private Companion of Young Married People. London: Printed and Published by H. Smith [William Dugdale], c. 1845.

Fruits of Philosophy, or, The Private Companion of Young Married People. London: J. Watson, 1845.

Fruits of Philosophy: *An Essay on the Population Question*. London: Freethought Publishing Company, 1877.

von Krafft-Ebing, Richard. *Psychopathia Sexualis, with Especial Reference to Contrary Sexual Instinct: A Medico-Legal Study*, translated by Charles Gilbert Chaddock. London: F. J. Rebman, 1893.

Psychopathia Sexualis, with Especial Reference to Contrary Sexual Instinct: A Medico-Legal Study, translated by Charles Gilbert Chaddock. London: F. J. Rebman, 1899.

Lallemand, Francois C. *A Practical Treatise on the Causes, Symptoms, and Treatment of Spermatorrhoea*, translated by H. J. McDougall. 2nd ed. London: Churchill, 1851.

La'Mert, Samuel. *Self-Preservation: A Medical Treatise on the Secret Infirmities and Disorders of the Generative Organs, Resulting from Solitary Habits, Youthful Excess, or Infection* ... London: Published by the Author, 1852.

The Silent Friend: Dr. Lamert's Science of Life [. . .]. Melbourne: Will Andrade, 1898.

La'Mert, Lima, and Samuel. *The Science of Life; or, Self-Preservation*. Melbourne: s.n., 1883.

Lankester, Edwin, ed. *Haydn's Dictionary of Popular Medicine and Hygiene*. London: Ward, Lock, 1874.

Lawrence, D. H. *Pornography and Obscenity*. London: Faber and Faber, 1929.

Lawrence, William. *Lectures on Surgery, Medical and Operative, as Delivered in the Theatre at St. Bartholomew's Hospital*. London: F. C. Westley, 1830.

Lewis, John A. *Controul of the Passions: A Popular Enquiry into the Duties and Obligations of the Married State* [. . .] *with Advice to those Suffering from Excessive Indulgence in a Secret Vice, or from Infection* [. . .]. [Liverpool?]: Published by the Authors, 1854.

The Life and Surprising Adlentures [*sic*] *of Bigenio, an Hermaphrodite, or Man-Woman, and Woman-Man*. [London]: Printed by H. Smith [William Dugdale], 37, Holywell-street, Strand, c. 1842.

The Limitation of Families. London: Malthusian League, [1878].

"List of Mr. Carrington's New and Forthcoming Works in English and French." In Jacobus X [pseud.], *The Ethnology of the Six Sense: Studies and Researches Into Its Abuses, Perversions, Follies, Anomalies, and Crimes*. Paris: Charles Carrington, 1899.

Little, Thomas [pseud.]. *The Beauty, Marriage Ceremonies and Intercourse in the Sexes of All Nations; to Which Is Added the New Art of Love (Grounded in Kalogynomia)*. London: J.J. Stockdale, 1824.

An Introduction to a Natural System of Anatomy, Pathology and Medicine, to Which Is Added a General View of Natural History. London: J. J. Stockdale, 1825.

Systems of the Physiology of Camper. London: J. J. Stockdale, 1825.

Lucas, C. J. and Co. *Manly Vigour: A Popular Inquiry into the Concealed Causes of Its Premature Decline with Instructions for Its Complete Restoration*. London: Published by the Authors, 1841.

The Lustful Turk [1828]. Olympia, WA: Olympia, 2006.

The Malthusian Handbook: Designed to Induce Married People to Limit Their Families within Their Means. London: W.H. Reynolds, 1898.

A Manual of the Etiquette of Love, Courtship and Marriage. London: Thomas Allman, 1853.

Marcus [pseud.]. *The Book of Murder! A Vade-Mecum for the Commissioners and Guardians of the New Poor Law throughout Great Britain and Ireland.* [London]: William Dugdale, 1839.

Mayo, Thomas. *Elements of the Pathology of the Human Mind*. Philadelphia, PA: Adam Waldie, 1839.

Merzbach, Georg. *Die krankhaften Erscheinungen des Geschlechtssinnes*. Wien: Hölder, 1909.

Milton, John L. *On a New Way of Treating Gonorrhoea*. London: John Churchill, 1852.

Moll, Albert. *Das Sexualleben des Kindes*. Leipzig: Vogel, 1908.

Moore, Theophilus. *Marriage Customs and Modes of Courtship of the Various Nations of the Universe*. London: John Bumpus, 1830.

Morison, John. *Counsels to a Newly Wedded Pair*. London: F. Westley and A.H. Davis, 1830.

My Secret Life. Amsterdam: Privately Printed For Subscribers, 1888.

The New Sprees of London; or, A Guide to All the Flash Cribs of the Metropolis. London: Printed and Published by H. Smith [William Dugdale], 1844.

"The Obscene M.D." Coloured Lithograph. *Morality of Modern Medicine Mongers*. London: British College of Health, 1852.

O'Donnoghue, Hallifield Cosgayne. *Marriage: The Source, Stability, and Perfection of Social Happiness and Duty*. London: V. Elkins, 1828.

An Old Bibliophile [Charles Carrington]. *Forbidden Books: Notes and Gossip on Tabooed Literature*. Paris: The Author and his Friends [Charles Carrington], 1902.

On the Use of Night Caps, or, Seven Years' Experience on the Practicality of Limiting the Number of a Family, by the Best Known Methods, Including Some Valuable and Novel Information, Never before Published, by a Married Man with Six Children! London: J. Turner [William Dugdale], [1844?].

Onania: or, The Heinous Sin of Self Pollution. 4th ed. London: Printed for the Author, 1725.

Owen, Robert Dale. *Moral Physiology: or, A Brief and Plain Treatise on the Population Question*. London: James Watson, 1842.

Palmer, J. H. *Individual, Family, and National Poverty*. London: E. Truelove, 1875.

Pancoast, Seth. *Porneio-Kalogynomia-Pathology: Boyhood's Perils and Manhood's Curse*. Philadelphia, PA: s.n., 1858.

Pardon, George Frederick. *The Popular Guide to London and Its Suburbs, Comprising Descriptions of all Its Points of Interest; with Historical, Literary, Statistical, and Useful Information*. London: Routledge, Warne, and Routledge, 1862.

Parker, Langston. *The Modern Treatment of Syphilitic Diseases*. London: John Churchill, 1839.

Perry, R. and L., & Co, *The Silent Friend: A Medical Work Treating of the Anatomy and Physiology of the Organs of Generation and Their Diseases*. London: R. and L. Perry & Co., 1847.

The Philosophy of Kissing, Anatomically and Physiologically Explained. London: H. Smith [William Dugdale], c. 1840.

Pickford, Percy. *On True and False Spermatorrhoea*. London: H. Baillière, 1852.

Place, Francis. *The Autobiography of Francis Place: 1771–1854*, edited by Marty Thale. Cambridge: Cambridge University Press, 1972.

To the Married of Both Sexes. [London]: s.n., n.d.

To the Married of Both Sexes of the Working People. [London]: s.n., n.d.

To the Married of Both Sexes in Genteel Life. [London]: s.n., n.d.

Pollack, Robert. *The Course of Time*. Edinburgh: William Blackwood and T. Cadell, 1827.

Poor Inquiry (Ireland). Appendix (H.) – Part II. London: W. Clowes and Sons, 1836.

Powell, Arthur. *The Law Specially Affecting Printers, Publishers, and Newspaper Proprietors*. London: Stevens and Sons, 1887.

Pulvermacher, J. L. *Medical Electricity: Its Use and Abuse; or How to Cure Rheumatic, Nervous, Muscular, and Functional Disorders by Self-Application*. London: J.L. Pulvermacher, 1873.

The Queen v. Charles Bradlaugh and Annie Besant (Specially Reported). London: Freethought Publishing Company, 1877.

The Queen v. Edward Truelove, for Publishing the Hon. Robert Dale Owen's "Moral Physiology," and a Pamphlet, Entitled "Individual, Family, and National Poverty." (Specially Reported). London: Edward Truelove, 1878.

Rackstrow's Museum, *A Brief Description of Those Curious and Excellent Figures of the Human Anatomy in Wax*. London: s.n., c. 1790.

Richerand, Anthelme. *The Elements of Physiology*, translated by Robert Kerrison. London: John Murray, 1803.

Roberton, John. *On the Generative System: Being an Anatomical and Physiological Sketch on the Parts of Generation, and a Treatise on Their Diseases*. 4th ed. London: J.J. Stockdale, 1817.

A Practical Essay on the More Important Complaints Peculiar to the Female. London: Printed for J.J. Stockdale, 1813.

de Roos, Walter. *Silent Hints on Certain Subjects; or Common Sense on Common Matters. A Guide to Health, or, Medical Mentor for the Million, Addressed to the Young, the Old, the Grave, the Gay* [. . .]. London: Published and Sold by the Author, [1852].

Roscaud, Count [pseud?]. *Human Gorillas: A Medical, Legal and Historical Study of Rape with Violence*. Paris: Charles Carrington, 1901.

Ryan, Michael. *The Philosophy of Marriage in Its Social, Physical, and Moral Relations*. London: John Churchill, 1837.

Prostitution in London: With a Comparative View of that of Paris and New York. Paris: Baillière, 1839.

Schrenck-Notzing, Albert von. *Therapeutic Suggestion in Psychopathia Sexualis (Pathological Manifestations of the Sexual Sense), with Especial Reference to Contrary Sexual Instinct*, translated by Charles Gilbert Chaddock. London: F. J. Rebman, 1895.

Sears, M. U. *The Female's Encyclopaedia of Useful and Entertaining Knowledge*. London: J. Sears, 1830

The Secrets of Nature Revealed; or, The Mysteries of Human Procreation and Copulation Considered and Explained. London: Printed for the Booksellers in Town and Country [William Dugdale], 1832.

Seduction by Chloroform: The Secret and Villanous Use of the Power of a New and Scientific Discovery Lately Introduced by Celebrated Doctors [. . .]. London: J. Turner [John Lambert Dugdale], [1850?]

The Sins of the Cities of the Plain; or, The Recollections of a Mary Ann. Olympia, WA: Olympia, 2006. First published 1881 by William Lazenby (London).

Smith, Henry. *The Warning Voice, or Private Medical Friend; A Treatise on the Causes, Symptoms, and Treatment of Nervous and Physical Debility* [. . .]. London: Published by the Author, 1860.

Smithers, Leonard. *Catalogue of Rare and Curious Books*, April 1895. London: Leonard Smithers, 1895.

Solomon, Samuel. *A Guide to Health, or, Advice to Both Sexes in a Variety of Complaints* [. . .]. London: Printed for the Author, c. 1797.

Stockdale, John Joseph. *Encyclopaedia for Youth; or, An Abridgement of All of the Sciences, for the Use of Schools of Both Sexes*. London: Printed for J. J. Stockdale by T. Gilet, 1807.

Stopes, Marie. *The Early Days of Birth Control*. London: G. P. Putnam, 1922.

Swaine, R. J. & Co. *Geneseology, or, The Physiology of Woman: A Medical Work, Treating on the Structure and Uses of the Generative Organs in the Female: with Medical Observations on the Urinary and Generative Organs, Pregnancy, Abortion, and Midwifery* [. . .]. London: Published and Sold by the Authors, 1850.

Sweeney, John. *At Scotland Yard: Being the Experiences during Twenty-Seven Years Service*. London: Grant Richards, 1904.

Tarnowsky, Benjamin [Veniamin Mikhaĭlovich Tarnovskiĭ]. *The Sexual Instinct and Its Morbid Manifestations from the Double Standpoint of Jurisprudence and Psychiatry*, translated by W. C. Costello and Alfred Allinson. Paris: Charles Carrington, 1898.

Taylor, Alfred Swaine. *A Manual of Medical Jurisprudence*. London: John Churchill, 1844.

Teevan, J. *An Exposure of the Most Nefarious and Heartless System of Swindling Ever Tolerated in any Civilized Community*. London: S.J. Cuckow, 1851.

Trall, Russell Thatcher. *Sexual Physiology: A Scientific and Popular Exposition of the Fundamental Problems in Sociology*. New York: Wood & Holbrook, 1866.

Venette, Nicolas. *Conjugal Love; or, The Pleasures of the Marriage Bed Considered in Several Lectures on Human Generation*. London: Printed for the Booksellers, c. 1750.

Vogel, Julius. *The Pathological Anatomy of the Human Body*, translated by George E. Day. London: Baillière, 1847.

Walker, Alexander. *Beauty: Illustrated Chiefly by an Analysis and Classification of Beauty in Women*. London: Effingham Wilson, 1836.

Intermarriage; or, The Mode in Which, and the Causes Why, Beauty, Health and Intellect, Result from Certain Unions, and Deformity, Disease, and Insanity, From Others. London: John Churchill, 1838.

Woolf, Virginia. "The Censorship of Books." *The Nineteenth Century and After* 105 (1929): 446–447.

X, Jacobus [pseud.]. *Untrodden Fields of Anthropology: Observations on the Esoteric Manners and Customs of Semi-Civilized Peoples; Being a Record of Thirty Years Experience in Asia, Africa, America and Oceania*. 2 vols. Paris: Librairie de Médicine, Folklore, et Anthropologie [Charles Carrington], 1896.

Untrodden Fields of Anthropology: Observations on the Esoteric Manners and Customs of Semi-Civilized Peoples; Being a Record of Thirty Years Experience in Asia, Africa, America and Oceania. 2nd rev. ed. 2 vols. Paris: Librairie de Médicine, Folklore, et Anthropologie [Charles Carrington], 1898.

The Yokel's Preceptor: or, More Sprees in London! Being a Regular and Curious Show-Up of All the Rigs and Doings of the Flash Cribs in this Great Metropolis. London: H. Smith [William Dugdale], c. 1844

2 Secondary Sources

Adcock, John. *Yesterday's Papers*, accessed February 19, 2014, https://john-adcock.blogspot.com/.

Alberti, Samuel. *Morbid Curiosities: Medical Museums in Nineteenth-Century Britain*. Oxford: Oxford University Press, 2011.

Altick, Richard Daniel. *The Shows of London*. Cambridge, MA: Harvard University Press, 1978.

Arondekar, Anjali. *For the Record: On Sexuality and the Colonial Archive in India*. Durham, NC: Duke University Press, 2009.

Baines, Paul, and Pat Rogers. *Edmund Curll, Bookseller*. Oxford: Oxford University Press, 2007.

Baisel, Nicola Kay. *Imperiled Innocents: Anthony Comstock and Family Reproduction in Victorian America*. Princeton, NJ: Princeton University Press, 1998.

Baldwin, Melinda. *Making Nature: The History of a Scientific Journal*. Chicago: University of Chicago Press, 2015.

Barker, Hannah. "Medical Advertising and Trust in Late Georgian England." *Urban History* 36, no. 3 (2009): 379–398.

Barker, Hannah. "Stockdale, John (c.1749–1814)." In *Oxford Dictionary of National Biography*, Oxford: Oxford University Press, 2004; online ed., 2011. https://doi.org/10.1093/ref:odnb/26541.

Barker, Juliet. *The Brontës*. London: Weidenfeld and Nicholson, 1994.

Bartrip, Peter. "The British Medical Journal: A Retrospect." In *Medical Journals and Medical Knowledge: Historical Essays*, edited by W. F. Bynum, Stephen Lock, and Roy Porter, 126–145. London: Routledge, 2019.

Mirror of Medicine: A History of the British Medical Journal. Oxford: Oxford University Press, 1990.

Bates, A. W. "Dr. Kahn's Museum: Obscene Anatomy in Victorian London." *Journal of the Royal Society of Medicine* 99 (2006): 618–624.

"Anatomy on Trial: Itinerant Anatomy Museums in Mid Nineteenth-Century England," *Medical History* 9, no. 2 (2016): 188–204.

Bauer, Heike. *English Literary Sexology: Translations of Inversion, 1860–1930*. Basingstoke: Palgrave Macmillan, 2009.

ed. *Sexology and Translation: Cultural and Scientific Encounters across the Modern World*. Philadelphia, PA: Temple University Press, 2015.

Bauer, Heike, and Ivan Crozier. "Sexology, Historiography, Citation, Embodiment: A Review and (Frank) Exchange," *Book Reviews* (blog), *History of the Human Sciences*, June 27, 2017, www.histhum.com/category/book-reviews/.

Beccalossi, Chiara. *Female Sexual Inversion: Same-Sex Desires in Italian and British Sexology, c. 1870–1920*. Basingstoke: Palgrave Macmillan, 2012.

Berger, Doreen. *The Jewish Victorian: Genealogical Information from the Jewish Newspapers, 1871–1880*. Whitney: Robert Boyd, 1999.

Berkowitz, Carin. "The Beauty of Anatomy: Visual Displays and Surgical Education in Early-Nineteenth-Century London," *Bulletin of the History of Medicine* 85, no. 2 (2011): 248–278.

Berridge, Virginia. "Popular Journalism and Working Class Attitudes, 1854–1886: A Study of Reynolds Newspapers and Lloyd's Weekly Paper." PhD thesis, University of London, 1976.

Bettley, James. "Post Voluptatem Misericordia: The Rise and Fall of the London Lock Hospitals." *The London Journal* 10, no. 2 (1984): 167–175.

Bourdieu, Pierre. *Language and Symbolic Power*, translated by Gino Raymond, and Matthew Adamson. Cambridge, MA: Harvard University Press, 1991.

Bowler, Peter J., and Iwan Rhys Morus. *Making Modern Science: A Historical Survey.* Chicago: University of Chicago Press, 2005.

Boyle, Thomas. *Black Swine in the Sewers of Hampstead: Beneath the Surface of Victorian Sensationalism*. New York: Viking, 1989.

Brady, Sean. *John Addington Symonds and Homosexuality: A Critical Edition of Sources*. Basingstoke: Palgrave Macmillan, 2012.

Masculinity and Male Homosexuality in Britain, 1861–1913. 2nd ed. London: Springer, 2016.

Brake, Laurel, and Marysa Demoor, eds. *Dictionary of Nineteenth-Century Journalism in Great Britain and Northern Ireland*. London: Academia, 2009.

Brody, Howard, Zahra Meghani, and Kimberly Greenwald, eds. *Michael Ryan's Writings on Medical Ethics*. London: Springer, 2009.

Brome, Vincent. *Havelock Ellis: Philosopher of Sex: A Biography.* London: Routledge, 1979.

Brooks, Ross. "Bad Sexology: The Scientific Publications of the University Press (Watford and London), 1897–1901." *Social History of Medicine* 36, no. 4 (2023): 615–641.

Brown, Michael. "Medicine, Quackery, and the Free Market: The "War" against Morison's Pills and the Construction of the Medical Profession, c. 1830–c. 1850." In *Medicine and the Market in England and Its Colonies, c. 1450–c. 1850*, edited by Mark S. R. Jenner and Patrick Wallis, 238–261. Basingstoke: Palgrave Macmillan, 2007.

Performing Medicine: Medical Culture and Identity in Provincial England, c. 1760–1850. Manchester: Manchester University Press, 2011.

"'Bats, Rats and Barristers': The *Lancet*, Libel and the Radical Stylistics of Early Nineteenth-Century English Medicine." *Social History* 39, no. 2 (2014): 182–209.

Bull, Sarah. "Content Generation in the Age of Mechanical Reproduction." *Book History* 26, no. 2 (2023): 324–361.

"A Purveyor of Garbage? Charles Carrington and the Marketing of Sexual Science in Late-Victorian Britain." *Victorian Review* 38, no. 1 (2012): 55–76.

Burmeister, Maritha. "Popular Anatomical Museums in Nineteenth-Century England." PhD diss., Rutgers University, 2000.

Bush, M. L. *What Is Love? Richard Carlile's Philosophy of Sex*. London: Verso, 1998.

Bynum, W. F. *Science and the Practice of Medicine in the Nineteenth Century*. Cambridge: Cambridge University Press, 1994.

"Treating the Wages of Sin: Venereal Disease and Specialism in Eighteenth Century Britain." In *Medical Fringe and Medical Orthodoxy, 1750-1850*, edited by W.F. Bynum and Roy Porter, 5–28. London: Croom Helm, 1987.

Bynum, W. F., and Janice C. Wilson. "Periodical Knowledge: Medical Journals and Their Editors in Nineteenth-Century Britain." In *Medical Journals and Medical Knowledge: Historical Essays*, edited by W. F. Bynum, Stephen Lock, and Roy Porter, 29–48. London: Routledge, 2019.

Bynum, W. F., and Roy Porter, eds. *Medical Fringe and Medical Orthodoxy, 1750–1850*. London: Croom Helm, 1987.

Bynum, W. F., Stephen Lock, and Roy Porter, eds. *Medical Journals and Medical Knowledge: Historical Essays*. London: Routledge, 2019. First published 1992 by Routledge (London).

Calder-Marshall, Arthur. *Havelock Ellis: A Biography*. London: Hart-Davis, 1959.

Carnevale, Andrea, Denise McGuire, and Johanna Kelly. "'Removes All Obstacles': Abortifacients in Nineteenth-Century Toronto and Beyond." *International Journal of Historical Archaeology* 20 (2016): 743–767.

Carroll, Jordan S. *Reading the Obscene: Transgressive Editors and the Class Politics of US Literature*. Stanford, CA: Stanford University Press, 2021.

Chandrasekhar, Sripati. *Reproductive Physiology and Birth Control: The Writings of Charles Knowlton and Annie Besant*. London: Routledge, 2018.

Chard, Leslie. "Joseph Johnson: Father of the Book Trade." *Bulletin of the New York Public Library* 79, no. 1 (1975): 51–82.

Charnock, Hannah, Sarah L. Jones, and Ben Mechen. "Sexpertise: Sexual Knowledge and the Public in the Nineteenth and Twentieth Centuries." *Social History of Medicine* 36, no. 4 (2024): 585–591.

Cheshire, Jim. *Tennyson and Mid-Victorian Publishing: Moxon, Poetry, Commerce*. Basingstoke: Palgrave Macmillan, 2016.

Clark, Anna. *Desire: A History of European Sexuality*. London: Routledge, 2019.

Cocks, Harry G. "Review: The Growing Pains of the History of Sexuality." *Journal of Contemporary History* 39, no. 4 (2004a): 657–666.

"Saucy Stories: Pornography, Sexology and the Marketing of Sexual Knowledge in Britain, c. 1918–70." *Social History* 29, no. 4 (2004b): 465–484.

Colligan, Colette. *The Traffic in Obscenity from Byron to Beardsley: Sexuality and Exoticism in Nineteenth-Century Print Culture*. Basingstoke: Palgrave Macmillan, 2006.

A Publisher's Paradise: Expatriate Literary Culture in Paris, 1890–1960. Amherst, MA: University of Massachusetts Press, 2014.

"Digital Discovery and Fake Imprints: Unmasking Turn-of-the-Century Pornographers in Paris." *Book History* 22, no. 1 (2019): 249–279.

Cohen, Patricia Cline, Timothy J. Gilfoyle, and Helen Lefkowitz Horowitz. *The Flash Press: Sporting Male Weeklies in 1840s New York*. Chicago: University of Chicago Press, 2008.

Cook, Hera. *The Long Sexual Revolution: English Woman, Sex, and Contraception, 1800–1975*. Oxford: Oxford University Press, 2004.

Cook, Matt. *London and the Culture of Homosexuality, 1885–1914*. Cambridge: Cambridge University Press, 2003.

Cordell, Ryan, and Avery Blankenship. "Reprinting Wright." Prepublication release from *Going the Rounds: Virality in Nineteenth-Century Newspapers*. Minneapolis, MN: University of Minnesota Press, forthcoming, https://manifold.umn.edu/projects/going-the-rounds.

Cox, David J., Kim Stevenson, Candida Harris, and Judith Rowbotham. *Public Indecency in England, 1857–1960: 'A Serious Growing Evil'*. London: Routledge, 2015.

Crane, Mary Thomas. *Framing Authority: Sayings, Self, and Society in Sixteenth-Century England*. Princeton, NJ: Princeton University Press, 1993.

Cray, Ed. "Introduction." In *Bawdy Songbooks of the Romantic Period: Items Published by William West (1836–42)*, edited by Ed Cray, xxix–xxxvi. London: Routledge, 2022.

Creager, Angela N. H., Mathias Grote, and Elaine Leong. "Learning by the Book: Manuals and Handbooks in the History of Science." *BJHS Themes* 5 (2020): 1–13.

Cressy, David. *Birth, Marriage, and Death: Ritual, Religion, and the Life-Cycle in Tudor and Stuart England*. Oxford: Oxford University Press, 1997.

Crozier, Ivan. "The Medical Construction of Homosexuality and Its Relation to the Law in Nineteenth-Century England." *Medical History* 45, no. 1 (2001): 61–82.

"Introduction: Havelock Ellis, John Addington Symonds and the Construction of Sexual Inversion." In *Sexual Inversion: A Critical Edition*, edited by Ivan Crozier, 1–95. Basingstoke: Palgrave Macmillan, 2008a.

"Nineteenth-Century British Psychiatric Writing about Homosexuality before Havelock Ellis: The Missing Story." *Journal of the History of Medicine and Allied Sciences* 63, no. 1 (2008b): 65–102.

"Pillow Talk: Credibility, Trust, and the Sexological Case History." *History of Science* 46, no. 4 (2008c): 375–404.

Crowther, M. Anne, and Marguerite W. Dupree. *Medical Lives in the Age of Surgical Revolution*. Cambridge: Cambridge University Press, 2007.

Cryle, Peter, and Elisabeth Stephens. *Normality: A Critical Genealogy*. Chicago: Chicago University Press, 2017.

Csiszar, Alex. *The Scientific Journal: Authorship and the Politics of Knowledge in the Nineteenth Century*. Chicago: University of Chicago Press, 2018.

Daly, Nicholas. *The Demographic Imagination and the Nineteenth-Century City: Paris, London, New York*. Cambridge: Cambridge University Press, 2015.

D'Arcy, F. "The Malthusian League and the Resistance to Birth Control Propaganda in Late Victorian Britain." *Population Studies* 31, no. 3 (1977): 429–448.

Darnton, Robert. *The Literary Underground of the Old Regime*. Cambridge, MA: Harvard University Press, 1982.

"First Steps toward a History of Reading." *Australian Journal of French Studies* 51, no. 2/3 (2014): 152–177.

Dawson, Gowan. *Darwin, Literature, and Victorian Respectability*. Cambridge: Cambridge University Press, 2007.

Derkatch, Colleen. *Bounding Biomedicine: Evidence and Rhetoric in the New Science of Alternative Medicine*. Chicago: University of Chicago Press, 2016.

Desmond, Adrian. *The Politics of Evolution: Morphology, Medicine, and Reform in Radical London*. Chicago: Chicago University Press, 1989.

Digby, Anne. *Making a Medical Living: Doctors and Patients in the English Market for Medicine, 1720–1911*. Cambridge: Cambridge University Press, 1994.

Dolan, Brian, ed. *Malthus, Medicine, & Morality: "Malthusianism" after 1798*. London: Brill, 2016.

DuMaurier, Daphne. *The Infernal World of Branwell Brontë*. Garden City, NY: Doubleday, 1961.

Durbach, Nadja. *Spectacle of Deformity: Freak Shows and Modern British Culture*. Berkeley, CA: University of California Press, 2009.

Eliot, Simon. "Books and Their Readers: Part I." In *The Nineteenth-Century Novel: Realisms*, edited by Delia da Sousa Correa, 5–39. London: Routledge, 2000.

"Some Patterns and Trends in British Book Production, 1800–1919." *Occasional Papers of the Bibliographical Society* 8 (1994): 59–77.

Fisher, Kate. "Modern Ignorance." In *Reproduction: Antiquity to the Present*, edited by Nick Hopwood, Rebecca Fleming, and Lauren Kassell, 471–484. Cambridge: Cambridge University Press, 2018.

Fisher, Kate, and Jana Funke. "'Let Us Leave the Hospital; Let Us Go on a Journey around the World': British and German Sexual Science and the Global Search for Sexual Variation". In *A Global History of Sexual Science, 1880–1960*, edited by Veronika Fuechtner, Douglas E. Haynes, and Ryan M. Jones, 51–69. Berkeley, CA: University of California Press, 2017.

"'Are We to Treat Human Nature as the Early Victorian Lady Treated Telegrams?' British and German Sexual Science, Investigations of Nature and the Fight against Censorship, ca. 1890–1940." *Journal of the History of Sexuality* 32, no. 1 (2024): 79–101.

Fisher, Kate, and Rebecca Langlands. "General Introduction." In *Sex, Knowledge, and Receptions of the Past*, edited by Kate Fisher and Rebecca Langlands, 1–25. Oxford: Oxford University Press, 2015.

Fissell, Mary. "Making a Masterpiece: The *Aristotle* Texts in Vernacular Medical Culture." In *Right Living: An Anglo-American Tradition of Self-Help Medicine*, edited by Charles E. Rosenberg, 59–87. Baltimore, MD: Johns Hopkins University Press, 2003.

"The Marketplace of Print." In *Medicine and the Market in England and Its Colonies, c. 1450-c. 1850*, edited by Mark S. R. Jenner and Patrick Wallis, 108–132. Basingstoke: Palgrave Macmillan, 2007.

"Popular Medical Writing." In *The Book in the Renaissance*, edited by Andrew Pettegree, 297–318. New Haven, CT: Yale University Press, 2010.

Fissell, Mary, and Roger Cooter. "Exploring Natural Knowledge: Science and the Popular." In *The Cambridge History of Science*. Vol. 4, *Eighteenth-Century Science*, edited by Roy Porter, 129–158. Cambridge: Cambridge University Press, 2003.

Flint, Kate. *The Woman Reader, 1837–1914*. Oxford: Clarendon, 1993.

Foucault, Michel. *The History of Sexuality: An Introduction, Volume I*, translated by Robert Hurley. New York: Vintage, 1990.

Frampton, Sally. "'A Borderland in Ethics': Medical Journals, the Public, and the Medical Profession in Nineteenth-Century Britain." In *Science Periodicals in Nineteenth-Century Britain: Constructing Scientific Communities*, edited by Gowan Dawson, Bernard Lightman, Sally Shuttleworth and Jonathan R. Topham, 311–336. Chicago: Chicago University Press, 2020.

"The Medical Press and Its Public." In *The Edinburgh History of the British and Irish Press*. Vol. 2, *Expansion and Evolution, 1800–1900*, edited by David Finkelstein, 438–456. Edinburgh: Edinburgh University Press, 2022.

Frampton, Sally, and Jennifer Wallis, eds. *Reading the Nineteenth-Century Medical Journal*. London: Routledge, 2020.

Funke, Jana, Kate Fisher, Jen Grove, and Rebecca Langlands. "Illustrating Phallic Worship: Uses of Material Objects and the Production of Sexual Knowledge in Eighteenth-Century Antiquarianism and Early Twentieth-Century Sexual Science." *Word & Image* 33, no. 3 (2017): 324–337.

Fyfe, Aileen. *Steam-Powered Knowledge: William Chambers and the Business of Publishing, 1820–1860*. Chicago: University of Chicago Press, 2012.

Fyfe, Aileen, Noah Moxam, Julie McDougall-Waters, and Camilla Mørk Røstvik. *A History of Scientific Journals: Publishing at the Royal Society, 1665–2015*. London: UCL Press, 2022.

Gamer, Michael. "Genres for the Prosecution: Pornography and the Gothic." *PMLA* 114, no. 5 (1999): 1043–1054.

Genette, Gerard. *Paratexts: Thresholds of Interpretation*, translated by Jane Lewin. Cambridge: Cambridge University Press, 1997.

Gettmann, Royal A. *A Victorian Publisher: A Study of the Bentley Papers* [1960]. Cambridge University Press, 2010.

Gibson, Ian. *The Erotomaniac: The Secret Life of Henry Spencer Ashbee*. Boston, MA: Da Capo Press, 2001.

Gieryn, Thomas F. *Cultural Boundaries of Science: Credibility on the Line*. Chicago: University of Chicago Press, 1999.

Gill, Phoebe Letitia. "The Production, Circulation, and Reception of Sexual Knowledges in Published Advice Literature in Britain and Ireland, 1918–1987." PhD thesis, University of Birmingham, 2023.

Glass, David Victor. *Population Policies and Movements in Europe*. 2nd ed. London: A.M. Kelly, 1967.

Glass, Loren. *Counterculture Colophon: Grove Press, the Evergreen Review, and the Incorporation of the Avant-Garde*. Stanford, CA: Stanford University Press, 2013.

Golby, David J. *Instrumental Teaching in Nineteenth-Century Britain*. London: Routledge, 2017.

Golden, Catherine J. *Posting It: The Victorian Revolution in Letter-Writing*. Gainesville, FL: University Press of Florida, 2009.

Gray, Donald J. "Early Victorian Scandalous Journalism: Renton Nicholson's *The Town* (1837–42)." In *The Victorian Periodical Press: Samplings and Soundings*, edited by Joanne Shattock and Michael Wolff, 317–348. Toronto: University of Toronto Press, 1982.

Green, Jonathon and Nicholas J. Karolides, eds. *Encyclopedia of Censorship*. London: Infobase, 2014.

Green, Monica Helen. "'Diseases of Women' to 'Secrets of Women': The Transformation of Gynecological Literature in the Later Middle Ages." *The Journal of Medieval and Renaissance Studies* 30, no. 1 (2000): 5–40.

Gregory, James. *On Victorians and Vegetarians: The Vegetarian Movement in Nineteenth-Century Britain*. London: Taurus Academic Studies, 2007.

Grosskurth, Phyllis. *Havelock Ellis: A Biography*. New York: Knopf, 1960.

Guacamole, Howard [pseud.]. *Charles Carrington (1867–1921): Bibliographie eines Verlags*. Norderstedt: Ars Amandi in Kommission, 2005.

Hall, Lesley A. "Forbidden by God, Despised by Men: Masturbation, Medical Warnings, Moral Panic, and Manhood in Great Britain, 1850–1950." *Journal of the History of Sexuality* 2, no. 3 (1992): 365–387.

"'The English Have Hot-Water Bottles': The Morganatic Marriage between Sexology and Medicine in Britain Since William Acton." In *Sexual Knowledge, Sexual Science: The History of Attitudes to Sexuality*, edited by Roy Porter and Mikulas Teich, 350–366. Cambridge: Cambridge University Press, 1994.

"Malthusian Mutations: The Changing Politics and Moral Meanings of Birth Control in Britain," In *Malthus, Medicine, and Morality: "Malthusianism" after 1798*, edited by Brian Dolan, 141–163. London: Clio Medica, 2000.

"The Victorians: Our Others, Our Selves?" In *Sex, Knowledge, and Receptions of the Past*, edited by Kate Fisher and Rebecca Langlands, 160–176. Oxford: Oxford University Press, 2015.

Sex, Gender and Social Change in Britain since 1880. 2nd ed. London: Bloomsbury, 2017.

Hall, Robert G. "A Bookshop of their Own: Reading and Print in Chartism, 1838–1850." *The English Historical Review* 136, no. 581 (2021): 894–917.

Hallam, Elizabeth. *The Anatomy Museum: Death and the Body Displayed*. London: Reaktion, 2008.

Hamblin, Kimberly A. *From Eve to Evolution: Darwin, Science, and Women's Rights in Gilded Age America*. Chicago: University of Chicago Press, 2014.

Hanley, Anne R. *Medicine, Knowledge, and Venereal Diseases in England, 1886–1916*. Basingstoke: Palgrave Macmillan, 2016.

Harrison, Stephen, and Christopher Stray, eds. *Expurgating the Classics: Editing Out in Latin and Greek*. Bristol: Bristol Classical, 2012.

Hartley, Lucy. "Walker, Alexander (1779–1852)." In *Oxford Dictionary of National Biography*. Oxford: Oxford University Press, 2004; online ed., 2011. https://doi .org/10.1093/ref:odnb/56049.

Harvey, Karen. *Reading Sex in the Eighteenth Century: Bodies and Gender in English Erotic Culture*. Cambridge: Cambridge University Press, 2004.

Haycock, David Boyd, and Patrick Wallis. "Quackery and Commerce in Seventeenth-Century London: The Proprietary Medicine Business of Anthony Daffy." *Medical History* 25 (2005): 1–36.

Heath, Deana. *Purifying Empire: Obscenity and the Politics of Moral Regulation in Britain, India and Australia*. Cambridge: Cambridge University Press, 2010.

Hewitt, Martin. *The Dawn of the Cheap Press in Victorian Britain: The End of 'Taxes on Knowledge,' 1849–1869*. London: Bloomsbury, 2013.

Himes, Norman E. "Charles Knowlton's Revolutionary Influence on the English Birth Rate." *New England Journal of Medicine* 199, no. 10 (1928): 461–465.

Medical History of Contraception. New York: Schocken, 1970. First published 1936 by Williams & Wilkins (Baltimore).

Hobbs, Andrew. *A Fleet Street in Every Town: The Provincial Press in England, 1855–1900*. Cambridge: Open Book, 2018.

Howell, Phillip. "Sex and the City of Bachelors: Sporting Guidebooks and Urban Knowledge in Nineteenth-Century Britain and America." *Ecumene* 8, no. 1 (2001): 20–50.

Howsam, Leslie. *Kegan Paul: A Victorian Imprint*. Toronto: University of Toronto Press, 1998.

Hunt, Lynn. *The Invention of Pornography: Obscenity and the Origins of Modernity, 1500–1800*. New York: Zone Books, 1993.

Jackson, Lee. *Palaces of Pleasure: From Music Halls to the Seaside to Football, How the Victorians Invented Mass Entertainment*. New Haven, CT: Yale University Press, 2019.

Janssens, Leon. "Erotische Censuur. De Seksuele Revolutie in Gecensureerde Pornografische Filmposters in België (1971–1980)." *Tijdschrift voor Geschiedenis* 133, no. 2 (2020): 347–66.

"Pornography on Rails: Trains and Belgium's 'War on Pornography,' 1880–1891." *Journal of the History of Sexuality* 32, no. 3 (2023): 269–287.

Johns, Adrian. *The Nature of the Book: Print and Knowledge in the Making*. Chicago: University of Chicago Press, 1998.

Piracy: The Intellectual Property Wars from Gutenberg to Gates. Chicago: University of Chicago Press, 2009.

Jones, Claire L. "Under the Covers? Commerce, Contraceptives, and Consumers in England and Wales, 1880–1960." *Social History of Medicine* 29, no. 4 (2015): 734–756.

The Medical Trade Catalogue in Britain, 1870–1914. London: Routledge, 2016.

The Business of Birth Control: Contraception and Commerce in Britain before the Sexual Revolution. Manchester: Manchester University Press, 2020.

Jones, Sarah L. "'As though Miles of Ocean did not Separate us': Print and the Construction of a Transatlantic Free Love Community at the Fin de Siècle." *Journal of Victorian Culture* 25, no. 1 (2020): 95–109.

Johnson, Dale A. "Popular Apologetics in Late Victorian England: The Work of the Christian Evidence Society." *Journal of Religious History* 11, no. 4 (1981): 558–577.

Jordanova, Ludmilla J. *Sexual Visions: Images of Gender in Science and Medicine between the Eighteenth and Twentieth Centuries*. Madison, WI: University of Wisconsin Press, 1993.

Joudrey, Thomas J. "Penetrating Boundaries: An Ethics of Anti-Perfectionism in Victorian Pornography." *Victorian Studies* 57, no. 3 (2015): 423–432.

Jütte, Robert. *Contraception: A History*. Cambridge: Polity, 2008.

Kearney, Patrick. *The Private Case: An Annotated Bibliography of the Private Case Erotica Collection in the British (Museum) Library*. London: J. Landesman, 1989.

Kelly, Laura. *Irish Medical Education and Student Culture, c.1850–1950*. Oxford: Oxford University Press, 2017.

Kendrick, Walter. *The Secret Museum: Pornography in Modern Culture*. Berkeley, CA: University of California Press, 1996. First published 1987 by Penguin (New York).

Kennedy, Dane. *The Highly Civilized Man: Richard Burton and the Victorian World.* Cambridge, MA: Harvard University Press, 2000.

Knight, Patricia. "Women and Abortion in Victorian and Edwardian England." *History Workshop* 4, no. 1 (1977): 57–68.

Kronick, D. A. "Medical 'Publishing Societies' in Eighteenth-Century Britain." *Bulletin of the Medical Library Association* 82, no. 3 (1994): 277–282.

Kuhn, Phillip. "The Sexual Life of Our Time: Medical Censorship in Early-20th-Century England." *History of Psychology* 23, no. 1 (2020): 40–61.

Lake, Elizabeth. "Medicine." In *The Oxford History of the Irish Book.* Vol. IV, *The Irish Book in English, 1800–1891*, edited by James H. Murphy, 576–584. Oxford: Oxford University Press, 2011.

Lang, Birgit. "The Shifting Case of Masochism: Leopold von Sacher-Masoch's Venus im Pelz (1870)." In *A History of the Case Study: Sexology, Psychoanalysis, Literature*, edited by Birgit Lang, Joy Damousi, and Alison Lewis, 19–54. Manchester: Manchester University Press, 2017.

Lansbury, Coral. "Gynaecology, Pornography, and the Antivivisection Movement." *Victorian Studies* 28, no. 3 (1985): 413–437.

Lavine, Matthew. "'Advanced Marriage Technique': Sex as a Perfectible Skill in Mid-Twentieth-Century American Marriage Manuals." *Journal of Family History* 46, no. 4 (2021): 460–482.

Leckie, Barbara. *Culture and Adultery: The Novel, the Newspaper, and the Law, 1857–1914*. Philadelphia, PA: University of Pennsylvania Press, 1999.

Ledbetter, Rosanna. *A History of the Malthusian League*. Columbus, OH: Ohio State University Press, 1976.

Lee, Maurice S. *Overwhelmed: Literature, Aesthetics, and the Nineteenth-Century Information Revolution*. Princeton, NJ: Princeton University Press, 2019.

Legman, Gershon. "The Lure of the Forbidden." In *Libraries, Erotica, and Pornography*, edited by Martha Cornog, 36–68. Phoenix, AZ: Oryx Press, 1991.

Leng, Kirsten. *Sexual Politics and Feminist Science: Women Sexologists in Germany, 1900–1933*. Ithaca, NY: Cornell University Press, 2018.

Leonard, Sarah L. "Pornography and Obscenity." In *Palgrave Advances in the Modern History of Sexuality*, edited by H. G. Cocks and Matt Houlbrook, 180–205. Basingstoke: Palgrave Macmillan, 2006.

Lightman, Bernard. *Victorian Popularizers of Science: Designing Nature for New Audiences*. Chicago: University of Chicago Press, 2007.

Loudon, Irvine. *Medical Care and the General Practitioner, 1750–1850*. Oxford: Oxford University Press, 1986.

Lubey, Kathleen. "Making Pornography, 1749–1968: The History of The History of the Human Heart." *ELH* 82, no. 3 (2015): 897–935.

What Pornography Knows: Sex and Social Protest since the Eighteenth Century. Stanford, CA: Stanford University Press, 2022.

Lupton, Deborah. *The Imperative of Health: Public Health and the Regulated Body.* London: Sage, 1995.

Mackintosh, Alan. *The Patent Medicines Industry in Georgian England: Constructing the Market by the Potency of Print*. Basingstoke: Palgrave Macmillan, 2018.

Manchester, Colin. "Obscenity Law and Its Enforcement in the Nineteenth Century." *Journal of Legal History* 2, no. 1 (1981): 45–61.

"Lord Campbell's Act: England's First Obscenity Statute." *Journal of Legal History* 9, no. 2 (1988): 223–241.

Manion, Jen. *Female Husbands: A Trans History*. Cambridge: Cambridge University Press, 2020.

Marsh, Joss. *Word Crimes: Blasphemy, Culture, and Literature in Nineteenth-Century England*. Chicago: University of Chicago Press, 1998.

Mason, Michael. *The Making of Victorian Sexual Attitudes*. Oxford: Oxford University Press, 1994.

Maxwell, Alexander, Carol Harrington, and Sarah Bracey. "Scientific Eroticism, Beauty Theorists, and the Borders of the Erotic: John Roberton's *Kalogynomia* and Alexander Walker's *Beauty*." *Porn Studies* 8, no. 2 (2021): 138–153.

McCalman, Iain. *Radical Underworld: Prophets, Revolutionaries, and Pornographers in London, 1795–1840*. Cambridge: Cambridge University Press, 1988.

McGill, Meredith. *American Literature and the Culture of Reprinting, 1834–1853*. Philadelphia, PA: University of Pennsylvania Press, 2013.

McGillen, Petra S. *The Fontane Workshop: Manufacturing Realism in the Industrial Age of Print*. London: Bloomsbury, 2019.

McGrath, Roberta. *Seeing Her Sex: Medical Archives and the Female Body*. Manchester: Manchester University Press, 2002.

McKitterick, David. "Publishing for the Trades and Professions." In *The Cambridge History of the Book in Britain*. Vol. 6, edited by David McKitterick, 500–530. Cambridge: Cambridge University Press, 2010.

McLaren, Angus. "Abortion in England, 1890–1914." *Victorian Studies* 20, no. 4 (1977): 379–400.

Birth Control in Nineteenth-Century England. London: Croom Helm, 1978.

Sexual Blackmail: A Modern History. Cambridge, MA: Harvard University Press, 2002.

Mendes, Peter. *Clandestine Erotic Fiction in English 1800–1930: A Bibliographical Study* [1993]. London: Routledge, 2016.

Merkle, Denise. "When Expurgation Constitutes Ineffective Censorship. The Case of Three Vizetelly Translations of Zola." In *Translation and Meaning, Part 5. Proceedings of the Maastricht Session of the 3rd International Maastricht-Lodz Duo Colloquium, held in Maastricht, The Netherlands, 26–29 April 2000*, edited by B. Lewandowska-Tomaszczyk, and M. Thelen, 285–293. Maastricht: Maastricht School of Translation and Interpreting, Hogeschool Maastricht, 2001.

"The Lutetian Society." *TTR: traduction, terminologie, redaction* 16, no. 2 (2003): 73–101.

Meynell, G. G. *The Two Sydenham Societies: A History and Bibliography of the Medical Classics Published by the Sydenham Society and the New Sydenham Society (1844–1911)*. Folkestone: Winterdown, 1985.

Miller, Elizabeth Carolyn. *Slow Print: Literary Radicalism and Late-Victorian Print Culture*. Stanford, CA: Stanford University Press, 2013.

Mort, Frank. *Dangerous Sexualities: Medico-Moral Politics in England Since 1830*. 2nd ed. London: Routledge, 2000.

Moulds, Alison. "'Making your Mark' in Medicine: The Struggling Young Practitioner and the Search for Success in Britain, 1830s–1900s." *History* 104, no. 359 (2019): 83–104.

Mullin, Katherine. *James Joyce, Sexuality, and Social Purity.* Cambridge: Cambridge University Press, 2003, 6–10.

"Poison More Deadly Than Prussic Acid: Defining Obscenity after the 1857 Obscene Publications Act (1850–1885)." In *Prudes on the Prowl: Fiction and Obscenity in England, 1857 to the Present Day*, edited by David Bradshaw and Rachel Potter, 11–29. Oxford: Oxford University Press, 2013.

"Unmasking *The Confessional Unmasked*: The 1868 *Hicklin* Test and the Toleration of Obscenity." *ELH* 85, no. 2 (2018): 471–499.

Myers, Robin. "The London Scots." In *The Edinburgh History of the Book in Scotland.* Vol. 3, *Ambition and Industry, 1800–1880*, edited by Bill Bell, 396–408. Edinburgh: Edinburgh University Press, 2007.

Nead, Lynda. *Victorian Babylon: People, Streets, and Images in Nineteenth-Century London*. New Haven, CT: Yale University Press, 2000.

Nelson, James G. *Publisher to the Decadents: Leonard Smithers in the Careers of Beardsley, Wilde, Dowson*. Philadelphia, PA: Pennsylvania State University Press, 2000.

Newman, Harry. "'[P]rophane fidlers': Medical Paratexts and Indecent Readers in Early Modern England." In *Medical Paratexts from Medieval to Modern: Dissecting the Page*, edited by Hannah C. Tweed and Diane G. Scott, 15–42. Cham: Palgrave Macmillan, 2018.

Ngai, Sianne. *Theory of the Gimmick: Aesthetic Judgement and Capitalist Form*. Cambridge, MA: Harvard University Press, 2020.

Noakes, Richard. "Punch and Comic Journalism in Mid-Victorian Britain." In *Science in the Nineteenth-Century Periodical: Reading the Magazine of Nature*, edited by Geoffrey Cantor, Gowan Dawson, Graeme Gooday et al., 91–122. Cambridge: Cambridge University Press, 2004.

O'Connell, Lisa. "'Matrimonial Ceremonies Displayed': Popular Ethnography and Enlightened Imperialism." *Eighteenth-Century Life* 26, no. 3 (2002): 99–116.

O'Connor, Ralph. "Reflections on Popular Science in Britain: Genres, Categories, and Historians." *Isis* 100, no. 2 (2009): 333–345.

Östling, Johan, David Larsson Heidenblad, Erling Sandmo, Anna Nilsson Hammar, and Kari H. Nordberg. "The History of Knowledge and the Circulation of Knowledge" In *Circulation of Knowledge: Explorations in the History of Knowledge*, edited by Johan Östling, David Larsson Heidenblad, Erling Sandmo, Anna Nilsson Hammar, and Kari Nordberg, 9–33. Lund: Nordic Academic Press, 2018.

Oxford English Dictionary Online, s.v. "quacksalver, n," accessed September 23, 2020, www.oed.com/view/Entry/155643.

Parkes, Adam. *Modernism and the Theater of Censorship*. Oxford: Oxford University Press, 1996.

Peakman, Julie. *Mighty Lewd Books: The Development of Pornography in Eighteenth-Century England.* Basingstoke: Palgrave Macmillan, 2003.

Pease, Allison. *Modernism, Mass Culture, and the Aesthetics of Obscenity.* Cambridge: Cambridge University Press, 2000.

Peel, John. "The Manufacture and Retailing of Contraceptives in England." *Population Studies* 17, no. 2 (1963): 113–125.

Piggott, Jan. *Palace of the People: The Crystal Palace at Sydenham, 1854–1936.* London: Hurst, 2004.

Porter, Roy. *Health for Sale: Quackery in England, 1660–1850*. Manchester: Manchester University Press, 1989.

"The Rise of Medical Journalism in Britain to 1800." In *Medical Journals and Medical Knowledge: Historical Essays*, edited by W. F. Bynum, Stephen Lock, and Roy Porter, 6–28. London: Routledge, 2019.

Porter, Roy, and Lesley Hall. *The Facts of Life: The Creation of Sexual Knowledge in Britain, 1650–1950*. New Haven, CT: Yale University Press, 1995.

Potter, Rachel. *Obscene Modernism: Literary Censorship and Experiment, 1900–1940*. Oxford: Oxford University Press, 2013.

Price, Leah. *How to Do Things with Books in Victorian Britain*. Princeton, NJ: Princeton University Press, 2012.

Qureshi, Sadiah. "Displaying Sara Baartman, the 'Hottentot Venus'." *History of Science* 42, no. 2 (2004): 233–257.

Rectenwald, Michael. *Nineteenth-Century British Secularism: Science, Religion, and Literature*, Basingstoke: Palgrave Macmillan, 2016.

Richards, Evelleen. *Darwin and the Making of Sexual Selection*. Chicago: University of Chicago Press, 2017.

Richardson, Ruth. *The Making of Mr. Gray's Anatomy: Bodies, Books, Fortune, Fame*. Oxford: Oxford University Press, 2009.

Roberts, M. J. D. "The Society for the Suppression of Vice and Its Early Critics, 1802–1812." *History Journal* 26, no. 1 (1983): 159–176.

"Making Victorian Morals? The Society for the Suppression of Vice and Its Critics, 1802–1886." *Australian Historical Studies* 21, no. 83 (1984): 157–173.

"Morals, Art, and the Law: The Passing of the Obscene Publications Act, 1857." *Victorian studies* 28, no. 4 (1985): 609-629.

"The Politics of Professionalization: MPs, Medical Men, and the 1858 Medical Act." *Medical History* 53 (2009): 37–56.

Rose, Jonathan. *The Intellectual Life of the British Working Classes*, 2nd ed. New Haven, CT: Yale University Press, 2010.

Rosenberg, Anat. *The Rise of Mass Advertising: Law, Enchantment, and the Cultural Boundaries of British Modernity*. Oxford: Oxford University Press, 2022.

Rosenman, Ellen Bayuk. *Unauthorized Pleasures: Accounts of Victorian Erotic Experience*. Ithaca, NY: Cornell University Press, 2003.

Rovere, Richard H. *Howe and Hummel: Their True and Scandalous History*. New York: Farrar, Strauss, 1947.

Rowbotham, Judith, and Kim Stevenson, eds. *Criminal Conversations: Victorian Crimes, Social Panic, and Moral Outrage*. Columbus, OH: Ohio State University Press, 2005.

Royle, Edward. *Victorian Infidels: The Origins of the British Secularist Movement, 1791–1866*. Manchester: Manchester University Press, 1974.

Radicals, Secularists, and Republicans: Popular Freethought in Britain, 1866–1915. Manchester: Manchester University Press, 1980.

Salesa, Damon Ieremia. *Racial Crossings: Race, Intermarriage, and the Victorian British Empire*. Oxford: Oxford University Press, 2019.

Schaeffer, Neil. *The Marquis de Sade: A Life*. Cambridge, MA: Harvard University Press, 1999.

Schaffner, Anna Katherina. "Fiction as Evidence: On the Uses of Literature in Nineteenth-Century Sexological Discourse." *Comparative Literature Studies* 48, no. 2 (2011): 165–199.

Schwatz, Laura. *Secularism, Religion, and Women's Emancipation, England 1830–1914*. Manchester: Manchester University Press, 2015.

Searle, Geoffrey Russell. *Morality and the Market in Victorian Britain*. Oxford: Clarendon, 1998.

Secord, James A. "Talking Origins." In *Reproduction: Antiquity to the Present*, edited by Nick Hopwood, Rebecca Fleming, and Lauren Kassell, 375–389. Cambridge: Cambridge University Press, 2018.

Seville, Catherine. *Literary Copyright Reform in Early Victorian England: The Framing of the 1842 Copyright Act*. Cambridge: Cambridge University Press, 1999.

Shuttleworth, Sally. "Female Circulation: Medical Discourse and Popular Advertising in the Mid-Victorian Era." In *Body/Politics: Women and the Discourses of Science*, edited by Mary Jacobus, Evelyn Fox Keller, and Sally Shuttleworth, 47–68. New York: Routledge, 1989.

Sigel, Lisa Z. *Governing Pleasures: Pornography and Social Change in England, 1815–1914*. Rutgers, NJ: Rutgers University Press, 2001.

"Censorship in Inter-War Britain: Obscenity, Spectacle, and the Workings of the Liberal State." *Journal of Social History* 45, no. 1 (2011): 61–83.

Making Modern Love: Sexual Narratives and Identities in Interwar Britain. Philadelphia, PA: Temple University Press, 2012.

Simon, Josep. *Communicating Physics: The Production, Circulation and Appropriation of Ganot's Textbooks in France and England, 1851–1887*. London: Routledge, 2016.

Slauter, Will. *Who Owns the News? A History of Copyright*. Stanford, CA: Stanford University Press, 2020.

Soloway, Richard A. *Birth Control and the Population Question in England, 1877–1930*. Durham, NC: University of North Carolina Press, 1982.

Squires, Clare. *Marketing Literature: The Making of Contemporary Writing in Britain*. Basingstoke: Palgrave Macmillan, 2007.

St. Clair, William. *The Reading Nation in the Romantic Period*. Cambridge: Cambridge University Press, 2004.

Stephens, Elizabeth. "Pathologizing Leaky Male Bodies. Spermatorrhea in Nineteenth-Century British Medicine and Popular Anatomy Museums." *Journal of the History of Sexuality* 17, no. 3 (2008): 421–438.

Anatomy as Spectacle: Public Exhibitions of the Body from 1700 to the Present. Liverpool: Liverpool University Press, 2011.

Stoler, Ann Laura. *Race and the Education of Desire: Foucault's History of Sexuality and the Colonial Order of Things*. Durham, NC: Duke University Press, 1995.

Stoops, Jamie. "Class and Gender Dynamics of the Pornography Trade in Late Nineteenth-Century Britain." *The Historical Journal* 58, no. 1 (2015): 137–156.

The Thorny Path; Pornography in Early Twentieth Century Britain. Montreal: McGill-Queens University Press, 2018.

Strachan, John. *Advertising and Satirical Culture in the Romantic Period*. Cambridge: Cambridge University Press, 2011.

Straight, Sheryl. *The Erotica Bibliophile*, accessed February 19, 2024, www.eroticabibliophile.com/.

Stuart, Ann Elisabeth F. "The Case of Dr. Allbutt." M.Phil diss., University of Cambridge, 2000.

Szreter, Simon, and Kate Fisher. *Sex before the Sexual Revolution: Intimate Life in England, 1918–1963*. Cambridge: Cambridge University Press, 2010.

Takács, Judit. "The Double Life of Kertbeny." In *The Past and Present of Radical Sexual Politics: Working Papers: Fifth Meeting of the Seminar "Socialism and Sexuality," Amsterdam, October 3–4, 2003*, edited by G. Hekma, 51–62. Amsterdam: Mosse Foundation, 2004.

Tanselle, Thomas G. "Bibliography and Science." *Studies in Bibliography* 27 (1974): 55–89.

Thomas, Kate. *Postal Pleasures: Sex, Scandal, and Victorian Letters*. Oxford: Oxford University Press, 2011.

Tomes, Nancy. "'Not Just for Doctors Anymore': How the *Merck Manual* Became a Consumer Health 'Bible'." *Bulletin of the History of Medicine* 95, no. 1 (2021): 1–23

Tone, Andrea. *Devices and Desires: A History of Contraceptives in America*. New York: Hill and Wang, 2001.

Toulalan, Sarah. *Imagining Sex: Pornography and Bodies in Seventeenth-Century England*. Oxford: Oxford University Press, 2007.

"Pornography, Procreation and Pleasure in Early Modern England." In *The Cambridge Companion to Erotic Literature*, edited by Bradford K. Mudge, 105–122. Cambridge: Cambridge University Press, 2017.

Traub, Valerie. *Thinking Sex with the Early Moderns*. Philadelphia, PA: University of Pennsylvania Press, 2015.

Turner, James Grantham. *Schooling Sex: Libertine Literature and Erotic Education in Italy, France and England, 1534–1685*. Oxford: Oxford University Press, 2003.

Ueyama, Takahiro. *Health in the Marketplace: Professionalism, Therapeutic Desires, and Medical Commodification in Late-Victorian London*. Palo Alto, CA: Society for the Promotion of Science and Scholarship, 2010.

Waits, Robert. "Gustave Flaubert, Charles Dickens, and Isaac Pulvermacher's 'Magic Band'." *Progress in Brain Research* 205 (2013): 219–239.

Walker, Rachel E. *Beauty and the Brain: The Science of Human Nature in Early America*. Chicago: University of Chicago Press, 2022.

Walkowitz, Judith R. *Prostitution and Victorian Society: Women, Class, and the State*. Cambridge: Cambridge University Press, 1982.

Wånggren, Lena. *Gender, Technology, and the New Woman*. Edinburgh: Edinburgh University Press, 2017.

Weedon, Alexis. *Victorian Publishing: The Economics of Book Production for the Mass Market, 1836–1916*. London: Ashgate, 2003.

Weeks, Jeffrey. *Sex, Politics and Society: The Regulation of Sexuality since 1800*. 4th ed. London: Routledge, 2017.

Werbel, Amy. *Lust on Trial: Censorship and the Rise of American Obscenity in the Age of Anthony Comstock*. New York: Columbia University Press, 2018.

White, Brenda M. "Medical Police. Politics and Police: The Fate of John Roberton." *Medical History* 27, no. 4 (1983): 407–422.

Whiteley, Rebecca. "Spratt's Flaps: Midwifery, Creativity, and Sexuality in Early Nineteenth-Century Visual Culture." *British Art Studies* 19 (2021): https://doi.org/10.17658/issn.2058-5462/issue-19/rwhiteley

Wickstead, Helen. "Sex in the Secret Museum: Photographs from the British Museum's Witt Scrapbooks." *Photography and Culture* 11, no. 3 (2018): 351–366.

Winter, Alison. *Mesmerized: Powers of Mind in Victorian Britain*. Chicago: University of Chicago Press, 2000.

Wood, Janice Ruth. *The Struggle for Free Speech in the United States, 1872–1915: Edward Bliss Foote, Edward Bond Foot, and Anti-Comstock Operations*. London: Routledge, 2008.

Wright, Maureen. *Elizabeth Wolstenholme Elmy and the Victorian Feminist Movement: The Biography of an Insurgent Woman*. Oxford: Oxford University Press, 2014.

Yeandle, Peter. "Exotic Bodies and Mundane Medicines: Advertising and Empire in the Late-Victorian and Edwardian Press." In *Paraphernalia! Victorian Objects*, edited by Helen Kingstone and Kate Lister, 244–264. London: Routledge, 2019.

Index

For EU product safety concerns, contact us at Calle de José Abascal, 56–1°,
28003 Madrid, Spain or eugpsr@cambridge.org.

www.ingramcontent.com/pod-product-compliance
Lightning Source LLC
LaVergne TN
LVHW011808200926
848484LV00005B/1106
* 9 7 8 1 0 0 9 5 7 8 0 7 3 *